Infection Control
in Clinical Practice

Infection Control in Clinical Practice

Jennie Wilson BSc RGN

Programme Leader, Laboratory of Hospital Infection,
Central Public Health Laboratory, Colindale, UK

Baillière Tindall
London Philadelphia Toronto Sydney Tokyo

Baillière Tindall
An imprint of Harcourt Publishers Limited
is a registered trademark of Harcourt Publishers Limited

© 1995 Baillière Tindall
© 1999 Harcourt Publishers Limited

Reprinted 1999

This book is printed on acid-free paper

A catalogue record for this book is available from the British Library

ISBN 0–7020–1722–1

Typeset by J & L Composition Ltd, Filey, North Yorkshire
Printed and bound in Great Britain by The Bath Press, Bath

Contents

A colour plate section can be found between pages 180–181.

Preface

The prevention and control of infection is fundamental to the provision of a safe environment for patients and forms an integral part of the practice of any health care professional working in a clinical setting. None the less it is a complex field, frequently difficult to understand and strongly influenced by ritual and tradition. My intention in this book is to overcome these barriers by providing a comprehensive guide to the principles of infection control, the research which supports them and the microbiology which forms their foundation. Throughout the text I have tried to make the information practical, relevant, readable and research-based. It is not within the scope of this book to comment on the theories or models of nursing in relation to infection and readers are expected to refer to the many excellent texts on nursing practice for this purpose.

Chapter 1 provides simple information about the properties of microbes and how they behave in a clinical environment. Chapter 2 explains how specimens are investigated in the microbiology laboratory and the interpretation of the results. Chapter 3 describes infections commonly encountered in hospital and discusses the precautions required to prevent their spread. Chapter 4 contains a simple explanation of how the body protects itself against invading micro-organisms and the principles of preventing infection in those whose immune system is damaged. Chapter 5 describes the use of antimicrobial agents to treat infections and their role in creating infection control problems such as MRSA. Chapter 6 examines the way that micro-organisms spread in both hospital and community settings and the factors which influence their transmission. The remaining chapters focus on major areas of practice related to infection prevention and control beginning in Chapter 7 with the basic principles; handwashing, protective clothing and waste disposal. Chapters 8, 9, 10 and 11 outline the factors which contribute to infection of wounds, intravascular devices, urinary catheters and the respiratory tract, and in each case describes the measures recommended to prevent infection and the supporting research. Chapter 12 describes the principles of food hygiene in the prevention of gastrointestinal infections and Chapter 13 the disinfection and sterilization of equipment. Chapter 14 describes procedures recommended to prevent the spread of infectious disease and Chapter 15 the measures required to treat ectoparasitic infections and infestations of the environment. References are provided at the end of each chapter and for those readers seeking more detailed information I have also made suggestions for further reading. A glossary of terms is included to facilitate the reading and there are appendices to Chapters 13 and 14 describing sterilization and disinfection methods and infection control precautions for commonly encountered infectious diseases. It is my intention that the reader should critically appraise the contents of the later chapters drawing from information contained in Chapters 1 to 6.

I anticipate that this book will be a useful reference for nurses practising in acute, long-term care and community settings, nurse educators and other health care professionals. It is also intended for use by nurses and medical support workers in training, particularly those following higher level NVQ, diploma or degree level courses. I hope that it will be of value both in the application of infection prevention and control in day-to-day practice and in providing a sound scientific basis for the formulation of policies and standards of care.

Jennie Wilson

Acknowledgements

I wish to take the opportunity to thank the many people whose support has made the production of this book possible. In particular, I would like to thank Dr Dinah Barrie for her invaluable advice and assistance and Phyllada Breedon for being her usual source of inspiration. My thanks must also go to Peter Hoffman, Professor Robert Pratt, Larry Baker, Dr John Maunder and Lynda Taylor for their helpful suggestions and my editor, Sarah James for her words of encouragement.

Finally, I would like to thank my family – Philip, Sarah and Josie, who have endured my long absences at the word processor with only a few complaints!

Figure Acknowledgements

Figs 1.11, 1.13, 2.1, Plates 2.4, 2.5, 2.6, 2.7, 2.8, 2.10, 3.1, 3.2, 3.3, 3.4, 3.5, 3.7, 7.1, 8.1 were reproduced with kind permission of Dr D Barrie, Charing Cross and Westminster Medical School, London, UK.

Figs 2.3, 2.4 were redrawn from Ayton M (1982) Microbiological investigations. *Nursing* **2**(8): 226–30 with permission of Mark Allen Publishing.

Figs 3.2 and 4.11 are Crown Copyright and were redrawn with permission from Controller of Her Majesty's Stationery Office.

Fig 7.2 reprinted from Taylor L (1978) An evaluation of handwashing techniques. *Nursing Times*, **74**: 108–10.

Figs 7.3, 12.2, 13.3, 14.5 reprinted with kind permission of Glenys Griffiths.

Figs 7.7, 7.9 were reproduced with permission of Riverside Health Authority, original artwork by Linda Foreman.

Fig 9.1 was reproduced with kind permission from Elliot TSJ (1988) Intravascular device infections. *J. Med. Micro.* **27**, 161–7.

Fig 15.1 reprinted with kind permission of Dr J. Lane, London School of Hygiene and Tropical Medicine.

Fig 15.2 was redrawn with permission from Kettle DS (1990) *Medical and Veterinary Entomology*, CAB International, from an original drawing by HJ Hawthorne.

Figs 15.3, 15.4, 15.5 were reproduced with kind permission of Mr L Baker.

List of Colour Plates

Plate 1.1 *Candida albicans*. When incubated in serum the cells produce characteristic outgrowths called germ tubes.

Plate 1.2 A filamentous fungi. Tubular hyphae with groups of spores.

Plate 1.3 *Entamoeba histolytica*. These protozoa cause amoebic dysentry. The black dots are red blood cells which have been engulfed. The nucleus can be seen in the lower right of the cell.

Plate 2.1 There are four main groups of bacteria: (a) Gram-positive cocci, (b) Gram-positive bacilli (rods), (c) Gram-negative cocci, and (d) Gram-negative bacilli (rods).

Plate 2.2 Cerebrospinal fluid from two cases of meningitis. (a) Large mononuclear cells and neutrophils can be seen with a number of small Gram-negative rods. Provisional diagnosis: *Haemophilus influenzae* meningitis. (b) Cerebrospinal fluid containing large numbers of pus cells. Some neutrophils contain small Gram-negative diplococci. Provisional diagnosis: *Neisseria meningitidis* meningitis.

Plate 2.3 Large colonies of *Bacillus cereus*.

Plate 2.4 *Staphylococcus aureus*.

Plate 2.5 *Streptococcus* Group A. Haemolysins produced by *Streptococcus* lyse the red blood cells in blood agar, producing a clear area around the colonies.

Plate 2.6 *Pseudomonas aeruginosa*. The colonies of *Ps. aeruginosa* appear green when grown on nutrient agar.

Plate 2.7 *Serratia marcescens*. The colonies of *S. marcescens* have a characteristic red coloration.

Plate 2.8 Mixed growth of organisms. Specimens often contain more than one type of bacteria, illustrated by the different forms of colony on this plate.

Plate 2.9 API galleries. The colour change in each chamber of the gallery helps to identify the species of bacteria present.

Plate 2.10 Antibiotic sensitivity testing. Antibiotics in each disc diffuse into the agar. Bacteria cannot grow around the discs unless they are resistant to the antibiotic in the disc.

Plate 2.11 Sputum from a case of suspected pneumonia. Gram-positive cocci, mostly in pairs, can be seen amongst the numerous, large, pus cells. Provisional diagnosis: pneumococcal pneumonia.

Plate 2.12 Tubercle bacilli appear as clumps of fine rods.

Plate 2.13 Biohazard label.

Plate 3.1 Staphylococcal infection of the eyes.

1

Introduction to Microbiology and Infection Control

Introduction

Microbiology is the study of living organisms so small that they cannot be seen with the naked eye. This generally includes any organism of between 0.1 and 1 mm in diameter, which although just visible require magnification to see detail. Organisms of less than 0.1 mm cannot be seen at all without a microscope.

Investigation of the world of the **microbe** began in the seventeenth century with the invention of the **microscope** by a Dutch merchant, Antony Van Leeuwenhoek, who like many great scientists of his time made astounding discoveries in his spare time. Although modern microscopes bear little resemblance to those designed by Leeuwenhoek, they are based are broadly similar principles (Fig. 1.1).

Leeuwenhoek was the first to appreciate the variety and profusion of the microbial world as he indicated in one of his letters to the Royal Society of London:

I have had several gentlewomen in my house who were keen on seeing the little eels in vinegar; but some of them were so disgusted at the spectacle, that they vowed they'd never use vinegar again. But what if one should tell such people in future that there are more animals living in the scum on the teeth in a man's mouth, than there are men in a whole kingdom?

Fig.1.1
The principles of the light microscope (a) Leeuwenhoek's microscope. Magnification is achieved by means of a lens with a very short focal length which is capable of high magnification. The specimen is brought into focus by moving the position of the lens relative to the specimen. (b) A modern light microscope. Visible light is directed through the specimen and magnified by the lens and eyepiece.

(a) Leeuwenhoek's microscope

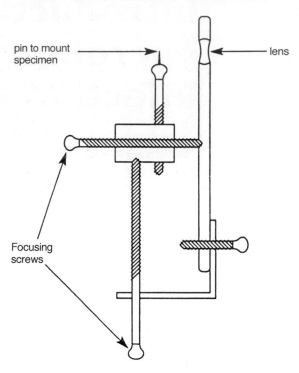

pin to mount specimen

lens

Focusing screws

(b) light microscope

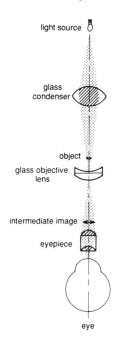

light source

glass condenser

object

glass objective lens

intermediate image

eyepiece

eye

Microbes are everywhere, they are able to survive in almost every conceivable environment, even in conditions where other plants or animals cannot. Some can withstand temperatures of more than 95°C and live in hot water springs, whilst others can grow at temperatures as low as −10°C. Some grow in the absence of oxygen and they can utilize almost any chemical substance as a source of energy.

They perform many useful functions in the ecological cycle, forming the first link in the aquatic food chain (e.g. plankton, algae) and fixing atmospheric nitrogen into the soil so that it can be used by plants. Microbes are responsible for the breakdown of dead plants and animals making their constituent chemicals available for use by others.

Many foods are produced by the activities of microbes; cheese, yoghurt, beer, wine, bread and vinegar and they are also used to manufacture drugs such as insulin, and hepatitis B **vaccine**.

Classification

A system of identifying individual organisms and their relationship to each other has been gradually developed since the mid-eighteenth century when Linnaeus established the first system of biological classification. Organisms are placed into groups according to similarities in their structure. Each is allocated two names, the first denotes the group or **genus** to which it belongs and the second gives it a specific name within that group, the **species**.

Bacteria of a species can often be further distinguished into different 'strains', according to slightly different characteristics. This subdivision of bacterial species usually requires complex laboratory techniques called typing based on the analysis of cellular **proteins** or susceptibility to bacterial viruses (**bacteriophages**).

In the early days, microbial science developed independently to other biological sciences and microbial cells were considered to be very different to plant or animal cells. By the mid-twentieth century it had become apparent that there were many similarities in the biochemistry of all living organisms and the study of microbes has helped our understanding of how all cells work at a molecular level.

As our knowledge and laboratory techniques have improved, organisms previously categorized together are found to be unrelated or more closely related to another genus. These **micro-organisms** sometimes change their name when they are re-classified (e.g. *Streptococcus faecum* has recently been re-named as an *Enterococcus*). Some micro-organisms are very difficult to classify as they have features of more than one genus. For example, *Pneumocystis carinii*, although currently classified as a **protozoa**, is actually very closely related to **fungi**.

Fig. 1.2
The structure of cells.
(a) A bacterial cell.
(b) A eucaryotic cell.

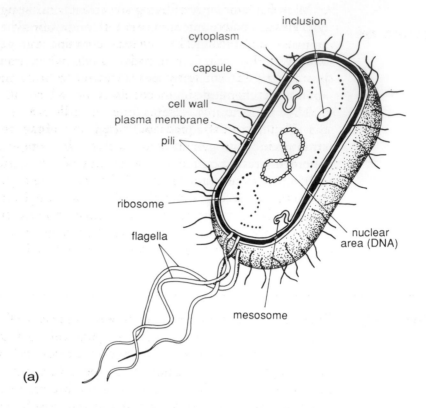

(a)

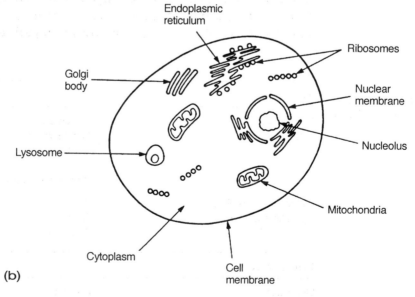

(b)

The Structure of Cells

A cell is the basic unit of living structures, consisting of a **nucleus** and **cytoplasm** enclosed in semipermeable membrane and, in some cases, an outer **cell wall**. The nucleus contains the genetic information unique to that cell, it is a code which, when translated, creates the specific proteins and **enzymes** necessary to build and operate the cell.

Although these basic mechanisms by which all cells function are broadly the same, two distinct types of cells can be identified (see Fig. 1.2). Plants, animals, protozoa, fungi and **algae** are all composed of **eucaryotic cells**. Plants and animals are composed of many cells, extensively differentiated so that groups of cells perform different tasks within the whole plant or animal. Protozoa and algae are much simpler organisms, consisting of single cells, whilst fungi can be unicellular or multicellular, but without any differentiation between the cells.

Procaryotic cells are less complex; they only form single-celled organisms and include all **bacteria** (see Table 1.1).

The Cell Wall

There are significant differences between the cell walls of procaryotic and eucaryotic cells. The shape of procaryotic cells is determined by a rigid cell wall made of a network of **carbohydrates** and **amino acids** called **peptidoglycan**. The amount of peptidoglycan in the cell wall determines the staining properties of the bacterial cell (see Chapter 2), and provides a method of identifying and classifying bacteria (see Fig. 1.3). **Gram-positive** organisms are surrounded by a cell wall made almost entirely of peptidoglycan. **Gram-negative** cells have a layer of

Table 1.1
Examples of eucaryotic and procaryotic organisms

Eucaryotic	
Multicellular (differentiated)	Vertebrates
	Invertebrates
	Seed-forming plants
	Ferns
	Mosses and liverworts
Multicellular/unicellular (undifferentiated)	Algae
	Fungi
	Protozoa
Procaryotic	
Unicellular	Bacteria
	Mycoplasma
	Rickettsia
	Chlamydia

Fig. 1.3
The structure of the cell wall of a Gram-negative bacteria. Both inner and outer membranes are made of phospholipid. The porins in the outer membrane enable substances to pass into the cell. The sugars and side chains attached to the outer membrane are antigenic. The layer of peptidoglycan between the membranes is not as thick in Gram-positive cells.

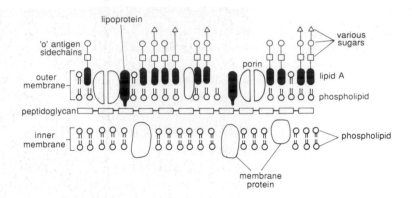

peptidoglycan sandwiched between two layers of **phospholipid** membrane. The outer membrane contains **lipopolysaccharides** – these are **endotoxins** and have harmful effects on the animal host. The chains of sugars which form part of the lipopolysaccharide are called O **antigens**. These are an important means of identification for Gram-negative bacteria. Penicillin and many other **antibiotics** destroy bacteria by interfering with the synthesis of peptidoglycan. Eucaryotic cells do not contain peptidoglycan therefore these drugs have no effect on the cells of the animal receiving treatment.

Eucaryotic cells are usually enclosed by a membrane rather than a cell wall, but if a cell wall is present then it is a simple structure composed of sugars or, in the case of algae and plant cells, cellulose.

Capsules

Most bacteria produce a layer of gelatinous material outside the cell wall which forms either a loose layer of slime or a more clearly defined **capsule**. This protects the cell against white blood cells and also helps it to adhere to a range of surfaces, including teeth, plastic catheters and prosthetic devices.

Spores and Cysts

Clostridium and *Bacillus* bacteria are able form **spores** by enclosing their cells in a resistant casing which is extremely difficult to destroy by chemicals or heat. The bacteria form spores when they are exposed to adverse environmental conditions e.g. no food source, high or low temperatures or oxygen (see Fig. 1.4). When conditions improve the spores germinate and the cell starts to multiply. Spores can survive for very long periods; spores of *Bacillus anthrax* could still be recovered from the soil of an island off the Scottish coast used to test biological weapons many years after they had been tested there.

Fig. 1.4
A Clostridium *cell showing a spore distending the middle of the rod (electronmicrograph).*

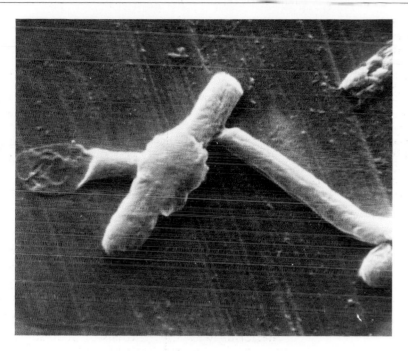

Some protozoa (e.g. *Giardia* and *Entamoeba*) change into **cysts** which enable them to survive for many months outside a host.

The Cytoplasm

The biochemical reactions that maintain the cell and enable it to reproduce all take place within the cytoplasm of the cell. The membrane that surrounds the cell is selectively permeable, it allows some substances to pass through but not others.

Eucaryotic cells have a complex cytoplasm with many tubules to enable the cytoplasm to move from one part of the cell to another. **Organelles** are also present; these are distinct structures in which various cellular activities take place. Unicellular organisms can take up nutrients from the environment easily because the surface area available for absorption is much greater than in multicellular organisms. The cytoplasm of prokaryotic cells is therefore much less complex because they do not need the same transport mechanisms; however, a few organelles are present (Table 1.2).

The Nucleus

In eucaryotic cells the nucleus contains more than one chromosome and is surrounded by a nuclear membrane. Procaryotic cells contain only one chromosome which is not enclosed in a membrane but lies in the cytoplasm.

	Eucaryotic cell
Endoplasmic reticulum	Parallel pairs of membranes where synthesis and transport of proteins, lipids, and other products takes place
Ribosomes	Sites of protein synthesis. They are found both on the endoplasmic reticulum and free in the cytoplasm
Mitochondria	These contain the enzymes responsible for the synthesis of ATP
Golgi complex	These are groups of vesicles which secrete synthesized substances such as lipids, enzymes and other proteins out of the cell
	Procaryotic cell
Mesosomes	These are formed by involution of the cell membrane. In some bacteria they contain enzymes responsible for respiration
Ribosomes	Many of these are found free in the cytoplasm. They are the site of protein synthesis and are smaller than those in eucaryotic cells
Inclusion bodies	These are for the storage of lipids

The Genetic Code

The chromosome is made of **deoxyribonucleic acid (DNA)** which carries the genetic information needed to operate all the activities within the cell. DNA is made of two complementary stands of **nucleotides** held together by **hydrogen bonds** and twisted together to form a double-**helix**. In bacterial cells the helix is further coiled and, although it may be 1000 times the length of the cell, it only takes up 10% of the cytoplasm. Nucleotides consist of a sugar molecule, attached to a phosphate molecule and one of four bases: **adenine**, **cytosine**, **guanine** and **thymine** (see Fig. 1.5). A **base** is a molecule which can accept a hydrogen ion and can connect with another base by forming a weak association or hydrogen bond. Adenine always bonds or pairs with thymine, whilst guanine always pairs with cytosine. Two chains or strands of nucleotides are held together by hydrogen bonds between the **pairs of bases** and are therefore mirror images of each other.

The sequence of bases form the code in which all the information needed to make the constituent molecules of the cell is stored. The code made by adenine, cytosine, guanine and thymine can be compared to making-up three-letter 'words' with A, C, G, and T. Each 'word' can be translated into one of the amino acids that are needed to make proteins (Table 1.3).

An average protein is composed of about 400 amino acids and corresponds to a sequence of 1200 bases along the nucleotide chain. Each section of DNA that codes for a protein is called a **gene**.

When cells divide, the chromosome of each new cell must contain both strands of DNA. To make an accurate copy of the DNA the two

Fig. 1.5
The structure of deoxyribonucleic acid (DNA). S, sugar molecule; P, phosphate molecule; C, cytosine; G, guanine; A, adenine; T, thymine; - - -, hydrogen bond.

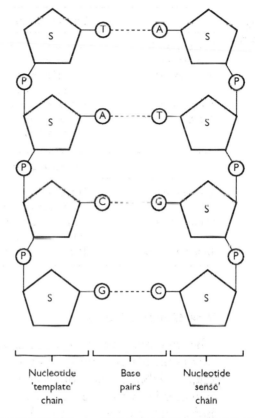

Nucleotide 'template' chain   Base pairs   Nucleotide 'sense' chain

Table 1.3
The genetic code

Sequence of bases on DNA	Equivalent amino acid
GCG	Alanine
TTC	Phenylalanine
CGC	Arginine
AAA	Lysine

strands are gradually separated and both then become a pattern against which a new strand is made. After replication, the two daughter chromosomes contain one strand from the parent and one new strand (see Fig. 1.6).

Plasmids

Many bacterial cells carry small circles of DNA called **plasmids** which are not incorporated into the main chromosome. Plasmid DNA can be replicated on its own and copied into each daughter cell. Plasmids do not contain any genes essential for cell viability and can be lost without damaging the cell. Plasmids often contain genes that confer resistance to antibiotics, synthesize **toxins** that enable the organism to harm its

Fig. 1.6
The copying of a chromosome.
(a) The two strands of DNA are
separated and a copy made of
each half. (b) The two identical
chromosomes.

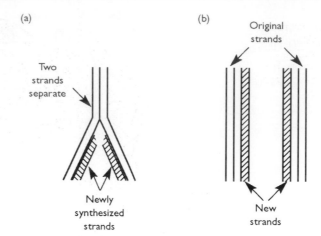

(a)

Two strands separate

Newly synthesized strands

(b)

Original strands

New strands

hosts (e.g. **haemolysins** which destroy red blood cells), or cause serious illness (e.g. diphtheria).

The Properties of Cells

The activities of all cells from the smallest bacteria to the largest mammal are controlled by enzymes (see Fig. 1.7). Enzymes catalyse or speed up a whole range of chemical reactions; they control energy-making reactions, enable the cell to synthesize complex materials from nutrients and to grow and divide into new cells.

Cell Metabolism

The chemical reactions that take place in all living cells are described as the **metabolism** of the cell. **Anabolism** is where new compounds are formed from simple molecules. **Catabolism** is where large and complicated compounds are broken down into their constituent molecules, releasing energy.

The protein structure of the cell and its enzymes are made up of amino acids and the main food reserves of the cell, carbohydrates and **fats**.

All living cells need energy to maintain the chemical and physical composition of their cytoplasm and to grow and replicate themselves. The original source of energy is solar energy from the sun. This is captured by plants and a few bacteria by a process called **photosynthesis**. Most bacteria and all animals then use plants as a source of nutrients and energy.

The biologically usable form of energy, which is present in all cells, is **adenosine triphosphate (ATP)**. Glucose is broken down in the cell and its energy is captured in the form of ATP. There are 10 chemical reactions used to convert one molecule of glucose to carbon dioxide and water,

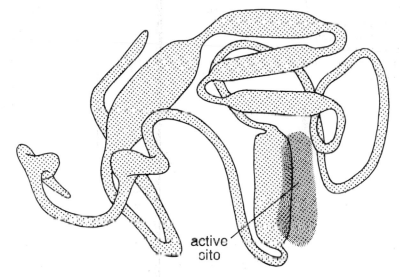

Fig. 1.7
The structure of an enzyme. The complicated folded structure of enzymes is essential for their activity. The active site is where molecules combine with the enzyme.

active site

and during these reactions 30 molecules of ATP are produced. ATP is then used by the cell to:

- make new cell components
- transport substances into the cell
- move the cell
- move the cell cytoplasm

When this energy-forming process involves the use of oxygen, it is called **respiration**. Some cells use **organic compounds** instead of oxygen and produce **alcohol** as the end product instead of water. This process is called **fermentation** and is characteristic of **anaerobic** bacteria.

Protein Synthesis

The synthesis of a string of amino acids begins with the creation of a short length of **ribonucleic acid (RNA)** corresponding to the sequence of bases on the DNA strand. RNA has a similar structure to DNA except that it is a single chain, the sugar is ribose not deoxyribose and the thymine is replaced by a very similar base, **uracil**. This 'messenger RNA' moves to the **ribosomes** where the code is read and the appropriate amino acids assembled into a chain. Amino acids are brought to the ribosome by a carrier called '**transfer RNA**' (tRNA). There is a specific tRNA for each type of amino acid (see Fig. 1.8).

Cell Division

Procaryotic cells multiply by dividing in two in a process called **binary fission**. When the cell has grown to a certain size, the single

Fig. 1.8
The synthesis of protein. A length of RNA is made from the DNA strand and moves to a ribosome. The amino acids corresponding to the code on the RNA are brought from the cytoplasm by transfer RNA and assembled into a protein.

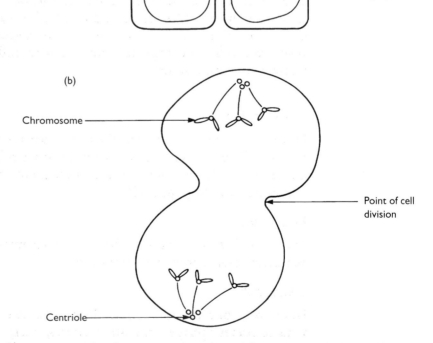

Alanine   Arginine   Lysine

Transfer RNA

G C G   C G C   A A A

C G C G C G U U U

Messenger RNA

Ribosome

Fig. 1.9
Simple cell division (meiosis). (a) A bacterial cell. The chromosome replicates, a new cell wall forms and divides the original cell into two. (b) A eucaryotic cell. The chromosome replicates, one set is then distributed to each end of the cell which then divides into two.

(a)

Cell wall

Nuclear area

Cytoplasm

(b)

Chromosome

Point of cell division

Centriole

chromosome divides into two identical copies and the cell wall and membrane grow inwards forming a new cell wall across the cell. Eventually it splits the cytoplasm into two cells, each with a chromosome (see Fig 1.9). Often the two cells do not completely separate from each other but remain together as clumps (e.g. staphylococci), in chains (e.g. streptococci) or in pairs (e.g. pneumococci).

Eucaryotic cells can divide by simple division, or **mitosis**, in a similar way to procaryotes. All the DNA is copied and each set enclosed in a nuclear membrane. The cytoplasm then divides to form two identical cells. This type of division will occur as the plant or animal makes new cells to grow or to repair damaged tissue.

Sexual Reproduction

Sexual reproduction describes the process of mixing genetic information from more than one individual together and is a method of introducing variation into the population. Variation is important because it enables a species to adapt to its environment and gradually evolve.

Eucaryotes

In eucaryotic cells sexual reproduction is achieved by fusing two cells from different individuals together. Since this would result in one cell with double the usual number of chromosomes, a special type of cell division called **meiosis** is required. Instead of replicating the chromosomes, the pairs are separated and one half of each pair placed in each cell, each cell has half the usual number of chromosomes. At **fertilization**, two cells fuse together and the new cell will contain the full number of chromosomes.

Procaryotes

Procaryotic cells do not multiply by sexual reproduction. However, transfer of genetic material between bacterial cells occurs but always in one direction, from a donor cell to a recipient cell. Transfer happens in one of three ways (Fig. 1.10):

Transformation

Strands of free DNA outside the cell are absorbed through the cell wall and incorporated into the chromosome.

Transduction

DNA from one bacteria is introduced into another cell by a bacterial virus or bacteriophage. Like other viruses, phages must incorporate into the host DNA in order to replicate. Sometimes some of the host's DNA is copied with the virus DNA by mistake and ends up being taken out of the cell with the phage. This is the method by which some bacteria acquire resistance to antibiotics.

Fig. 1.10
Methods used by bacteria to exchange genetic information.
(a) Transformation.
(b) Transduction.
(c) Conjugation.

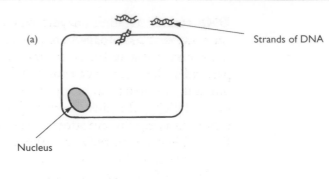

(a)

Strands of DNA

Nucleus

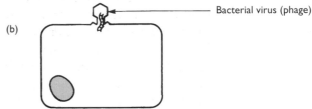

(b)

Bacterial virus (phage)

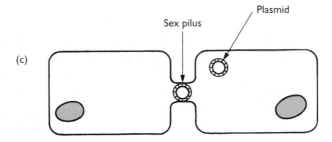

Plasmid

Sex pilus

(c)

Conjugation

This is the transfer of plasmid DNA from one bacterial cell to another through a small tube or **sex pilus**. The pilus of one cell must attach to the **sex pilus** of another cell. The plasmid DNA then replicates and one copy enters the recipient cell. Plasmids commonly carry genes conferring resistance to antibiotics or toxin production, so conjugation is of major importance in the spread of these abilities between strains of bacteria.

Genetic Engineering

Although the term genetic engineering can sound very threatening, it has enabled tremendous advances to be made both in our understanding of the **genetic code**, in particular the human chromosome, and in the synthesis of substances useful in medicine and industry.

Genetic engineering depends on the activity of **nucleases**, which are enzymes that cut the DNA strand. **Restriction endonucleases** are special types of nuclease that recognize specific sequences of bases in

DNA strands. As each enzyme will always recognize the same sequence, the same sections of DNA are always obtained from a particular chromosome and it is possible to separate a single gene known to synthesize a particular chemical. If the same endonuclease is then used to cut a DNA plasmid, the gene cut from the chromosome can be inserted into the plasmid. The plasmids are mixed with bacterial cells and the plasmid DNA, carrying the introduced gene, enters the bacteria by **transformation**. When the bacteria are cultured they synthesize the substance coded for by the introduced gene.

This method has been used to manufacture substances used in the treatment of human disease by inserting genes from the human chromosome into bacteria. For example, the gene coding for human insulin has been inserted into a bacteria and human insulin can now be manufactured by the culture of these bacteria. Fragments of DNA from the hepatitis B virus have also been incorporated into a plasmid, which is inserted into a yeast. The viral proteins produced by the yeast as it multiplies are purified and made into a vaccine against hepatitis B virus.

Cell Motility

Many bacteria are not capable of independent movement. Some have appendages called **flagella** which, by rotating like a propeller, enable them to swim (see Fig 1.11). These motile bacteria swim towards chemicals such as nutrients that they are attracted to, and swim away from toxic substances. Many Gram-negative bacteria such as *Escherichia coli* and *Pseudomonas* have flagella and are motile. Motile bacteria thrive in

Fig. 1.11
Flagella on a bacterial cell.

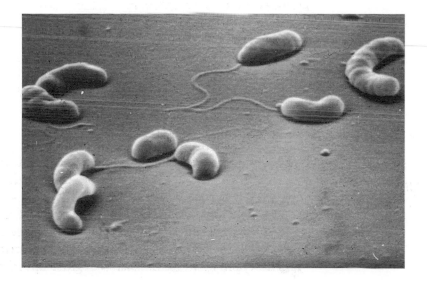

moist conditions where the ability to swim is an advantage, whilst non-motile bacteria are able to survive in dry environments.

Eucaryotic cells may also have flagella or **cilia** but with a much more complex structure.

The Growth and Multiplication of Bacteria

Since bacteria live in an enormous range of environments, it is not surprising that the nutrients they need vary widely from species to species. A bacteria supplied with all the nutrients it needs will divide, on average once every 15 min and will continue to grow at this rate until the supply of nutrients is exhausted. There are certain basic substances that are essential to support the growth of all bacteria:

Energy Source

Energy is generally obtained from the breakdown of organic carbon-containing compounds, although some bacteria are able to capture the energy of the sun in the same way as plants.

Carbon Source

Carbon is necessary to form the compounds that make up the structure of the cell. Most bacteria obtain carbon from organic compounds such as glucose, but some use carbon from the atmosphere in the form of carbon dioxide (CO_2).

Nitrogen Source

Nitrogen is also found in many of the cell structures, for example proteins. Nitrogen can be obtained in the form of ammonia (NH_4) or nitrates (NO_3) and some microbes can use atmospheric nitrogen.

Inorganic Ions

Sodium, potassium, magnesium, chloride, sulphate and phosphorus are needed both to form the structure of the cell and to operate some of its machinery.

Some bacteria will grow in very simple media containing only these substances, although usually they will grow very slowly. Most of the bacteria which cause disease in humans depend on the presence of additional 'growth factors' available in the host tissue. These are usually **amino acids** or vitamins that the bacteria cannot make themselves.

Other chemicals, or **trace elements** such as iron or zinc, may be required to make enzymes.

We can help to prevent the multiplication of bacteria in the clinical environment by removing potential sources of nutrients. For example, body fluid spilt on to equipment, furniture or floors will support the growth of bacteria and should be removed as soon as possible; baths or washbowls that are not properly cleaned will retain a coating of skin scales and soap on their surface which provides plentiful supply of nutrients for the growth of bacteria (Greaves, 1985).

Environmental Factors

Environmental conditions also have a very important effect on the growth of bacteria. Bacteria that cause disease usually grow most rapidly under the environmental conditions found in the human body.

Water

Water is an essential requirement for the growth of bacteria and most die rapidly in the absence of water. The moisture-loving Gram-negatives, in particular, will thrive in damp places. They are particularly vulnerable to desiccation and will only survive for a short time on dry surfaces. The susceptibility of many bacteria to a lack of water provides us with a very useful infection control measure; we can prevent bacteria multiplying by keeping surfaces clean and dry and by drying equipment thoroughly before it is stored. Equipment should not be immersed in liquids for prolonged periods as bacteria can even grow in **disinfectants**. Thermometers stored in disinfectant solutions or mops lingering in buckets of dirty water are commonly encountered infection hazards (Werry *et al.* 1988). Equipment such as nebulizers or ventilator equipment which are in contact with water are particularly hazardous because bacteria can multiply rapidly in the moisture (Botman and de Krieger, 1987; Cefai *et al.*, 1990).

Other bacteria are more resistant to drying out (e.g. staphylococci and *Mycobacterium*) or are able to form spores (e.g. *Clostridium difficile*). They may be able to survive for hours or even months, recommencing multiplication if a supply of water is resumed. These organisms may survive in dust and thus preventing the accumulation of dust on surfaces and floors can be an important infection control measure (Casewell, 1986; Cartmill *et al*, 1994).

Oxygen

Most bacteria can grow with or without oxygen and are called facultative anaerobes. Some bacteria will grow only in the presence of oxygen and they are called **aerobes**. Bacteria that will not grow if oxygen is present are called anaerobes and they are found inside body cavities such as the intestines and vagina. Anaerobic bacteria such as *Clostridium perfringens* can cause serious infection in wounds where the tissue is extensively damaged or **necrotic** and poorly supplied with oxygen. Wounds that have a good blood supply will be well oxygenated and unlikely to support the growth of anaerobic bacteria.

Temperature

Most bacteria will grow within a wide range of temperatures but those that grow in association with humans grow most rapidly at around body temperature. Some bacteria are known for their ability to multiply even at very low temperatures. *Listeria monocytogenes*, for example, multiplies even at 5°C and can therefore spoil refrigerated food.

pH

The pH of a solution reflects the concentration of hydrogen ions. Most bacteria prefer approximately neutral solutions, but some can survive in very **acidic** environments and others in very **alkaline**.

Concentration of Solution

Molecules that are dissolved in a solution are called **solutes**. The membrane surrounding the cell prevents the passage of solutes into the cell. If the cell is in a solution where the concentration of solutes is greater than in the cytoplasm of the cell, then there is a tendency for water to diffuse out of the cell into the solution in order to equilibrate the concentrations. If the concentration of solutes in the cytoplasm is greater than outside the cell then the water will diffuse into the cell. This process is known as **osmosis**. Like all cells, bacteria have transport mechanisms operating at the membrane to make sure that the level of solutes in the cytoplasm remains at the desired concentration regardless of the concentration in their environment. In fact, the bacterial cell wall is able to withstand a wide range of very strong and dilute solutions.

The common practice of adding salt to a patient's bath to 'clean' wounds is of no actual value. The salt would need to be added in enormous quantities to achieve a final concentration in the bathwater sufficient to disrupt bacterial cells and simply adding a cupful of salt to a bath of water has no antibacterial effect at all (Ayliffe *et al.*, 1975; Austin, 1988).

Fungi

Fungi are plants. They have eucaryotic cells but lack the green pigment, **chlorophyll**, which other plants use for photosynthesis. Most fungi grow as filamentous, branching tubes and are described as **moulds**. Others grow as single, ovoid cells or **yeasts**. Often one species can grow as either a yeast or a mould depending on the temperature and the availability of oxygen and nutrients. Mycology is the term used to describe the study of fungi.

Yeasts

Yeast cells are between 20 and 100 times larger than a bacterial cell but can only be seen with the aid of a microscope. They can be grown on solid **agar** medium where, like bacteria, they appear as masses of cells or colonies (see Chapter 2). Yeasts multiply asexually by forming buds, where a new cell gradually grows out of the parent cell (Plate 1.1). They reproduce sexually by meiotic division of a single cell, which then forms two daughter cells or ascospores. Later two ascospores will fuse to form a new cell.

Yeasts are widely distributed in nature and commonly found on plants and in soil. Many species are extremely useful, for example in the fermentation of sugars to produce alcohol and carbon dioxide, a process used in brewing and bread making.

Filamentous Fungi

These fungi produce branching, tubular filaments or *hyphae* which form a mass called *mycelium*. Filaments act like roots, penetrating into the substance on which they are growing. In some species the filaments are separated into cells by transverse walls, although these are often perforated allowing for the movement of cytoplasm or nuclei. Filamentous fungi usually reproduce asexually by forming spores but they can also form buds like yeasts, or detach short segments of mycelium (Plate 1.2). Sexual reproduction occurs by fusion of cells in the mycelium to form spores but the exact mechanism varies in each species.

Moulds, like yeasts, are widely distributed in the environment and many live in soil, where they decompose organic matter. They can be grown on the same media as bacteria but because they can survive in relatively little moisture and in high osmolarity, they are often found growing on substances which will not support the growth of bacteria (e.g. jams and other preserved foods).

Protozoa

These are relatively large, but still microscopic eucaryotic cells (Plate 1.3). They have a tough outer cell membrane instead of a cell wall and can obtain nutrients by ingesting solid particles of food, a distinctive characteristic of animal cells. The cells multiply by dividing in two and some species differentiate between male and female cells. Many protozoa have life cycles; that is, a series of stages in their development. They are motile in at least one of these stages and some form thick-walled, dormant cysts which are important in transmission (e.g. *Entamoeba histolytica*).

Viruses

Viruses are not cells, they are simply a piece of **nucleic acid**, either DNA or RNA, protected by a protein coat and sometimes an envelope made of **lipids**. Viruses contain none of the structures necessary to synthesize the proteins or enzymes encoded by their nucleic acid. The smallest viruses contain enough nucleic acid to make three or four proteins, the largest several hundred proteins (Fig. 1.12).

Viruses are extremely small, ranging from 27 nm in diameter to about 200 nm, compared to an average bacterial cell of about 1000 nm in diameter, and are therefore too small to be seen with an ordinary light microscope. Instead they can be seen using an **electron microscope** which uses a beam of **electrons** instead of light to create an image of an object on a photographic plate. Figure 1.13 shows an electron micrograph of adenovirus.

Viral Replication

Viruses can only multiply inside living cells. Receptors on the protein coat recognize and attach to particular cells in their host. The viral nucleic acid then enters the nucleus of the host cell where it instructs the cell's own mechanism to copy the nucleic acids and translate its code into viral proteins. Many copies of the viral nucleic acid and proteins are made by the host cell in this way. The virus components are then assembled in the cytoplasm and new viruses are released from the cell either by budding out of the cell membrane or causing the cell to rupture (Figure 1.14). The host cells infected are usually destroyed by the virus,

Fig. 1.12
The structure of viruses

naked icosahedral (e.g. poliovirus)

KEY.

spikes (glycoprotein)
envelope (protein and lipids)

proteins making up
the capsid

nucleic acid

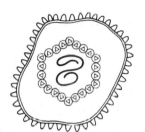

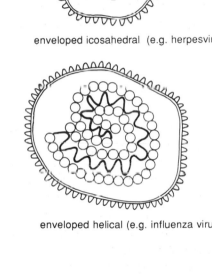

enveloped icosahedral (e.g. herpesvirus)

enveloped helical (e.g. influenza virus)

Fig. 1.13
*An electron micrograph of
adenovirus.*

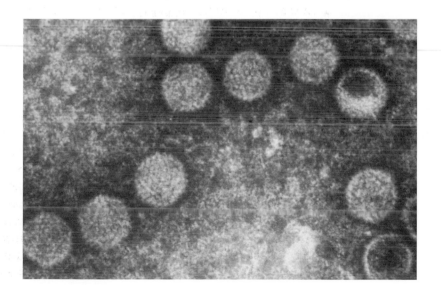

Fig. 1.14
The replication of viruses within a host cell.
The virus enters the host cell and its genome moves to a ribosome where it is transcribed, to make many copies of viral proteins and genome. The protein coats and genomes are assembled and then bud out of the cell, collecting part of the cell membrane of the host cell on the way out.

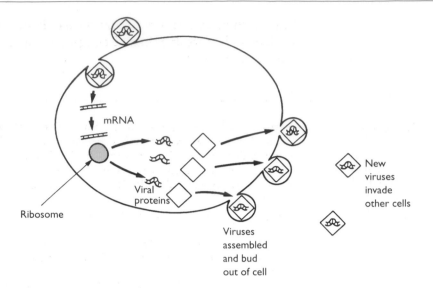

mRNA

Ribosome

Viral proteins

Viruses assembled and bud out of cell

New viruses invade other cells

but because the cells are rapidly replaced, most viral illnesses are short and recovery is complete. Some viral infections can cause permanent damage; for example the human immunodeficiency virus (HIV) so depletes the **T cells** of the immune system that the immune system becomes defective.

Some viruses insert all or part of their nucleic acids into the host cell's DNA, where it remains and causes the cell to become malignant by coding for unlimited cell division. This has been suggested as the mechanism by which viruses such as herpes simplex type 2 virus and human papilloma virus could cause cancer of the cervix (Mindel, 1989).

Viral Growth Requirements

Since viruses depend on living cells for their replication, it is not possible to grow them in artificial media in the same way as bacteria. Instead, viruses are grown in cultures of living cells and require an environment that will maintain the cells, including salts, amino acid and vitamins. A few viruses, for example rotavirus, cannot even be grown in these artificial cell cultures, and thus to experiment on them live animals must be used.

Most viruses are fragile and cannot survive outside a living cell for long. However, some viruses can survive for some time on surfaces or hands and from there are transmitted to a new host (Mahl and Sadler, 1975). Viruses are fairly resistant to the activity of some disinfectants such as phenol or chlorhexidine that are unable to disrupt their protein coat or lipid membrane. Outbreaks of viral gastrointestinal or respiratory infection occur frequently in hospital. Preventing outbreaks of infection by viruses can be extremely difficult; they are very small, can be exhaled on small respiratory droplets or be excreted in high numbers in faeces.

Transmission commonly occurs on hands and may potentially occur on inadequately decontaminated equipment such as commodes or bedpans (Ansari *et al.*, 1991).

References

Ansari SA, Springthorpe VS, Sattar SA *et al.* (1991) Potential role of hands in the spread of respiratory viral infections: Studies with Human Parainfluenza Virus 3 and Rhinovirus. 14 *J. Clin. Micro.* **29**: 2115–19.

Austin L (1988) The salt bath myth. *Nursing Times* **84** (9): 79–83.

Ayliffe G, Babb JR, Collins BJ (1975) Disinfection of baths and bathwater. *Nursing Times* **71** (37): 22–3

Bodey GP (1988) The emergence of fungi as major hospital pathogens. *J. Hosp. Inf.* **11** (Suppl. A): 411–26.

Botman MJ, de Krieger RA (1987) Contamination of small-volume medication nebulizers and its association with oropharyngeal colonisation. *J. Hosp. Inf.* **19**. 204–8.

Cartmill TDI, Parigrahi H, Worsley MA *et al.* (1994) Management and control of a large out break of diarrhoea due to *Clostridium difficile*. *J. Hosp. Inf.* **27**:1–16.

Caswell MW (1986) Epidemiology and control of the 'modern' methicillin resistant *Staphylococcus aureus*. *J. Hosp. Inf.* **7** (Suppl. A): 1–11.

Cefai C, Richards J, Gould FK *et al.* (1990) An outbreak of *Acinetobacter* respiratory tract infection resulting from incomplete disinfection of ventilatory equipment. *J. Hosp. Inf* **15**: 177–82.

Greaves A (1985) We'll just freshen you up, dear. *Nursing Times* **Mar 6** (suppl.). 3–8.

Mahl MC, Sadler C (1975) Virus survival on inanimate surfaces. *Canadian J. Micro.* **21**: 819–23.

Mindel A (1989) *Herpes Simplex Virus*. Springer-Verlag, London.

Walzer PD (1993) *Pneumocystis carinii*: recent advances in basic biology and their clinical application. *AIDS* **7**: 1293–305.

Werry C, Lawrence JM, Sanderson PJ (1988) Contamination of detergent cleaning solutions during hospital cleaning. *J. Hosp. Inf* **11**: 44–9.

Further Reading

Ackerman V, Dunk-Richards G (1991) *Microbiology – an Introduction for the Health sciences*. WB Saunders\Baillière Tindall, London.

Fuerst R (1983) *Frobisher and Fuerst's Microbiology in Health and Disease*, 15th edn. WB Saunders, London.

Kedzierski M (1991) Understanding virology. *Professional Nurse* Nov: 99–102.

Postgate J. (1992) *Microbes and Man*, 3rd edn. Cambridge University Press, Cambridge.

Stanier RY, Ingraham JL, Wheelis ML, Painter PR (1987) *General Microbiology*, 5th edn. Macmillan Education, London.

Stuke VA.(1993) *Microbiology for Nurses – Application to Patient Care*, 7th edn. Baillière Tindall, London.

Szekely M (1980) *From DNA to Protein*. Macmillan, London.

2 Understanding the Microbiology Laboratory

Introduction

In the modern age we rely extensively on antimicrobial agents to treat **infection**. It is easy to assume that at the first sign of fever we need only reach for an **antibiotic** to treat the infection and that identification and investigation of the causative organism are unnecessary. For minor infections it is reasonable to make an educated guess about the organism causing the infection, for example skin infections such as boils or septic spots are invariably caused by *Staphylococcus aureus*, and easily treated with flucloxacillin. However, the bacteria may be resistant to the antibiotic chosen, the bacteria may continue to multiply and the patient remains ill.

The function of the microbiology laboratory is to:

- assist in the diagnosis of infection
- identify the causative organism
- provide advice on the best antibiotic to treat the infection

The procedures used in the microbiology laboratory aim to reproduce the environmental conditions in which **pathogenic micro-organisms** grow and to identify the causative organism by separating out the different species present in the specimen.

Micro-organisms are found on every surface of the body as part of the normal flora (see Chapter 3) and they can therefore be isolated from almost any specimen. The microbiologist must be able to find the organism that is causing infection amongst all the other micro-organisms that normally live at the site or that may have contaminated the specimen.

The laboratory, as well as helping to interpret the results of specimens, can also provide advice on how the infection should be treated, the type of antibiotic to use and for how long. This advice is provided by medical microbiologists, doctors who, in addition to their medical qualification, have a specialist knowledge of microbiology. The infection control nurse can also provide a link between the laboratory and ward staff by helping to interpret results and advising on appropriate action.

The most common specimens received by a hospital microbiology laboratory include urine, faeces, blood, sputum, wound and throat swabs. Other laboratories, such as the Public Health Laboratories, specialize in identifying bacteria in food, water or other environmental samples; assist in the identification of uncommon organisms and advise on **outbreaks of infection** in hospitals or the community.

Identification of Bacteria
Microscopy

Examination of bacterial cells on glass slides under the **microscope** can reveal some important information about their structure and shape. The two main shapes of bacterial cells are round (cocci) or oblong (bacilli or rods), but other bacteria form curved rods (e.g. vibrios) or spirals (e.g. *Treponema*).

In 1884, Christian Gram developed a method of colouring cells with dyes in a technique now known as the **Gram stain**. A Gram stain only takes a few minutes to carry out and is the principal method used to divide bacteria into Gram-positive and Gram-negative organisms. **Gram-positive** cells absorb a dark blue dye and appear blue under the microscope. **Gram-negative** cells do not absorb the blue dye, but when counterstained with a red dye, stain pink (Plate. 2.1).

Microscopy and Gram-staining are often used to provide a provisional identification, particularly where the infection is life-threatening. For example, where meningitis is suspected examination of cerebrospinal fluid under the microscope may enable a provisional diagnosis to be made and appropriate antibiotic therapy started immediately (see Plate 2.2). **Fungi** can also have a characteristic appearance under the microscope, for example the *Candida albicans* illustrated in Plate 1.1.

Culture Methods

Unfortunately, bacteria cannot be reliably identified by their appearance under the microscope alone. Specimens are therefore grown in special media and a variety of tests used to identify the organism.

Solid media is made by mixing nutrients with **agar**, a gelling agent extracted from seaweed. The most commonly used medium in a hospital laboratory is blood agar, which contains horse blood. Changing the concentration of chemicals in the media can be used to reflect more closely the environment in which the pathogens are growing or to help pathogenic bacteria to grow in favour of the normal flora, making them easier to identify. For example, deoxycholate agar is used to isolate *Shigella* from stool specimens as it inhibits the growth of normal faecal flora such as *Escherichia coli*.

Bacteria which normally live on, or cause disease in, humans grow best in media that mimics the secretions or tissues of the human body. Some bacteria will grow in very simple media containing very few nutrients, others require complex media to supply most of their growth requirements.

Incubation at around body temperature encourages bacteria to grow rapidly, but it can still take between 24 and 48 h before there are enough cells for further testing. Some specimens will be cultured in special oxygen-free cabinets if potential pathogens are likely to be **anaerobes**, for example swabs taken from infected wounds.

The Appearance of Colonies

When bacteria are grown on solid medium, each bacterial cell will multiply many times and, after several hours, millions of bacteria will be present. The distinct group of cells appears as a **colony** and these can be seen on the agar without a microscope. Their size, colour and shape vary quite markedly between different species of bacteria and an experienced microbiologist can identify some bacteria from the appearance of their colonies on different types of media. Some bacteria such as *Bacillus cereus* (Plate 2.3) produce characteristically large colonies, whilst others such as *Staphylococcus* are smaller (Plate 2.4). **Enzymes** produced by certain bacteria lyse the red blood cells in blood agar, causing clear areas to form around the colonies (Plate 2.5). Other bacteria produce colonies of characteristic colour such as the green pigment of *Pseudomonas aeruginosa* (Plate 2.6) or red of *Serratia marcescens* (Plate 2.7).

Commonly, specimens contain a mixture of different bacteria and the skills of the microbiologist are needed to separate and identify each one (Plate 2.8).

Tests to Identify the Organism

Once the micro-organisms in a specimen have been **cultured**, further tests may have to be conducted to establish the exact species present. Commercially prepared kits are available which are used to distinguish bacteria by their ability to break down a range of substances. These kits enable a quick and accurate identification to be made. They are **inoculated**, incubated overnight and the subsequent colour change in each chamber used to make the identification (see Plate 2.9).

Sensitivity to Antibiotics

It is also important to establish whether different antibiotics have an effect on the organism to ensure that the right antibiotic is selected for treatment of the infection. Antibiotic sensitivity is tested by spreading the organism evenly over the surface of an agar plate, placing small circles of paper impregnated with different antibiotics onto the surface and incubating the plate overnight. The antibiotic diffuses from the paper into the agar and prevents sensitive bacteria growing in the area around the paper. Bacteria that are not affected by an antibiotic will be able to grow right up to the impregnated paper and hence are resistant to the antibiotic (see Plate 2.10).

Serology

Laboratories use a range of known antibodies that are specific to **antigens** on known **species** of micro-organism. The bacteria to be identified are mixed with the known **antibodies**. If they are of corresponding species, the specific antibody will bind to the bacterial cells and this reaction will be apparent as a clumping or **agglutination** of bacterial cells.

Typing of Bacterial Strains

In outbreaks of infection further, more specialized tests or 'typing' may be used to establish how closely related are bacteria isolated from different patients, and to indicate whether they have been acquired as a result of cross-infection. This usually involves sending the specimen to a specialist Public Health Laboratory which will distinguish discrete strains of bacteria by their susceptibility to bacterial viruses (**bacteriophages**), production of inhibitory substances or possession of specific antigens.

Identification of Viruses

There are two different approaches to the identification of viral infections. The first is the culture of virus or direct detection of virus particles, the second is the detection of specific antibodies in blood by **serological** testing.

Virus Culture

Unlike bacteria, viruses cannot be grown on artificial media but can only be cultured in living cells; that is, tissue cultures. Sheets of cells are grown in nutrient medium on glass or plastic. Viruses present in clinical specimens grown in the culture will alter the appearance of the cells in a characteristic manner (e.g. Herpes simplex). Not all viruses will grow in tissue culture. Some are diagnosed by special staining techniques or by **electron microscopy**. Provided sufficient viral particles are present these very powerful microscopes can be used to detect particles as small as $0.0001\mu m$ in size (Fig. 2.1). Detection of virus in samples of body fluid can resemble the search for a needle in a haystack and the absence of virus under the electron microscope should not be considered conclusive evidence of the absence of infection.

Serological Tests

Infection by a virus may be followed by the appearance of antibodies to the virus in the blood. The detection of these antibodies is the basis of serological testing and is used extensively to diagnose viral infections. There are several methods of diagnosing viral illnesses based on the same principle of detecting antibodies. The most widely used method is the **enzyme-linked immunosorbent assay (ELISA)**. **Antigen** specific to the antibody to be detected is placed into small wells on special plates and incubated with **serum** from the patient. If an antibody specific to the antigen in the well is present in the blood it will bind to it. Then an enzyme attached to an antibody which recognizes and binds to other antibodies is added and attaches to those wells containing the patient's antibody. This reaction is detected by a colour change caused by the enzyme.

The different tests used to identify viral infections are summarized in Table 2.1.

Serum Antibodies

Different types of antibody appear in the blood during the course of an infection (see Chapter 4). The type of antibody detected in the blood indicates whether the person has had the infection in the past or is recovering from the infection. This method is used to diagnose several viral infections including rubella and hepatitis. In the case of hepatitis B,

Fig. 2.1
Electron micrograph of rotavirus.

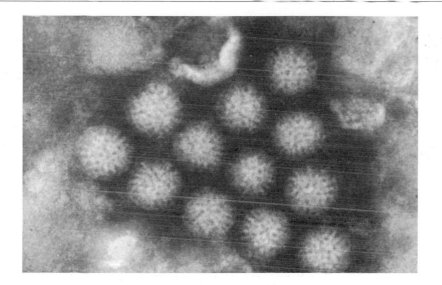

identification of the types of antibody present is used to indicate whether infection has persisted and the patient is a chronic **carrier** of the virus (see Chapter 3). Relating symptoms of an infection to a particular virus is difficult if only one sample of the patient's blood is examined. Antibodies to the virus may already be present as the result of a previous infection. A second sample of blood, taken about 10 days after the first, can be examined to see if the level of antibodies is greater than in the first sample. If a considerable increase in antibodies is found this is evidence that the virus is causing the infection. This test is described as *paired sera.*

The Collection of Specimens for Microbiological Investigation
Urine

Bladder urine is sterile but is easily contaminated during collection by bacteria which colonize the perineum. Contamination can be reduced by discarding the first few millilitres of urine and collecting the mid-stream of urine in a sterile container. Cleaning the perineum before the specimen is collected is of questionable value in reducing the risk of contamination (Holliday *et al.*, 1991).

If the patient has a urinary catheter, the specimen must always be withdrawn from the designated sampling sleeve on the tubing with a sterile needle and syringe (Fig. 2.2). Urine obtained from the catheter bag will provide misleading results as bacteria may have multiplied in the stagnant urine (Bradley *et al.*, 1986). The bag must not be disconnected from the catheter to obtain a specimen as this is likely to introduce bacteria into the system (Platt *et al.*, 1983). A urine sample of between 5 and 10 ml is usually sufficient for microbiological examination.

Table 2.1
*Some methods of
identifying viral infections*

Infection	Specimen	Test	Viruses
Respiratory tract infection	Throat swab nasopharyngeal washings	Culture	Influenza, para-influenza, RSV
	Paired sera	Serology	Influenza, para-influenza, RSV adenovirus, mumps
Vesicular skin lesions	Fluid from lesion	Electron microscopy, culture, serology	Herpes simplex, varicella zoster
Erythematous skin rash	Paired sera	Serology	Measles, rubella
Hepatitis	Serum	Serology	Hepatitis B, hepatitis A
Eye infections	Conjunctival scrapings	Culture	Herpes simplex, adenovirus
Gastroenteritis	Faeces	Electron microscopy	Rotavirus, calicivirus, small round virus

Paired sera = serum from two samples of blood taken 10 days apart.

Fig. 2.2
*The collection of a
specimen of catheter urine*

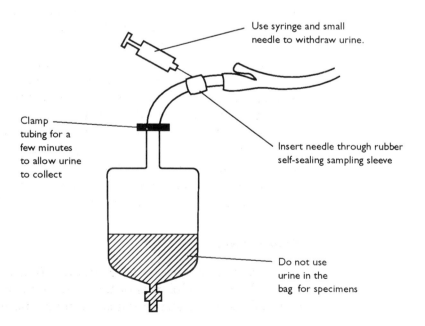

Use syringe and small needle to withdraw urine.

Clamp tubing for a few minutes to allow urine to collect

Insert needle through rubber self-sealing sampling sleeve

Do not use urine in the bag for specimens

Urine specimens easily support the growth of bacteria and their multiplication in specimens stored at room temperature can produce misleading results. The specimen should therefore be examined in the laboratory within 2 h, but if refrigerated can be stored for up to 24 h. The microbiologist investigates the number of white blood cells present in the specimen. Large numbers of white cells suggest that the body is mounting an immune response to infection and help to confirm that an organism present in the urine is actually causing infection. The number of bacteria present in the urine is calculated by culturing a drop of urine on solid media. If the patient has a urinary tract infection the specimen will probably contain at least a hundred thousand bacterial cells per millilitre and several white cells will be visible on examination under the microscope.

In the presence of a catheter, bacteria commonly **colonize** the bladder but do not necessarily invade the tissue to cause infection. In catheterized patients several species of bacteria are commonly present, although their significance is difficult to establish and antibiotic treatment is often unnecessary in the absence of clinical signs of infection such as pain or fever (Garibaldi, 1993).

Sputum

The lower part of the respiratory tract is normally sterile but the upper respiratory tract, mouth and nose are colonized by large numbers of different bacteria, some of which are able to cause **pneumonia**. A diagnosis of respiratory tract infection is therefore made by a combination of clinical examination history, chest X-ray and microbiological examination of sputum to confirm the diagnosis and identify the causative organism.

Specimens of saliva are of no value so it is important to ensure that the specimen is mucoid or mucopurulent. The physiotherapist may be able to help a patient who is having difficulty producing a specimen of sputum. Sputum specimens should be sent to the laboratory immediately as respiratory pathogens will not survive for prolonged periods.

The laboratory will examine the specimen for organisms likely to cause respiratory tract infection. If large numbers are present then identification can sometimes be assisted by **Gram-staining** and viewing under the microscope prior to culture (Plate 2.11).

Tuberculosis

The organism that causes tuberculosis, *Mycobacterium tuberculosis*, grows extremely slowly. Colonies of the bacteria do not appear before a minimum of a week of incubation and can take up to 6 weeks. Microscopic examination of sputum is therefore used to make an initial tentative diagnosis of tuberculosis. The numbers of *Mycobacterium* in the sputum may be quite low and to increase the chance of detection three separate specimens should be examined (Plate 2.12).

Mycobacterium have particularly resistant **cell walls**; they are stained using a special dye (hot carbol fuchsin) which cannot be removed by acid or alcohol. This method is used to detect *Mycobacterium* under the microscope, thus the term 'acid-fast bacilli' or AFB. Atypical mycobacterial infections caused by other species, for example *Mycobacterium avium intracellulare* (MAI), cannot be distinguished from tuberculosis under the microscope and therefore several weeks of incubation are necessary before the species causing the infection can be identified.

Faeces

Faeces normally contains millions of micro-organisms. The detection of the bacteria or viruses responsible for diarrhoea or gastroenteritis is therefore not easy as pathogens need to be distinguished from **normal flora** before identification is possible. Faecal specimens can therefore take the laboratory 3–4 days to process and more than one specimen may be required to eliminate infection as a cause of diarrhoea.

If *Clostridium difficile* is isolated from a specimen then additional tests are necessary to establish whether it is a pathogenic, **toxin**-producing **strain**.

Viruses which cause gastrointestinal infections cannot be cultured but are detected by examination of faeces under the electron microscope. Faecal specimens are often not automatically examined for viruses, therefore if infection is suspected as the cause of diarrhoea two specimens should be sent to the laboratory; one requesting examination for bacteria, the second for viruses.

A walnut-sized sample of faeces, or approximately 15 ml of a liquid stool, is sufficient for microbiological investigation. It should be examined within 12 h, unless faecal **parasites** are suspected when a fresh, warm stool is required.

Wound Swabs

Wounds should be swabbed before they are cleaned whilst the maximum number of bacteria are still present, and the swab should be taken directly from the area suspected to be infected. If **pus** is present it can be drawn up in a sterile syringe and transferred to a sterile container. Most types of swab are accompanied by a tube of transport medium, this will prolong the survival of micro-organisms for several hours. In the laboratory, the swab is wiped over an agar plate and the most likely cause of infection is assessed from the numbers of bacteria present.

A wound infection is defined by the presence of clinical signs of infection rather than the isolation of bacteria from a wound swab. A wide range of bacteria able to cause infection may be grown from a wound swab, but many of these organisms may equally be harmless colonizers of the wound or the surrounding skin. Bacteria isolated from a wound swab should not be considered as infecting the wound unless there is also evidence of an infection process occurring in the wound; for example pus, inflammation, **erythema** or fever. A swab need only be taken where the wound exhibits these signs of infection. This is particularly the case in chronic wounds such as pressure sores or ulcers, where wounds may be colonized by several different bacteria with no adverse effect (Gilchrist and Reed, 1989).

It is extremely important to label the wound swab accurately, indicating the exact site from which it has been collected. This helps the laboratory predict the types of micro-organisms to expect in the swab and to identify the site of infection should the patient have more than one wound.

Other Swabs

Nose swabs are sometimes necessary to detect carriage of potential pathogenic bacteria such as antibiotic-resistant strains of *Staphylococcus aureus*. A standard swab can be used but should first be moistened in the transport medium or some sterile saline, and then rubbed inside the exterior nares. One swab can be used to sample both nostrils.

Pernasal swab of the nasopharynx is required where whooping cough is suspected and should be taken by a trained member of staff. The swab is fixed onto a long flexible wire and accompanied by charcoal transport medium (see Fig. 2.3).

Throat swabs should be taken by depressing the tongue and gently rubbing the swab over the pillars of the fauces (see Fig. 2.4). Care should be taken to avoid touching other parts of the mouth which may contaminate the swab with other bacteria. The laboratory will examine the swabs for the presence of known pathogens such as streptococci and diphtheria.

Swabbing exudate from the eye can be used to identify organisms responsible for 'sticky eye' in babies, but conjunctival scrapings are preferred for other infections of the eye (e.g. *Chlamydia*) and these are usually carried out in ophthalmology departments.

Infections of the outer ear can be swabbed carefully ensuring that the swab is introduced gradually and is not inserted very far. If infection of

Fig 2.3
Areas to be swabbed when sampling the nose.

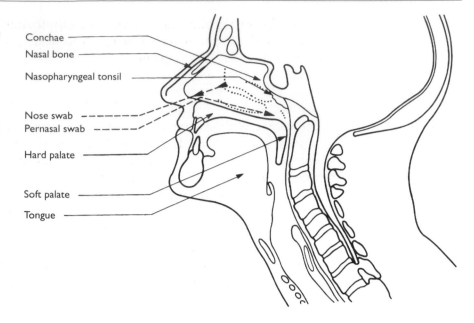

Conchae

Nasal bone

Nasopharyngeal tonsil

Nose swab – – – – –
Pernasal swab – – – –

Hard palate

Soft palate

Tongue

Fig. 2.4
Sampling the throat.

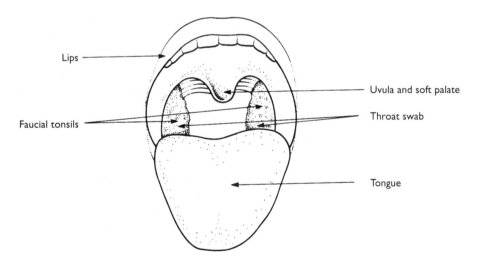

Lips

Uvula and soft palate

Throat swab

Faucial tonsils

Tongue

the inner ear is suspected a deeper swab is required which should be taken by medical staff using a speculum.

Vaginal swabs should be taken through a vaginal speculum and always sent to the laboratory in transport medium. Investigation for some sexually transmitted diseases requires special transport media.

Occasionally swabs of skin (e.g. groin, axilla) are requested to look for antibiotic-resistant strains of bacteria which may colonize the skin, particularly methicillin-resistant *S. aureus* (Chapter 5). Swabs should first be moistened in transport medium or sterile saline solution to improve the efficiency of sampling.

Swabs for the detection of virus in skin lesions should be broken off into a vial of special transport medium, obtained from the laboratory before the specimen is taken.

Blood Cultures

A patient with a high fever may have small numbers of the bacteria responsible for the infection circulating in the bloodstream. To identify bacteria in the blood, a sample must be taken very carefully to avoid contamination by skin flora, using a clean needle to inoculate the bottles. Blood is inoculated into two bottles, one to support the growth of anaerobic bacteria, the other **aerobic** bacteria. The bottles are incubated for at least a week but checked daily for signs of growth. Since bacteria are not normally present in the blood any growth from the bottle is usually significant. A **Gram-stain** will be performed immediately to provide early evidence of the cause of infection.

Cerebrospinal Fluid (CSF)

In suspected meningitis, specimens should be collected by a spinal tap as aseptically as possible, preferably before antibiotics are commenced. The specimen should be transported to the laboratory immediately to increase the chance of growing *Meningococcus* which is extremely fragile. Viral transport medium is not necessary for CSF specimens.

Sampling the Environment

Bacteria are normally present in the environment on all types of surface and in the air and usually present no risk to the patient. The results of sampling of the environment are difficult to interpret. Since the number of bacteria isolated is extremely variable and will depend on the exact area sampled. Little is known about what constitutes unacceptably high levels of contamination.

Routine sampling of equipment to demonstrate sterility is generally unnecessary, instead the efficiency of the decontamination process itself should be monitored.

Environmental sampling may be of value in outbreaks of infection where an environmental reservoir of infection may be contributing to spread of the organism (Ravn *et al.*, 1991; Lowbury et al 1992).

The air quality of operating theatres may sometimes need to be assessed, for example to test the efficacy of the ventilation in newly commissioned theatres. This requires the use of a microbiological air sampler which can measure the number of bacteria per cubic metre of air. Agar 'settle plates', although often used, are not easily interpreted and

(a)

Name : PARKER, Alice
Hosp. No. : (0000) T456378   Doctor : Malcolm, C
Age / D.o.B : 47 YRS 03/02/47   Sex : F   Location : Female Surgical

MICROBIOLOGY – Routine cultures

WOUND CULTURE   Collected: 20APR94
Source: WOUND SWAB
Lab No: MB-93-93678

-------------- Culture --------------

STAPHYLOCOCCUS AUREUS ; a heavy growth

-------------- Sensitivity --------------

S AUREUS

ERYTHROMYCIN   S
GENTAMICIN   S
FUSIDIC ACID   S
PENICILLIN   R
METH/FLUCLOX   S
VANCOMYCIN   S

(b)

Name : GREEN, James
Hosp. No. : (0000) T987654   Doctor : STRINGFELLOW, E
Age / D.o.B : 73 YRS 03/01/21   Sex : M   Ward : Medical unit

MICROBIOLOGY – Routine cultures

RESPIRATORY CULTURES   Collected: 30APR94
Source: SPUTUM
Lab No: MB-93-93675

-------------- Microscopy --------------

Acid Fast Bacilli seen

-------------- Preliminary report --------------

AFB cultures incubated, further report to follow.

(c)

Name : SMITH, Alexander
Hosp. No. : (0000) T345681   Doctor : Peters, D.
Age / D.o.B : 60 YRS 03/05/34   Sex : M   Location : Male Surgical

MICROBIOLOGY – Routine cultures

URINE CULTURE   Collected: 22APR94
Source: CATHETER URINE
Lab No: MB-93-93676

-------------- Microscopy --------------
>50 White blood cells/cmm
11–50 Red blood cells/cmm
<1 Casts/cmm

-------------- Culture --------------
KLEBSIELLA AEROGENES ; 10–100,000 organisms/ml

-------------- Sensitivity --------------

                    KLEB AER

AMP/AMOXY   R
CEPHALEXIN   R
NITROFURANTOIN   S
CO-TRIMOXAZOLE   S
GENTAMICIN   S
TRIMETHOPRIM   S

(d)

Name : BROWN, John
Hosp. No. : (0000) T987654   Doctor : Jones, B.
Age / D.o.B : 81 YRS 01/08/12   Sex M   Location : Care of the elderly

MICROBIOLOGY – Routine cultures

WOUND CULTURE   Collected: 30APR94
Source: SORE
Lab No: MB-93-93674

PRESSURE SORE

-------------- Culture --------------

STREPTOCOCCUS FAECALIS (ENTEROCOCCUS) ; a moderate growth
PROTEUS SPECIES ; a moderate growth
LACTOSE FERMENTING COLIFORM ; a scanty growth

do not accurately relect levels of contamination (Holton and Ridgeway, 1993).

Biohazard Labels

Laboratory staff regularly handle body fluids specimens containing pathogenic organisms and are therefore at particular risk of acquiring infection.

The use of biohazard labels is recommended to indicate, both to staff who transport the specimens and the laboratory, specimens which may contain particularly hazardous pathogens (Health Services Advisory Committee, 1991) (Plate 2.13). The indication for use of biohazard labels may vary between hospitals but usually they should be applied to specimens known or suspected to contain blood borne viruses or tuberculosis (DOH, 1990).

Transport of Specimens

Potentially infectious material presents a hazard when it is being transported and care must be taken to ensure that risk to other people is kept to a minimum. The Health Services Advisory Committee (1991) recommends procedures for the safe transport of specimens which include carriage in leak-proof boxes and a procedure for dealing with spillages.

The member of staff who collects the specimen has a responsibility to ensure the following:

- the specimen container is leak-proof and securely sealed
- all traces of body fluid have been removed from the outside of the container
- the specimen container is not overfilled
- biohazard labels are placed on the container and form where appropriate
- the specimen is accompanied by a fully completed request form in a separate pocket
- the container is sealed inside a plastic bag

Fig. 2.5
Interpretation of a laboratory request form. (a) The heavy growth of S.aureus in this wound indicates that this is the most likely cause of infection. In common with most hospital isolates of this organism it is resistant to penicillin. The exact site of the wound has not been indicated on the request form and this may cause some confusion if the patient has more than one wound. (b) This patient has pulmonary tuberculusis and requires isolation to minimize the risk of cross-infection. Isolation can be discontinued after 2 weeks of treatment, repeat specimens of sputum are not usually necessary. The specimen will now be cultured to determine the species of mycobacterium and antibiotic sensitivities. (c) The presence of Klebsiella and a large number of white cells in a specimen of catheter urine is not necessarily unusual. Treatment would be indicated if the patient has signs of infection, for example a pyrexia. The organism is resistant to ampicillin and cephalexin and these antibiotics should not be used to treat the infection. (d) It is not unusual to isolate several different species of bacteria from a chronic wound. Treatment for infection would only be indicated if clinical signs such as pus or inflammation were present.

Information on Request Forms

The request form provides a very important source of information for the laboratory staff. It assists them in the identification of the causative organism and indicates factors which may influence the identification process. The request form should therefore always be completed accurately.

Of particular importance is an accurate indication of the site of the specimen. Some bacteria may form part of the normal flora in one site of the body and yet be pathogenic if isolated elsewhere. If the patient is receiving antibiotic therapy, antibiotic present in the specimen may inhibit the growth of bacteria in laboratory cultures and produce misleading results. Ampicillin-resistant *Klebsiella*, an unlikely cause of respiratory tract infection, is commonly isolated from the sputum of patients receiving ampicillin for a chest infection because ampicillin present in the specimen inhibits the growth of the causative organism. The date and time of specimen collection indicates whether prolonged storage has occurred which may result in the death of certain bacteria or the overgrowth of others. A relevant history, including symptoms of infection or suspected site of infection can assist in the interpretation of the results. For example, information on the nature and frequency of vomiting and diarrhoea should accompany a specimen of faeces.

Interpretation of Laboratory Reports

The results of a microbiological examination must always be interpreted in combination with a clinical evaluation, without this the microbiological data are often meaningless. Some bacteria isolated from a specimen may be there as part of the normal flora and not capable of causing infection e.g. diphtheroids in a wound swab. Sometimes bacteria may be present in a specimen as a result of contamination during its collection but, in the absence of clinical signs of infection, antibiotic treatment is not indicated. For example, *Staphylococcus epidermidis* in a blood culture is often significant but in about 25% of cases organisms from the skin contaminate the blood culture bottle and if the patient is not pyrexial then treatment would not be indicated. Where treatment is indicated the laboratory report provides information on suitable antibiotics to prescribe. Some examples of laboratory report forms are shown in Fig. 2.5.

Advice and information about the interpretation of microbiology laboratory forms can be obtained from the Consultant microbiologist.

References

Ayton M (1982) Microbiological investigations. *Nursing* **2**(8):226–30.

Bradley C, Babb J, Davies J *et al.* (1986) Taking precautions. *Nursing Times* **5th March**: 70–3.

Department of Health – Advisory Committee on Dangerous Pathogens (1990) *Categorisation of Pathogens According to Hazard and Categories of Containment.* HMSO, London.

Garibaldi RA (1993) Hospital-acquired urinary tract infections. In *Prevention and Control of Nosocomial Infections*, 2nd edn (RP Wenzel, Ed.), pp. 600–613. Williams and Wilkins, Baltimore MD.

Gilchrist B, Reed C (1989) The bacteriology of leg ulcers under hydrocolloid dressings. *Br. J. Dermatol.* **121**: 337–44.

Health Services Advisory Committee (1991) *Safe Working and Prevention of Infection in Clinical Laboratories.* HMSO, London.

Holliday G, Strike PW, Masterton RG (1991) Perineal cleansing and midstream urine specimens in ambulatory women. *J. Hosp. Inf.* **18**: 71–6

Holton J, Ridgway GL (1993) Commissioning operating theatres. *J. Hosp Inf.* **23**: 153–60.

Lowbury EJL, Ayliffe GAJ, Geddes AM, Williams JD (Eds) (1992) *Control of Hospital Infection – a Practical Handbook*, 3rd Edn. Chapman & Hall. London.

Platt R, Polk BF, Murdock B, Rosner B (1983) Reduction of mortality associated with nosocomial urinary tract infection. *Lancet* **i**: 893–7.

Ravn P, Lundgren JD, Kjaeldgaard *et al.* (1991) Nosocomial outbreak of cryptosproridiosis in AIDS patients. *BMJ* **302**: 277–80.

Further Reading   Chambers S (1986) Microbiology. *Nursing* **4**: 121–8.

Glenister H. (1983) Diagnosis of the patient and specimen collection. *Nursing* **2**: 6–7.

McFarlane A. (1989) Using the laboratory in infection control. *Prof. Nurse* **4**(8): 393–7.

McKune I (1989) Catch or bag your specimen? A comparative study of the contamination rates between clean-catch and bag specimens of urine in children aged two years and under. *Nursing Times* **85**(37): 80–2.

Sleigh JD, Timbury MC (1990) *Medical Bacteriology*, 3rd edn. Churchill Livingstone, London.

3 Micro-organisms and their Control in Hospital

- Introduction
- Terminology
- Bacterial Infections
- Fungal Infections
- Protozoal Infections
- Viral Infections
- References and Further Reading

Introduction

There are many different **species** of bacteria, types of virus and other micro-organisms, but only a very small proportion cause disease or **infection**.

This chapter provides a brief outline of some micro-organisms commonly encountered in hospital. It focuses on the infection control implications of each organism and the precautions that the nurse may need to use when he or she encounters a patient with these infections.

Terminology

Every surface of the body is densely populated by a wide variety of micro-organisms which are described as the **normal flora** and which vary according to the local availability of nutrients, humidity, temperature and competition with other species (Table 3.1). These microbes are **commensals**; that is, they do not harm their hosts and could even be described as **symbiotic** because they benefit their host by preventing other, harmful micro-organisms from occupying the surfaces. Commensal micro-organisms are harmless in their normal site but may cause disease if they are transferred to a different part of the body (e.g. *Escherichia coli* from the intestine causes urinary tract infection) or when the hosts, normal defences are impaired (e.g. *Staphylococcus aureus* in the nose may cause infection if transferred to damaged skin).

Infection occurs when micro-organisms invade tissue, multiply and

Table 3.1
The normal flora of body
surfaces

Site of body	Common commensal micro-organisms
Skin	S. epidermidis, Streptococcus spp., Corynebacterium spp., Candida
Throat	Strep. viridans, Neisseria spp., diptheroids
Mouth	Strep. viridans, Neisseria catarrhalis, Actinomyces spp., spirochaetes
Respiratory tract	Strep. viridans, Neisseria spp., diptheroids, micrococci
Vagina	Lactobacilli, diptheroids, streptococci, yeasts
Intestines	Bacteroides spp., anaerobic streptococci, Cl. perfringens, E. coli, Klebsiella spp., Proteus, Strep. faecalis

cause adverse effects. The adverse effects in the tissue are recognized as symptoms of infection and may also be accompanied by fever and malaise (see Table 3.2).

Micro-organisms that cause disease are called **pathogens**. They account for only a small proportion of the total microbial population but are difficult to define accurately because the ability of some to cause disease depends on the susceptibility of the host. Those that only cause infection in people with impaired defences against infection are called **opportunistic pathogens**, for example *Pneumocystis carinii*, a **protozoan** found in the respiratory tract, which causes disease in the immunocompromised.

Potential pathogens can be present on the body but not cause adverse effects in the tissues or symptoms of infection. This is described as **colonization** and the colonized individual, a **carrier**. The carriage may be short-lived or may continue indefinitely. In some situations the carrier spreads infection to others. Patients in hospital colonized with **antibiotic**-resistant bacteria act as a reservoir, enabling the organism to spread easily to other patients. In extreme examples a carrier can spread infection to many other people; in the late nineteenth century, 'Typhoid Mary', a carrier of *Salmonella typhi*, infected 54 people over a period of 10 years through her employment as a cook.

The term **infectious** or **contagious** is applied to diseases caused by micro-organisms which are transmitted easily from person to person.

The **virulence** of an organism is a measure of its ability to cause disease and to transmit from person to person. Some pathogens have particular features that enable them to resist host defences, for example **capsules** or

Table 3.2
Symptoms of some
common infections

System of the body	Symptoms of infection
Skin	Inflammation, Pain, Swelling, Heat
Respiratory tract	Increased respiratory secretions Cough
Urinary tract	Pain (cystitis), Frequency, Urgency
Central nervous system	Confusion, Drowsiness, Stiff neck, Headache
Gastrointestinal tract	Abdominal pain, Vomiting, Diarrhoea

enzymes that coagulate or **haemolyse** blood. Others produce **toxins** that damage host cells. **Exotoxins** are substances produced by the cell which diffuse into their surrounding environment. They are mostly produced by Gram-positive bacteria and have a specific and often extremely toxic effect on the host. Some bacteria cause disease solely by the production of toxin without invading the host e.g. Botulism food poisoning is caused by the ingestion of a minute amount of toxin produced by *Cl. perfringens* when it multiplies in food. Other bacteria damage tissue by both invasion and toxin production e.g. a toxin produced by Streptococci causes the rash of scarlet fever. **Endotoxins** are parts of the bacterial cell released into the tissues when the cell dies and disintegrates. They are usually associated with Gram-negative bacteria e.g. Salmonella, *Pseudomonas aeuruginosa*, and have non-specific effects on their host, such as pyrexia, leucopenia, haemorrhage and necrosis of internal organs. The susceptibility of the host to infection will also vary; some individuals may acquire infection through exposure to a smaller number, or dose, of the same organism than others. Patients with an impaired immune system are very vulnerable to infection.

Bacterial Infections
Gram-positive Cocci

Staphylococci

The staphylococci are differentiated into 'coagulase positive' and 'coagulase negative' species, depending on whether they produce the **enzyme coagulase**, which clots **plasma**.

Staphylococcus aureus

Staphylococcus aureus is a coagulase-positive staphylococcus. It is commonly found colonizing normal skin, particularly warmer parts such as the axillae, groins, perineum and nose. It causes a range of superficial infections of the skin (Plate 3.1); septic spots, boils, abscesses and impetigo and is responsible for around one third of hospital-acquired wound infections (Meers *et al.*, 1981). *S. aureus* can also cause more serious infections; osteomyelitis, septicaemia, endocarditis and pneumonia. Some strains of *S. aureus* produce a toxin that attacks cells in the skin, causing it to split and desquamate. Infections sometimes occur in neonates where they cause 'scalded skin syndrome', characterized by large, red weeping areas where the skin has desquamated. Some strains of *S. aureus* produce a toxin that has widespread effects on the body and causes a condition known as toxic shock syndrome. Other strains produce an enterotoxin which interfere with electrolyte transfer in the gut and cause acute gastroenteritis if eaten with food.

Fig. 3.1
Staphylococcus epidermidis
adhering to a plastic
intravenous cannula.

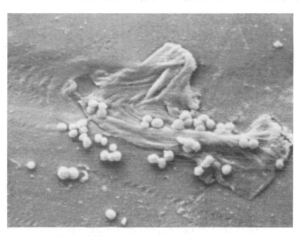

Staphylococcus epidermidis

S. epidermidis is a coagulase-negative staphylococcus. It colonizes the skin and used to be considered as non-pathogenic but is increasingly recognized as a major cause of infection acquired in hospital. It produces extracellular slime which enables it to adhere to and multiply on plastics and metals (Fig. 3.1). It is therefore able to cause infections associated with invasive plastic or metal devices; including peritoneal dialysis catheters, arterial grafts, cardiac prosthetic valves and prosthetic orthopaedic joints. It is also frequently responsible for **septicaemia** associated with intravenous devices. Immunosuppressed patients are particularly vulnerable and the natural resistance of *S. epidermidis* to many antibiotics, makes the infections it causes difficult to treat (Hamory and Parisi, 1987).

Infection control precautions Staphylococci are disseminated on skin scales and will collect in dust, where they may survive for several hours (Skaliy *et al.*, 1964). Regular cleaning will reduce the risk of dissemination. Staphylococci present on skin are able to gain access and cause infection in damaged skin sites such as wounds and cannula insertion sites. It is often difficult to establish whether the source of infections is the skin of the patient or of staff. Aseptic technique should always be used to handle invasive devices. Occasionally outbreaks of surgical wound infection are caused by a member of staff in the operating theatre who is heavily colonized with staphylococci and releases large numbers of the organism into the air on skin scales. Identification and treatment of the staff member is necessary to prevent further spread.

Cross-infection between patients occurs and outbreaks of infection caused by *S. epidermidis* and by *S. aureus* have been frequently reported (Hamory and Parisi, 1987; French *et al.*, 1990). Staphylococci are most frequently transmitted on the hands and clothing of staff and equipment as the classic experiments of Mortimer *et al.* (1966) eloquently demonstrated. Although airborne spread on skin scales is possible, it is probably overestimated as a route of transmission (Crossley *et al.*, 1979; Reybrouck, 1983).

Scrupulous handwashing is usually sufficient to prevent spread and isolation of patients infected with *S. aureus* is usually not necessary unless the infected wounds are extensive or the strain is resistant to several antibiotics. The management of antibiotic-resistant strains of *S. aureus* is discussed in more detail in Chapter 5.

Streptococci

Streptococci are divided into Lancefield groups A to S. The Group A streptococcus, *Streptococcus pyogenes* is associated with the most serious infections and causes pharyngitis, skin infections and **puerperal sepsis**. It produces several toxins which help it to spread through tissue, for example scarlet fever – a pharyngitis together with a generalized rash induced by a streptococcal toxin. Occasionally acute rheumatic fever or acute glomerulonephritis occur 1–4 weeks after a Group A streptococcal infection. These represent a hypersensitivity reaction, the streptococcus **antibodies** recognizing and destroying tissues in the body by mistake. Streptococci can invade damaged skin; surgical wounds, burns, ulcers and can cause skin infections, impetigo, erysipelas or cellulitis (Plate 3.2). Rarely, virulent strains of group A streptococcus cause invasive infections in tissue, destroying muscle or the sheath that surrounds it (necrotizing fasciitis). The damage is probably caused by toxins produced by these strains, which destroy tissue by breaking down **protein** (Nowak, 1994). Puerperal sepsis is a septicaemia which originates from the uterus infected by *Strep. pyogenes* during childbirth. It was a frequent complication of childbirth prior to the introduction of antibiotics and more hygienic approach to delivery. Now it is an uncommon, but still serious, infection.

Group B streptococci are normal inhabitants of the intestine and sometimes the vagina. They can cause **meningitis** and septicaemia in the neonate who is exposed to the bacteria in the vagina during delivery.

Group C and G streptococci are similar to the group A streptococci and although associated with less serious infection can cause skin infections, tonsilitis and septicaemia.

The viridans group of Streptococcus includes at least five species which are prevalent amongst the normal flora. They are associated with bacterial **endocarditis** in patients with previously damaged heart valves if they enter the bloodstream during dental procedures. *Strep. milleri* can cause deep abscesses.

Strep. pneumoniae are normal inhabitants of the respiratory tract but also an important cause of meningitis and **pneumonia**, **otitis media** and sinusitis. Resistance to the infection amongst the general population is high but is reduced by underlying heart or lung disease, influenza or **immunodeficiency**, and **epidemics** may occur in overcrowded conditions. Pneumococcal pneumonia is transmitted by respiratory droplets or by contact with oral secretions and several episodes of cross-infection amongst elderly or immunocompromised patients have been described (Denton *et al.*, 1993). Penicillin is the antibiotic of choice for pneumococcal infection and penicillin-resistant *Strep. pneumoniae* strains can be difficult to treat.

Infection control precautions Reports of outbreaks of infection in hospital due to streptococci A, B, C and G have been described (Efstratiou, 1989; Burnett and Norman, 1990; Denton *et al.*, 1993). The bacteria may be acquired on the hands of staff by contact with colonized or infected wounds and skin, and transferred to vulnerable sites on other patients. Isolation of patients with streptococcal infection is therefore recommended until the patient has received appropriate antibiotic therapy for 48 h (see Chapter 14). Longer periods of isolation may be necessary for infections in chronic wounds where the organism is more difficult to eradicate.

Patients with penicillin-resistant strains of *Strep. pneumoniae* should be isolated, especially in a ward with a high proportion of elderly or **immunocompromised** patients (Pallett and Strangeways, 1988; Ridgeway *et al.*, 1991).

Enterococcus

The main pathogens in the **genus** are *Enterococcus faecalis* and *E. faecium*, which are normal inhabitants of the bowel but are increasingly reported as a cause of hospital-acquired infection (Korten and Murray, 1993). They mostly cause urinary tract and wound infections especially in seriously ill patients. Occasionally they cause meningitis in neonates and pneumonia.

Resistance to many antibiotics provides enterococcus with an advantage over other bacteria in the hospital environment. Increasingly resistant strains are emerging and cause serious problems because of the limited options of antibiotics to treat the infections.

Infection control precautions Until recently, it was thought that enterococcus were acquired from the patient's own bowel flora. It is now recognized that they can be spread from patient to patient on the hands of staff and that reservoirs of the organism in the environment may also be involved, such as electronic thermometers (Livornese *et al.*, 1992). Outbreaks may be controlled by isolating infected or colonized patients, stringent handwashing and identification of potential environmental reservoirs.

The emergence of multiresistant strains can be discouraged by the prudent use of antibiotic therapy.

Gram-positive Bacilli

Bacillus

These are **aerobic** bacteria which form **spores**. They are widely distributed in soil, water and dust. The main pathogen is *Bacillus anthracis*, which causes anthrax, an infection of animals, especially sheep and cattle, and occasionally affects people whose work brings them into contact with animals or animal carcasses. It is spread by spores which can survive in soil for many years.

B. cereus causes food poisoning and is usually associated with foods that have been kept for prolonged periods (e.g. rice). It has occasionally been associated with surgical wound infections (Barrie *et al.*, 1992).

Clostridia

The clostridia are **anaerobic** bacteria which form spores. They are mostly found in soil where they have an important role in the decomposition of **organic** materials, and many species are normal commensals of the gut. The pathogenic species cause disease by producing potent toxins that have profound effects on the host.

Tetanus

Clostridium tetani is present in the intestinal tract of herbivores and in soil. Tetanus occurs when a wound is contaminated by *Cl. tetani* spores and the conditions in the tissues are sufficiently anaerobic for them to germinate, multiply and produce toxin. The toxin stimulates motor nerve cells and causes convulsive muscle contractions, beginning near to the site of the wound but spreading progressively throughout the body.

Tetanus is most likely to occur in wounds contaminated with soil or a foreign body, in deep puncture wounds or those with extensive tissue damage. It is associated with a high incidence and mortality in countries without **immunization** programmes or anti-tetanus prophylaxis treatment. In the UK all children should receive immunization and a single booster of toxoid vaccine will protect immune individuals who are at risk of tetanus infection from a potentially contaminated wound. Elderly people are less likely to have been immunized and are at greater risk of acquiring tetanus. Tetanus is not spread from one person to another.

Gas Gangrene

Gas gangrene is usually caused by *Cl. perfringens*, although it can also be caused by other species of clostridia, and before the introduction of antisepsis was a frequent complication of surgery. *Cl. perfringens* is a normal inhabitant of the human intestine and is sometimes isolated from wounds with no adverse effects. Gas gangrene occurs only when wounds are contaminated by soil or faecal material, or where there is extensive tissue damage or an impaired blood supply, creating the anaerobic conditions necessary for the organism to multiply in muscle tissue. These conditions are usually associated with war wounds, road accidents or other major injuries.

Gas gangrene is not infectious and does not spread from patient to patient. The organism is acquired **endogenously** from the gut or from the environment, and gas gangrene develops only if the conditions in the wound are suitable for its multiplication.

Clostridium difficile

Cl. difficile is commonly found in the human intestine where it is carried asymptomatically. It was not recognized as a cause of disease until the late 1970s when it was identified as a cause of hospital-acquired gastrointestinal infections, ranging from mild diarrhoea to a severe and sometimes fatal **pseudomembraneous colitis**. The infection usually occurs when the normal gut flora is altered by antibiotic therapy, especially ampicillin and cephalosporins (Nye, 1993). *Cl. difficile* multiplies in the absence of competition from other organisms, producing a toxin which is responsible for the symptoms and causes necrosis of the lining of the gut. The diagnosis is confirmed by the presence of the organism and its toxin in faeces but asymptomatic carriage of *Cl. difficile* is not uncommon.

A number of outbreaks of *Cl. difficile* have been reported, particularly amongst elderly patients, and it is clear that the organism can be transmitted between patients (Cartmill *et al.*, 1994). The main route of transmission is probably on the hands of staff but spores, disseminated in high numbers from infected patients, can survive for several months in the environment. In outbreaks of infection extensive contamination of the environment has been implicated as an important factor in its spread and it has been recovered from toilets, bedpans, bedding and mops (Fekerty *et al.*, 1981; Hoffman, 1993).

Infection control precautions Patients with toxin-producing stains of *Cl. difficile* in their faeces should be isolated whilst they have diarrhoea. Excreta should be discarded promptly into bedpan washer, macerator or toilet and hands washed after any contact with the patient. The standard of cleaning should be closely monitored and spillages of excreta promptly removed and the area thoroughly cleaned (Worsley, 1993).

Corynebacteria

Many species are commensals which colonize the upper respiratory tract, mucous membranes and skin. They occasionally cause serious postopera tive infections following cardiac surgery or other infections in immuno-compromised patients. The main human pathogen is *Corynebacterium diphtheriae*, the cause of diphtheria. *C. diphtheriae* can be carried in the nose or throat of a healthy person. In susceptible individuals, the organism infects the pharynx and larynx, forming membranes which can obstruct the airway. Sometimes, the organism infects the skin and causes cutaneous diphtheria. The toxin that the organism produces causes serious damage to heart, kidney and nerves. In the UK, routine immunization of children has ensured that cases of diphtheria are now extremely rare. A patient with diphtheria requires isolation and close contacts would be investigated for the presence of carriage or infection.

Listeria

Listeria monocytogenes is the main pathogen of this genus and is commonly found in soil and in the faeces of a variety of animals. It usually causes a mild influenza-like illness. However, infection during pregnancy can cause premature delivery and septicaemia and meningitis in the neonate. Cross-infection in neonatal units has been reported and extensive environmental contamination may occur following the delivery of an infected baby (Schlech, 1991). Serious infections may also occur in immunocompromised patients. The incidence of infection is low with around 130 cases reported annually (Newton *et al.*, 1992). It can be acquired through contact with live animals and raw meat, but most infections are acquired by consumption of contaminated food. Soft cheese, coleslaw, fruit, vegetables, ice-cream and salami have all been associated with outbreaks of infection (Jones, 1990). Listeria has been found in a variety of chilled foods and can survive and even multiply below normal refrigeration temperatures.

Infection control precautions Immunocompromised patients or pregnant women are most at risk of listeriosis and they should eat fresh and well-cooked or thoroughly reheated food. Food likely to contain listeria should be avoided (e.g. soft cheese, paté and coleslaw; DHSS, 1989). Isolation of infected patients is only necessary in neonatal units.

Mycobacteria

Mycobacteria, although **Gram-positive** bacteria, are characterized by their unusual staining properties. They are termed acid-fast **bacilli** (AFB) because, unlike most bacteria, they retain the stain after treatment with strong acids. There are many different species, some are found in animals and birds, others in soil and water. The main human pathogens are *Mycobacterium tuberculosis* and *M. leprae*, which cause tuberculosis and leprosy respectively.

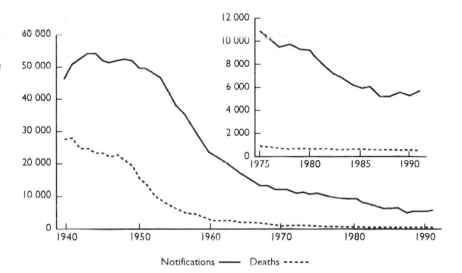

Fig. 3.2
*Incidence of tuberculosis:
notifications (——) and deaths
(- - -)-in England and Wales.
Crown copyright. Reproduced
with the permission of the
Controller of Her Majesty's
Stationery Office.*

Notifications —— Deaths - - - - -

Tuberculosis

Most cases of tuberculosis are caused by *M. tuberculosis* and a few by *M. bovis* but the incidence of the disease has declined during the last century as a result of the improvements in living conditions and effective chemotherapy (Fig. 3.2). In the past, over 90% of children living in cities would develop tuberculosis, although in most the infection would resolve spontaneously with no long-term adverse effects. At present, in the UK, about 5000 new cases are reported every year, especially from areas that have a high proportion of immigrants from the Indian subcontinent, where tuberculosis is common.

Tuberculosis is a chronic, progressive infection which most commonly affects the lungs, but which may also affect other organs or tissues such as the kidney, intestine, skin and bone. The primary infection of the lung is often asymptomatic but may be associated with general malaise, weight loss, fever and cough. Many cases resolve spontaneously, but others progress to bronchopneumonia, meningitis or invade other tissues such as kidney, bone and, particularly, the spine. Miliary tuberculosis occurs when tubercle bacilli are carried in the blood and cause small foci of infection the size of millet seeds around the body.

The tubercle bacilli are unusual in that they are ingested by **phagocytic** cells but, instead of being destroyed, multiply within them. The body must therefore respond to the infection by **cell-mediated immunity** and by the production of specially activated **macrophages** that are able to kill the phagocytes containing the mycobacteria. This response is called delayed hypersensitivity and is the basis of the tuberculin skin tests used to establish whether an individual has active tuberculosis or is immune to infection. A small amount of protein derived from mycobacteria is inoculated under the skin. If after a few days the area is inflamed and blistered, the individual probably has active tuberculosis. A slight response to the tuberculin indicates **immunity** to tuberculosis, whilst no response indicates non-immunity (Joint Tuberculosis Committee, 1990).

Outbreaks of infection in hospital have been reported and infection is particularly likely to spread amongst immunosuppressed patients (George *et al.*, 1986). People with HIV infection are at greater risk of developing tuberculosis. The impairment of the immune system caused by HIV infection enables dormant *M. tuberculosis* to reactivate (Watson, 1991). Outbreaks of multi-drug resistant strains have occurred amongst patients with HIV infection in the USA. In the UK the incidence of drug resistant *M. tuberculosis* is currently very low but is closely monitored (Uttley and Pozniak, 1993).

Other species of mycobacteria rarely cause tuberculosis in humans, but immunocompromised people, especially those with AIDS, are susceptible to a disseminated tuberculosis caused by *M. avium intracellulare* (MAI) and *M. kansaii*. Infections caused by these atypical bacteria are extremely difficult to treat.

Infection Control Precautions Patients with sufficient numbers of *M. tuberculosis* in their sputum for bacteria to be seen under the microscope are infectious and are described as having 'open' tuberculosis. If the bacilli cannot be seen in three separate sputum specimens, the patient may still have tuberculosis but is not exhaling enough mycobacteria to be considered infectious. The non-pulmonary forms of tuberculosis are also not infectious.

Transmission occurs by the inhalation of tubercle bacilli in airborne droplets expelled from the lungs of an infected person. Patients with open tuberculosis are usually treated at home but if nursed in the hospital, extensive isolation precautions are not necessary since prolonged close contact is usually required for transmission of infection to healthy people. The patient should be segregated from other patients in a single room for the first 2 weeks of chemotherapy. Gowns and masks are unnecessary and no special precaution are needed for crockery or linen (Joint Tuberculosis Committee, 1990). The main risk is to other patients with an impaired immune system who are particularly susceptible to infection (Joint Tuberculosis Committee, 1992).

The risk of health care workers acquiring infection from patients is extremely small and is minimized by the Occupation Health Department who ensure that all staff who have close contact with potentially infected patients or specimens are tuberculin tested and given vaccination where necessary (Thornbury, 1985).

The family and other close contacts of the patient should be investigated for the presence of active tuberculosis. This 'contact tracing' is co-ordinated by the Local Authority Proper Officer (Consultant in Communicable Disease Control).

Gram-negative Cocci

Neisseria spp.

Neisseria characteristically occur as pairs of cells called diplococci. There are a number of harmless species that form part of the normal flora of the mucous membranes, including the upper respiratory and genital tracts. The two main pathogens are *N. gonorrhoeae* (gonococcus) and *N. meningitidis* (meningococcus).

Gonorrhoea

This sexually transmitted disease is caused by *N. gonorrhoeae*. It is a very delicate organism that is susceptible to cold and lack of moisture. It is therefore unable to survive for long outside the body and is very unlikely to be transmitted by any route other than sexual intercourse. Newborn infants may be infected from the mother's birth canal at the time of delivery and subsequently develop conjunctivitis. *N. gonorrhoeae* causes acute urethritis in males but infection of the cervix in females can remain asymptomatic for long periods facilitating spread of the infection.

Meningococcal infection

N. meningitidis is carried in the upper respiratory tract of about 10% of healthy people. The organisms from the nasopharynx invade the blood-stream, causing meningococcal septicaemia, or the meninges, causing meningococcal meningitis. Both infections can be rapidly fatal if not treated with antibiotics. *N. meningitidis* dies rapidly outside the human host and transmission requires direct contact with respiratory secretions.

Meningococcal disease is most common amongst children and young adults. Sporadic epidemics of infection are usually associated with crowded conditions such as schools or army barracks, although some parts of the country have an unusually high incidence of infection.

Infection control precautions Isolation of infected patients for the first 24 h of antibiotic therapy is usually recommended but the risk of transmission is low. Prophylactic antibiotic therapy is recommended for all close contacts. Health care workers are at risk of infection *only* if they are intimately exposed to respiratory secretions (e.g. mouth–to–mouth resuscitation) and prophylactic antibiotics are rarely necessary (Benenson, 1990).

Aerobic Gram-negative Bacilli

The Coliforms

Coliforms is a general term given to a broad group of organisms capable of growing in the gut. They can survive in either aerobic or anaerobic environments under a wide range of different temperatures. They are commonly associated with warm, moist environments. Outbreaks of infection are sometimes related to contaminated equipment such as portable suction and ventilator tubing (Davies and Blenkharn, 1987; Gorman *et al.*, 1993).

The coliform bacteria primarily responsible for infections in hospital are *Escherichia coli*, *Klebsiella* spp., *Serratia* spp., *Proteus* spp. and *Enterobacter* spp. They often colonize sites where the normal defence mechanisms are breached, for example intravenous cannulae, urinary catheters and endotracheal or tracheostomy tubes. They can also cause severe infections including **peritonitis**, wound infection and urinary tract infection especially in the seriously ill, **immunosuppressed** or neonate. Certain strains of *E.coli* cause gastroenteritis by invading the epithelial cells of the gut or by the production of toxins. They are occasionally associated with outbreaks of infection on paediatric wards and neonatal units (Shanson, 1989).

Outbreaks of infection caused by coliforms resistant to many antibiotics, particularly *Serratia*, *Klebsiella* and *Enterobacter*, are also frequently reported. Infections caused by these strains can be difficult to treat.

Infection control precautions   The hands of staff are often implicated as the route of transmission of **Gram–negative** coliforms and organisms can remain on hands for prolonged periods (Casewell and Phillips 1977, Casewell and Desai, 1983). Colonized or infected patients may have the organism in their faeces and respiratory secretions, as well as in a variety of skin sites and wounds. The opportunity for transmission between patients is therefore high. Hands may also be contaminated by coliforms acquired from the environment, for example by handling towels, wash bowls, bed linen and equipment in the sluice (Sanderson and Weissler, 1992).

Transmission between patients should be prevented by the use of simple infection control precautions such as handwashing after contact with every patient or potentially contaminated equipment, and the wearing of gloves to handle body fluids. However, some antibiotic-resistant strains appear to spread readily and are not completely removed by handwashing with soap and water. Outbreaks of infection with these strains may need to be controlled by isolating infected or colonized patients. In some circumstances disinfectant solutions for handwashing may be recommended. (Wade *et al.*, 1991).

Antibiotic-resistant strains are a particular problem in intensive care or neonatal units where the patients are more susceptible to infection and where frequent staff contact facilitates their spread. Ventilator circuits are prone to contamination from respiratory secretions and hands should be washed after any contact (Gorman *et al.*, 1993).

Salmonella spp.

Salmonellae are found in the intestines of both humans and animals. Two species, *Salmonella typhi* and *S. paratyphi*, are human pathogens and cause enteric fever, a severe illness with symptoms of septicaemia, rather than gastroenteritis. After clinical or **sub-clinical** infection some people continue to excrete the organism in their faeces and a small number do so for many years. The disease is usually transmitted on food which has not been thoroughly cooked or has been contaminated by an animal source or human carrier. Outbreaks have also been associated with contaminated water and shellfish grown in polluted estuaries.

There are other species of *Salmonella* that cause gastroenteritis (salmonella food poisoning), for example *S. enteritidis* and *S. typhimurium*. Infections are mainly associated with foods derived from poultry, which are frequently contaminated and may cause illness if the *Salmonella* are not destroyed by adequate cooking. Infection can also occur if contaminated raw food cross-contaminates other food which is then eaten without further cooking. *S. enteritidis* in particular has recently been linked to the consumption of eggs (De Louvois, 1993), particularly food containing raw shell eggs, for example mayonnaise or lightly cooked eggs.

Infection control precautions Safe handling of food and strict attention to hygiene in the kitchen is essential to prevent transmission of *Salmonella* by hospital food. Immunosuppressed people should only eat eggs cooked until the yolk is solid and avoid eating food containing raw eggs. The principles of food hygiene are discussed in greater detail in Chapter 12. Handwashing after defecation and before handling food is an important measure to prevent transmission of infection.

Person-to-person transmission of infection has been reported in outbreaks of hospital-acquired *Salmonella* (DHSS, 1986; Joseph and Palmer, 1989) but can be prevented by the use of simple infection control precautions such as handwashing and the use of protective clothing for direct contact with faeces. Patients with *Salmonella* do not require isolation once they are asymptomatic.

Shigella spp.

These are the cause of bacillary dysentery, a gastrointestinal infection characterized by bloody, mucopurulent stools. Epidemics are associated with low standards of hygiene and, since very few organisms are necessary to cause infection, transmission frequently occurs through direct physical contact where hands have not been washed after defecation. Transmission also occurs indirectly by the contamination of food, and flies may transfer the organism from faeces to food. *Shigella sonnei* causes most cases in the UK and sometimes causes outbreaks in children in nursery schools. *Shigella* is not associated with long-term carriage in the faeces after the acute infection.

Infection control precautions Prevention of transmission of infection requires the use of gloves and aprons to handle excreta and thorough handwashing after contact with the patient. Control of outbreaks in schools and nurseries is a particular problem because standards of hygiene are poor and personnel may have frequent, close contact with each other. Staff with shigella infection should not work in these establishments or handle food until they have stopped excreting the organism (about 4 weeks after infection).

Pseudomonas spp.

Pseudomonas are aerobic, environmental organisms commonly found in soil and water but sometimes colonizing the intestines. The main patho-genic species is *Ps. aeruginosa*, which takes advantage of damaged host defences to establish infection in burns, wounds and urinary tract and it has consequently become a major cause of hospital-acquired infection. *Pseudomonas* is sometimes found in the bowel of healthy people but rapidly colonizes the gut of hospital patients. After a few weeks in hospital, up to 50% of patients will have *Pseudomonas* in their faeces (Olsen *et al.*, 1984). *Pseudomonas* is able to multiply in situations where very few nutrients are available such as moist equipment and solutions. Although commonly found in sinks and taps there is little evidence that organisms from these sources cause infection in patients (Levin *et al.*, 1984).

Infection control precautions Many infections caused by *Pseudomonas* are acquired from the patients' own intestinal colonization, although cross-infection on equipment and the hands of staff may occur. Respiratory therapy equipment is prone to contamination and can present a major risk of infection if not decontaminated appropriately and stored dry. Outbreaks of infection have been associated with humidifiers, temperature probes and irrigation tubing (Weems, 1993; Kolmos *et al.*, 1993).

Strains of *Pseudomonas* resistant to aminoglycoside antibiotics may cause outbreaks of infection which are difficult to treat, especially in intensive care or burns units. Preventing the spread of these antibiotic resistant strains may require the isolation of infected or colonized patients.

Haemophilus spp.

The main pathogenic species is *Haemophilus influenzae* which is also a normal inhabitant of the upper respiratory tract of most healthy people. It causes infection of the respiratory tract, particularly associated with chronic bronchitis and sometimes following viral influenza infection. It is also a major cause of meningitis in young children and can cause a potentially fatal **epiglottitis** although **vaccination** of all infants is now recommended (DOH, 1992a). Cross-infection in paediatric wards has been reported and may also occur with *H. influenzae* pneumonia on adult wards (Howard, 1991). Isolation of infected patients should be considered, particularly if the patient has contact with immunocompromised patients.

Legionella

There are several different species of *Legionella*, but the main human pathogen is *Legionella pneumophila* which causes a severe respiratory illness called legionnaires' disease. *Legionella* spp. normally live in water and infection is acquired by the inhalation of aerosols of contaminated water. Outbreaks of infection have been associated with air-conditioning systems, showers and whirlpools (Hutchinson, 1990). The organism is frequently isolated from the water supply but its multiplication and the subsequent outbreaks of infection can be prevented by correct cleaning and maintenance procedures, prevention of stagnation of water in the supply and by avoiding water temperatures that favour microbial growth (NHS Estates, 1993). There is no evidence that the infection can transmit from person to person and therefore isolation of patients with legionnaires' disease is not necessary.

Acinetobacter

Acinetobacter are aerobic bacteria which are found widely in the environment and are also part of the normal flora of the skin. Like the coliforms they can cause a range of infections in susceptible hospital patients, including pneumonia, meningitis, septicaemia and wound infection, and hospital strains are sometimes resistant to many antibiotics. They also have an affinity for warm, moist places and outbreaks of infection related to humidification equipment and damaged mattresses have been reported (Loomes, 1988; Cefai *et al.*, 1990). *Acinetobacter* are able to survive on dry surfaces for several days. Outbreaks of infection are increasingly reported in intensive care and burns units, where spread between patients on the hands of staff is the most likely route of transmission (Musa *et al.*, 1990). The same infection control precautions as those described for coliforms are required to prevent spread of *Acinetobacter*.

Anaerobic Gram-negative Bacilli

There are a number of strictly anaerobic Gram-negative bacteria of which the most commonly encountered are *Bacteroides*.

Bacteroides

These are normal inhabitants of the intestine, where they are present in considerable numbers, and they are also found in the mouth and genital tract. *Bacteroides fragilis* can cause appendicitis, pelvic inflammatory disease and puerperal sepsis. It may also be responsible for postoperative infection, usually in combination with other organisms, particularly following abdominal or gynaecological surgery. Infection occurs endogenously, rather than as a result of cross-infection.

Mycoplasma

Mycoplasma are very small bacteria which form a variety of cell shapes. They do not have cell walls and are therefore resistant to a range of antibiotics, including penicillins, which exert their effect on bacterial cell walls. Some species of *Mycoplasma* have been implicated as causes of non-specific urethritis. *M pneumoniae* causes respiratory tract infections which range from mild pharyngitis to pneumonia and **bronchitis**. Outbreaks of infection have been reported in crowded institutions and within families. Spread of infection occurs through close contact and in hospitals the principal risk is the transmission of infection from staff to patients. Staff suffering from the infection should not work (Kleemola and Jokinen, 1992).

Rickettsia

These are small bacteria that cannot grow outside the cells of their host and, except for Q fever, are transmitted by insects. They cannot be cultured on conventional bacterial culture medium but are grown in the yolk sac of chick embryos. The diagnosis is usually based on serological tests.

The main pathogen in the group is *Rickettsia prowazeki* which causes typhus. It is transmitted by the human louse, which acquires the organism when it feeds on the blood of an infected human. The microbe multiplies in the intestine of the louse, is excreted in the faeces on to the skin of a new host where it is introduced into the tissues by scratching. Typhus cannot be directly transmitted from person to person and epidemics are usually associated with unusual social conditions where the body louse is able to proliferate in the absence of regular washing of clothes, for example in wars and famines. Patients in hospital suffering with typhus do not require isolation.

Q-fever is an atypical pneumonia caused by the inhalation of *Rickettsia* from faeces, milk or placentae of farm animals.

Chlamydia

These are very small bacteria-like micro-organisms that cannot live outside the cells of their host. There are three main species. *Chlamydia trachomatis* is divided into several groups, one causing severe blinding conjunctivitis called trachoma, others causing genital tract infections, conjunctivitis and pneumonia in infants who acquire the organism from the mother's vagina.

C. psittaci is a parasite of parrots but is also found in other birds (e.g. pigeons, ducks, canaries). In humans it causes respiratory tract infection which can range from a mild or asymptomatic infection to a severe pneumonia with a high fatality rate. Infection is acquired through the inhalation of infected dust and faeces and usually occurs in people who have close contact with birds (e.g. bird breeders and pluckers). The risk of transmission of psittacosis to patients should be considered when parrots or other caged birds are kept as pets in ward areas.

C. pneumoniae is associated with **community-acquired** upper and lower respiratory tract infection, including pneumonia.

Fungal Infections

The successful treatment of immunocompromised patients involves the use of powerful antibiotics which, as a side-effect, destroy the bacteria that normally live on and in the body. Fungi take advantage of the lack of competition from the usual bacteria and have emerged as a major cause of serious, systemic infection in immunocompromised patients.

There are over 70 000 species of fungi, of which only a few are pathogenic. Diseases include superficial infections of the mucosa (e.g. thrush caused by yeasts) or infection by filamentous fungi of the skin, nails and hair (e.g. ringworm). More importantly they can invade the body to cause serious widespread disease which is often fatal (Bodey, 1988).

Candida

Ninety per cent of *Candida* infections in humans are caused by *Candida albicans* found in the normal flora of the mouth, intestinal tract and vagina. Superficial infection of mucous membranes may occur, particularly in neonates and in debilitated adults or those receiving antibiotic therapy which destroys the competing bacteria and enables the *Candida* to increase in numbers (Plate 3.3). **Systemic** infection may occur in people who are immunosuppressed. Although infection is usually **endogenous**, cross-infection may occur and the use of gloves for oral hygiene and handwashing after the procedure is important to prevent this (Burnie *et al.*, 1985).

Aspergillus

This filamentous fungi is found widely in the environment in dust and soil. It can cause infection in the lungs of people with underlying lung disease, for example cystic fibrosis, and systemic infection in people who are immunocompromised, for example following organ transplant. Outbreaks of infection in susceptible patients are often associated with high spore levels in the air derived from environmental sources (e.g. building sites) rather than person-to-person spread (Humphries *et al.*, 1991).

Cryptococcus

This yeast causes meningitis but is extremely rare, usually only occurring in patients with severe immunodeficiency. The main source of the organism is probably soil, although it has been associated with infected pigeon droppings, and infection is acquired through inhalation of dust.

Protozoal Infections

Protozoa are an unusual cause of infection in the UK although very common in other parts of the world. Malaria is caused by a protozoa transmitted by the mosquito in tropical and subtropical countries. *Amoeba* and *Giardia* cause gastrointestinal infections and are acquired through drinking water contaminated with faeces. Some protozoal infections have taken on a new significance because of their ability to cause serious disease in people with acquired immune deficiency syndrome (AIDS).

Toxoplasma

Toxoplasma gondii is a **parasite** of the cat family. The eggs of *T. gondii* are excreted in cat faeces and humans are infected by ingesting the eggs after handling cat faeces or soil contaminated by cat faeces and occasionally by ingesting eggs in raw or under-cooked meat. In most cases the infection is mild, although primary infection in early pregnancy can cause foetal death or brain damage. In the UK between 30 and 40% of the population has evidence of previous infection (Thomas, 1988). The **cysts** of the parasite can remain in the tissue after infection and can be reactivated in immunocompromised individuals to cause severe and often fatal disease. *Toxoplasma* are not directly transmitted from person to person and therefore no special infection control precautions are indicated.

Cryptosporidium

This causes profuse, watery diarrhoea although infection may be asymptomatic. It is found in the bowel of farm and domestic animals and is transmitted by contaminated food and water. Person-to-person spread may occur and outbreaks of infection have been reported (Benenson, 1990). Immunodeficient individuals may be unable to clear the organism from their bowel and response to antibiotic treatment is poor. Prolonged, serious disease may result.

Viral Infections

Numerous viruses infect humans. They are broadly grouped into families based on whether they have **DNA** or **RNA**, their general shape and the type of infection they cause (Table 3.3). This section discusses some of the viral infections commonly encountered in hospitals.

Herpes Viruses

These DNA viruses include Herpes simplex types 1 and 2, Epstein–Barr, varicella zoster and cytomegalovirus. An important feature of all herpes viruses is their ability to cause **latent infections** that may be reactivated subsequently.

Herpes Simplex Virus (HSV)

There are two types of this virus. Initial infection with HSV-1 usually occurs in infancy or early childhood, often asymptomatically, but it can produce acute gingivo-stomatitis and the vesicles turn to ulcers on the gums and oral mucosa. HSV-2 occurs much more infrequently. It causes genital herpes which affects the penis in the male and vulva, labia and cervix in the female. There is a correlation between HSV infection of the cervix and cervical cancer but HSV as a cause is not proven.

Table 3.3
Some important viral pathogens

Virus group	Disease	Route of entry
Adenoviruses	Respiratory tract infection Conjunctivitis	Respiratory tract
Rhinoviruses	Common cold	Respiratory tract
Orthomyxoviruses Influenza A & B	Influenza	Respiratory tract
Paramyxoviruses Para-influenza Respiratory syncytial virus Mumps Measles	Para-influenza Bronchiolitis Mumps Measles	Respiratory tract Respiratory tract Respiratory tract Respiratory tract
Herpes viruses Herpes simplex 1 Herpes simplex 2 Varicella zoster Cytomegalovirus Epstein–Barr	Herpetic skin lesions Genital herpes Chickenpox, shingles Febrile illness Glandular fever	Skin, mucosa Sexual intercourse Respiratory tract, lesions Mucosa Mucosa
Enteroviruses Polio Coxsackie A Coxsackie B Hepatitis A Echoviruses	Polio Hand, foot & mouth, Myo/pericarditis Hepatitis Meningitis	GIT GIT GIT GIT GIT
Papoviruses Papilloma	Warts, tumours	Skin
Reoviruses Rotavirus	Gastroenteritis	GIT
Hepatitis viruses	Hepatitis B, C, D	Blood, sexual intercourse
Retroviruses HIV	Immune deficiency	Blood, sexual intercourse
HTLV I	Leukaemia, lymphoma	

GIT, gastrointestinal tract.

Both viruses are transmitted by direct contact with lesions; HSV-1 by kissing or touching sores, genital herpes by sexual intercourse although it may also be carried asymptomatically in saliva. Infection with one type of HSV does not provide immunity against the other type.

During the primary infection, virus travels up the sensory nerves and lies dormant in the ganglia. It then periodically becomes reactivated, travels back down the nerves and replicates in the skin to cause new lesions at the site of the original infection.

Herpes simplex can also cause a mild self-limiting meningitis and more occasionally a more severe **encephalitis**. Herpetic whitlow occurs when virus contaminates abrasions on the fingers, particularly around the nail bed and is frequently encountered amongst health care workers (Plate 3.4).

Infection control precautions The main risk of transmission to health care workers is from asymptomatic salivary carriers and therefore the most important infection control precaution is the routine use of gloves for contact with oral secretions and for care of the mouth.

Varicella Zoster Virus

This virus causes chickenpox as a primary infection, mainly in children (Plate 3.5). Primary chickenpox in adults may be complicated by pneumonia which can cause serious illness. Virus is secreted in the characteristic vesicles on the skin but it is primarily an infection of the respiratory tract and large amounts of virus are found in respiratory secretions which provide the main route of transmission. It is extremely infectious and around 90% of people will have had chickenpox by the time they reach adulthood (DOH, 1992a). The virus travels along sensory nerves and remains dormant in the ganglion for prolonged periods. If reactivated, it travels back along the sensory nerve and erupts onto the surface of the skin along the nerve pathways appearing as vesicles. This is called shingles (Plate 3.6). It often causes severe, localized pain. Shingles cannot be caught from people with either shingles or chickenpox, it usually occurs in older adults or the immunosuppressed and represents a reactivation of the primary infection. The fluid from shingles vesicles contains varicella virus and therefore non-immune individuals can acquire chickenpox through contact with people with shingles.

Chickenpox acquired during the first 5 months of pregnancy may cause foetal abnormalities. A mother who acquires chickenpox a few days before delivery may transmit infection to her non-immune baby, who may subsequently develop severe illness (Cradock-Watson 1990).

Infection control precautions The main infection control problem presented by patients infected with chickenpox is the risk of transmission to immunocompromised patients (e.g. patients receiving immunosuppressive therapy, neonates, patients with HIV infection), who may develop serious and life-threatening disease.

When a patient or member of staff develops chickenpox, the infection control team should be notified so that they can identify other patients who may be at risk of infection and who may need protection by the inoculation of specific **immunoglobulin** if they are found to be non-immune. Immunity to chickenpox can be checked by looking for antibodies to the virus in blood. To minimize the risk of outbreaks of infection in high risk areas such as maternity units, some occupational health departments routinely check the immunity of health care workers without a history of prior infection.

Other Herpes Viruses

The Epstein–Barr virus causes glandular fever in teenagers and young adults, associated with fever, sore throat and enlarged lymph nodes. In parts of Africa it is associated with Burkitt's lymphoma and naso-pharyngeal cancer. It is not very infectious and is transmitted by saliva.

Cytomegalovirus (CMV) causes a mild disease, similar to glandular fever. It establishes a persistent latent infection which may be periodically reactivated throughout life, resulting in virus shedding in urine and other body fluids. It is a very common infection and 80% of the population have been infected by late middle-age (Tookey and Peckham, 1991). More serious infection occurs in the immunosuppressed, often as a result of the reactivation of the latent virus. Infection, either primary or reactivation, during pregnancy does not usually cause harm to the foetus but around 1% die or have severe congenital defects.

The virus is excreted in large amounts in saliva and urine and is transmitted by close contact and kissing; most patients excreting the virus will be asymptomatic.

Infection control precautions Most health care workers will be immune to primary CMV infection but may experience reactivation of a latent infection. There is no evidence that health care workers are more likely to acquire the virus at work. The routine use of gloves for handling body fluids and handwashing after the removal of gloves, minimizes the risk of CMV transmission and additional precautions are not recommended even for pregnant staff caring for infected patients (HSE, 1990; Tookey and Peckham, 1991).

Adenoviruses

There are many different types of these DNA viruses. Most cause mild, respiratory illness and establish persistent, latent infection in the adenoids and tonsils. Other types cause outbreaks of conjunctivitis and respiratory tract infection particularly amongst children. The main infection control problem associated with adenovirus is in neonatal intensive care units where they can cause severe viral pneumonia and may spread easily between babies (Piedra *et al.*, 1992). The spread of eye infections can be prevented by strict hygiene during eye examinations and the sterilization of equipment.

Other Respiratory Viruses

There are a number of other viruses commonly encountered in hospitals which, although not related, spread from person to person by respiratory droplets and by respiratory secretions carried on hands (Ansari *et al.*, 1991). Respiratory syncytial virus is one of the most important causes of respiratory tract infection in children and can be extremely severe in babies, causing bronchiolitis, croup and pneumonia. Outbreaks of infection may occur in paediatric units and infected children should therefore be isolated whilst symptomatic (Madge *et al.*, 1992). Measles (Plate 3.7), mumps and rubella are also commonly seen in paediatric units, although the incidence of all of these childhood diseases has declined since the introduction of the combined MMR **vaccine** in 1988 and around 90% of children now receive the vaccine (DOH, 1992a). Measures to reduce the spread of infection should be taken because a proportion of those infected may develop serious complications especially if they are immunocompromised, for example mumps, meningitis and encephalitis, otitis media and pneumonia associated with measles. If possible, infected patients should be discharged home and those that remain should be cared for by staff known to be immune to the infection to avoid secondary spread.

Enteroviruses

Enteroviruses are a large group of viruses which usually infect the gut although cause symptoms in other parts of the body.

Polio Viruses

There are three distinct types of polio virus. They generally cause a mild febrile illness but in a few cases cause meningitis and, in less than 1% of cases, degenerative changes in the spinal cord resulting in paralysis. In some countries, where standards of hygiene are low, the population overcrowded and there is no vaccination programme, the virus is **endemic** amongst children under 5 years. In the UK, about 90% of children are vaccinated and only 20 cases of polio have been reported between 1985 and 1991. The virus is transmitted by contact with faeces and pharyngeal secretions.

Approximately two cases of the vaccine strain of poliomyelitis a year are reported in association with polio vaccination. The **live-attenuated** virus is excreted in the faeces for up to 6 weeks after vaccination and people who have been recently vaccinated should wash hands thoroughly after defecation (DOH, 1992a).

Coxsackie Viruses

Coxsackie A virus causes 'hand, foot and mouth' disease where vesicles erupt on the mouth, hands and feet. Coxsackie B virus causes a

myocarditis and **pericarditis** from which most patients completely recover. Infection is mainly spread through contact with faeces and outbreaks occasionally occur in neonatal units.

Hepatitis A

Hepatitis A is a gastrointestinal infection characterized by nausea and abdominal pain followed after a few days by jaundice. It is generally a mild illness, often asymptomatic in children, lasting 1–2 weeks and not associated with any long-term adverse effects. The infection is spread by contact with faeces and is sometimes associated with poor sanitation. Hepatitis A can also be transmitted in food and water, particularly sandwiches and salads and also molluscs cultivated in contaminated water (Benenson, 1990). Hepatitis E causes a similar infection to hepatitis A and is spread by water contaminated with faeces and from person to person via the faecal–oral route.

Infection control precautions The transmission of infection can be prevented by the use of gloves to handle faeces or change nappies and by strict attention to hand hygiene after using the toilet by both staff and children. During outbreaks of infection in residential institutions or child day care centres, protection of staff by vaccination or with immunoglobulin may also be considered.

Other Gastro-Intestinal Viruses

Several other viruses cause gastrointestinal illness in both children and adults and may cause outbreaks of infection in hospital patients (Mitchell *et al.*, 1989). Infections are of greatest concern amongst the very young or the elderly who easily become severely dehydrated. Rotavirus causes a severe gastroenteritis associated with vomiting, watery diarrhoea and fever usually in children under 5 years, in whom it can cause severe dehydration. Most people acquire the infection during childhood and develop immunity to further infection, however immunity may diminish with age and outbreaks of rotavirus amongst the elderly also occur (Benenson, 1990). Other viruses associated with outbreaks of gastrointestinal illness in hospitals include the small round structured viruses (Norwalk group of viruses), some adenoviruses, astroviruses and caliciviruses. Outbreaks usually develop gradually and can spread extensively to both patients and staff (Reid *et al.*, 1990). Virus present in vomit may contribute to the spread of infection and virus is also frequently excreted in faeces for several days after the illness has resolved, particularly in the immunosuppressed (Benenson 1990; Chadwick and McCann, 1994).

Infection control precautions Outbreaks of infection should be controlled by isolation of patients until at least 48 h after symptoms have resolved. Virus may be particularly easily acquired on the hands through contact with excreta, vomitus, bedding and nappies. Rigorous handwashing and the use of gloves for contact with body fluids is therefore essential to prevent spread. Spills of vomit or faeces from affected patients should be treated with chlorine-based **disinfectants** to destroy any virus present (see Chapter 14).

Blood-borne Viruses

Viruses transmitted by blood and body fluid are of particular importance to health care workers who may be at risk of acquiring infection through contact with body fluid. The most important blood-borne viruses are hepatitis B, hepatitis C and human immunodeficiency virus (HIV). The hepatitis and HIV viruses are not related but will be considered together because the infection control implications are similar.

Viral Hepatitis

Hepatitis, or inflammation of the liver, has infectious and non-infectious causes. Most cases of viral hepatitis are caused by hepatitis A, B, C or E viruses. The hepatitis D virus is not a true virus but can cause a severe, acute hepatitis if it infects an individual already infected with, or carrying, hepatitis B virus. Other micro-organisms which can cause hepatitis include Epstein–Barr virus, cytomegalovirus, *Leptospires* and *Toxoplasma*. Non-infectious causes of hepatitis are drug induced, as a result of alcohol or toxic agents. Hepatitis causes malaise, nausea and, after a few days, jaundice.

Hepatitis B

The infection is often mild but can be severe and in a small number of cases may be fatal. The **incubation period** is usually between 2 and 3 months. A proportion of those infected do not completely eliminate the virus but continue to carry it their blood. Infants infected perinatally are particularly at risk of becoming long-term carriers. The carrier state of hepatitis B virus is associated with chronic hepatitis, cirrhosis and carcinoma of the liver. The prevalence of hepatitis B carriage varies in different parts of the world but in the UK is around 0.1%, although in some antenatal clinics in inner-city areas 1 in 100 women are found to carry the virus. Tests to detect viral components and antibodies formed against them in the blood are used to determine previous infection and the carrier state. The surface antigen HBsAg is found on the outer protein coat of the virus and its presence in blood indicates an active infection or carrier state with hepatitis B. Anti-HBs are antibodies formed to the surface antigen and if present in the blood indicate that the individual has been infected in the past but is no longer infectious. HBeAg or the 'e' **antigen** is part of the virus's nuclear material and its presence in blood indicates a high level of viral replication and a highly infectious patient.

Hepatitis B is transmitted when infected body fluids are inoculated through the skin, on instruments such as needles or through damaged or cut skin, or have contact with mucous membranes. The virus can be transmitted by sexual intercourse and perinatally from mother to baby.

The hepatitis B virus (HBV) has been isolated from virtually all body fluids but blood, semen and vaginal fluids are mostly implicated in transmission of the virus. Saliva has been found to contain the virus in much lower concentration than in blood, and although it does not appear to transmit infection through contact with mucous membranes, biting has been reported to transmit infection (Cancio-Bello *et al.*, 1982).

The incidence of hepatitis B carriage in a population varies throughout the world and may be as high as 15% in parts of Africa and Asia where infection is often acquired in childhood. In the UK, infection is more common amongst drug-users who share needles and people with multiple sexual partners (e.g. prostitutes, promiscuous male homo-sexuals). Health care workers are as much as five times more likely to become infected with hepatitis B than other workers because of their regular and close contact with body fluids. The rate of transmission following needlestick injury with HBeAg positive blood may be as high as 30% (RCP, 1992). Health care workers who are hepatitis B carriers may also transmit the virus to patients during invasive procedures such as surgery and obstetrical procedures (Heptonstall, 1991; RCP, 1992).

Hepatitis B immunization Vaccination is an effective method of protecting against infection and is recommended for health care workers who have direct contact with blood, blood-stained body fluids and tissues (UK Health Departments, 1993). A course of three injections over a period of 6 months confers protection in about 80–90% of individuals, although those over the age of 40 years are less likely to develop immunity. A booster dose is recommended after 3–5 years. Specific immunoglobulin (HBIG) can be used to provide immediate, temporary, protection against infection with hepatitis B but it must be administered within 48 h of an exposure.

Hepatitis C

This virus causes a similar, but milder, infection than hepatitis B and is often associated with subsequent chronic hepatitis. Hepatitis C transmission is associated with blood transfusions and intravenous drug users. Infection control precautions are the same as those described for hepatitis B. A diagnostic test for hepatitis C is now available and is used to screen blood for transfusion.

Human Immunodeficiency Virus (HIV)

HIV is a retrovirus. This means that the genetic information of the virus is made of RNA but it also has an enzyme, **reverse transcriptase**, which converts the RNA to DNA and then incorporates it into the DNA of the host cell.

The virus recognizes and infects cells in the body that carry a particular protein called CD4. The main target of the virus is the helper **T lymphocytes** of the immune system, but there are other cells which also carry CD4 and which can be invaded by the virus (e.g. macrophages, dendritic cells of the mucous membranes). Two distinct forms of HIV have been identified so far; HIV 1 occurs throughout the world, HIV 2 has been found primarily in West Africa.

After the virus enters the body the immune system mounts a response to the virus, but a few viruses survive inside the cells, gradually replicate, and eventually begin to damage the immune system. The virus has its greatest effect on the **cellular immune system**, whose main role is to destroy micro-organisms that invade host cells and cells that become malignant. Months or years may pass before the symptoms of infection, acquired immune deficiency syndrome (AIDS), become apparent. The underlying immunodeficiency enables a range of organisms normally held in check by the immune system to establish infection; for example *Pneumocystis carinii*, toxoplasmosis, *Cryptococcus*, disseminated herpes simplex and atypical forms of *Mycobacteria*.

HIV infection is diagnosed by detecting antibodies to the virus in the blood. These are not usually detectable until about 3 months after infection when the individual is said to have seroconverted. Infection with HIV will persist indefinitely. The infected person can transmit HIV to others soon after acquiring the infection, but probably becomes more infectious as immunodeficiency increases. HIV is transmitted by sexual intercourse; inoculation of infected body fluids; transplantation of tissues or organs and transfusion of contaminated blood. The virus is also transmitted from mother to baby, either through the placenta or during delivery; between 13 and 35% of infants born to HIV-infected mothers will acquire the infection (European Collaborative Study, 1991). Around one-third of the 8000 haemophiliacs in the UK acquired HIV from contaminated blood factor VIII. Blood products are now screened and heat-treated to eliminate the risk of HIV infection.

The greatest concentration of virus is found in blood or body fluid containing visible blood. The virus has also been found in semen, vaginal secretions, tissues, cerebrospinal fluid, amniotic fluid and synovial fluid. HIV is probably transmitted by breast milk although the risk is probably greatest in the colostrum and early milk which contains more macrophages, and in mothers who have developed AIDS (Mok, 1993). HIV has also been found in saliva and tears, although in much lower concentrations, and these fluids have not been associated with transmission of the infection (CDC, 1987).

Occupational transmission of HIV to health care workers has been reported (Table 3.4). The first documented case of a health care worker who acquired HIV occupationally was reported in 1984. By September 1993, 64 reports worldwide of health care workers who acquired HIV after a specific occupational exposure had been published in the literature, although this probably underestimates the actual number infected. (Heptonstall *et al.*, 1993) Occupational transmission of the virus to health care workers has followed inoculation of infected body fluid into the skin by a needle or other sharp instrument and contamination of damaged skin or mucous membranes by infected body fluids. Follow-up of health care workers exposed to HIV-infected body fluids indicates that the rate of transmission of HIV is much lower than hepatitis B. In studies following up health care workers exposed to HIV-infected blood through a needlestick injury, around 1% have acquired the infection. The greatest risk is thus associated with needlestick injury, and transmission depends on the infectivity of the patient and the volume of blood inoculated (CDC, 1988b; Heptonstall *et al.*, 1993).

Transmission of HIV from an infected dentist to five of his patients has been reported, although the exact route of transmission remains unclear (CDC, 1991).

There is no vaccine to the virus currently available. Zidovudine (azidothymidine or AZT) inhibits viral replication and has been administered to health care workers following needlestick injury from a known HIV positive source. It must be given within 1 h of the injury and even then there is no clear evidence that it prevents or reduces the risk of **seroconversion** (DOH, 1992b).

At present, the number of people infected with HIV in the UK is unknown and it is difficult to forecast how many will develop the

Table 3.4
Definite occupational transmission of human immunodeficiency virus. From Heptonstall et al. *(1993)*

Type of exposure	Health care workers infected
Percutaneous	35
Mucous membrane	2
Damaged skin	3
Source not reported	24
Total	**64**

infection in the future. Since 1982, 9161 cases of AIDS have been reported in the UK; 8414 of these cases are men, 747 women and 6187 are known to have died (CDR, 1994). Only 12 cases of HIV-2 have been identified in the UK and most had some connection with West Africa (Evans *et al.,* 1991). It has been estimated that by 1997 between 1945 and 3215 new cases of AIDS will be reported annually (Day *et al.,* 1993). Initial data from the unlinked anonymous seroprevalence studies suggest that at the moment the numbers are small but vary considerably between regions with the greatest number in London and the south-east (PHLS, 1993) (Table 3.5). The incidence of infection in the UK is highest among homosexual men, intravenous drug users and sexual partners of these groups. However, in other parts of the world the infection is more widely distributed amongst heterosexuals. The World Health Organization estimates that by the end of 1993 there were 3 million cases of AIDS in the world, two-thirds of these in Africa, and that by the year 2000 30–40 million people will be infected with HIV (WHO, 1993).

Infection control precautions for blood-borne viruses The screening of blood donors for hepatitis B, treatment of blood products and the targeting of high risk groups for immunization against hepatitis B, particularly infants born to infected mothers, has reduced the incidence of the infection in the UK (DOH, 1992a). The absence of a vaccine against HIV means that controlling the spread of infection depends on education to discourage behaviour that may transmit infection, such as

Table 3.5
Estimated incidence of infection with human immunodeficiency virus in England and Wales (1990–92). From PHLS (1993)

Source of specimens	Prevalence of HIV infection (%)
Genito-urinary clinics (London)	
Homo/bisexual men	21
Heterosexual men	1
Heterosexual women	0.6
Genito-urinary clinics (outside London)	
Homo/bisexual men	5
Heterosexual men	0.3
Heterosexual women	0.2
Injecting drug users (London)	6
Antenatal clinic attenders	
London	0.21
Outside London	0.01
London district hospitals (non-HIV specialties)	
men	0.6
women	0.2

unprotected sexual intercourse and the sharing of used needles to inject drugs.

Frequent contact with body fluids places many health care workers at particular risk of acquiring blood-borne viruses who may be infected in the following ways:

- inoculation of infected blood or body fluid through the skin on contaminated sharp instruments
- contamination of mucous membranes such as the eyes or mouth with infected blood or body fluid
- contamination of broken skin with infected blood or body fluid

Health care workers can avoid infection by the use of protective clothing in situations when exposure to body fluids is anticipated, keeping cut or damaged skin covered with a waterproof dressing and the careful use and disposal of sharp instruments (CDC, 1988a; Morgan, 1990; UK Health Departments 1990). Health care workers are often unaware of patients who are infected with hepatitis viruses or HIV and therefore any blood and most body fluids must be considered potentially infectious. The infection control precautions required to prevent the transmission of blood-borne viruses are discussed in more detail in Chapter 7.

Patients known to be infected with blood-borne viruses do not require isolation unless contamination of the environment is likely (e.g. profuse bleeding). Infection cannot be transmitted by social contact with patients. Protective clothing is only necessary for direct contact with blood or body fluids and not for the routine care of the patient. Patients with HIV may also be infected with other pathogens which present a risk to other patients, for example tuberculosis, salmonella. Isolation may be indicated for such patients for the duration of their illness with these secondary pathogens. Transmission of hepatitis B amongst renal dialysis patients was a major problem in the 1970s but improved infection control, particularly the management of sharps and equipment, has reduced the incidence of infection from around 5% in patients, 1.3% in staff to 0.3% and 0.1%, respectively (Polakoff, 1976).

Injury with a contaminated sharp instrument is the most likely route of transmission to health care workers and every hospital should have a policy outlining the procedures to be followed in the event of a needle-stick injury (see Fig 7.7). Equipment that enters a sterile area of the body or has close contact with mucous membranes (e.g. fibreoptic endoscope), has the potential to transmit blood-borne viruses between patients. Such equipment must be appropriately decontaminated after each use to prevent cross-infection. Chapter 13 discusses methods of disinfection and sterilization in more detail.

Transmission of blood-borne viruses from an infected health care worker to a patient can only occur during procedures in which injury to the health care worker could result in blood contaminating the patient's open tissue, for example when hands are in contact with sharp instruments, bone or teeth (DOH, 1993; UK Health Departments 1993). All health care workers who perform such procedures should be vaccinated against hepatitis B infection. Vaccination is also recommended for health care workers who have contact with blood or body fluid (DOH, 1992a; UK Health Departments 1993). Health care workers who think that they may be infected with a blood-borne virus should seek medical advice and may need to modify their practice or avoid performing invasive procedures.

Unconventional Virus-like Agents

A group of degenerative diseases of the brain associated with unidentified infectious agents, includes Creutzfeldt–Jakob disease in humans, scrapie in sheep and bovine spongiform encephalopathy in cattle. These virus-like particles can replicate and can be transmitted to other humans or animals although the exact mode of transmission is unknown. Creutzfeldt–Jakob disease is associated with a progressive dementia developing between the age of 40 and 70 years. The disease is not highly transmissible and the main risk is associated with neurosurgery, particularly the transplantation of brain tissue or corneas. Cases have also occurred after the injection of growth hormone prepared from human pituitary glands. The precautions advised for blood-borne viruses are sufficient to protect against infection. The Department of Health recommends prolonged sterilization procedures for suspected cases of Creutzfeldt–Jakob disease (DOH, 1984).

Haemorrhagic Fevers

A number of viral haemorrhagic fevers which do not occur in the UK are occasionally seen in patients recently returned from abroad, for example Lassa fever, Marburg and Ebola viruses. The viruses are transmitted to humans from animals such as rats and monkeys, but transmission to health care workers through handling of infected blood and body fluids has been reported. These haemorrhagic fevers are associated with a high fatality rate and when a case is suspected the patient must be transferred immediately to a special infectious disease unit in London, Liverpool or Glasgow, where they will be nursed under strict isolation (DOH 1986b).

References

Ansari SA, Springthorpe S, Sattar SA *et al.* (1991) Potential role of hands in spread of respiratory viral infections: studies with human parainfluenza virus 3 and rhinovirus 14. *J. Clin. Micro.* **29**: 2115–9.

Benenson AS (Ed.) (1990) *Control of Communicable Disease in Man*, 15th edn. Am. Public Health Ass. Washington. USA.

Barrie DB, Wilson JA, Hoffman PN *et al.* (1992) *Bacillus cereus* meningitis in two neurosurgical patients: an investigation into the source of the organism. *J. Inf.* **25**: 291–7.

Bodey GP (1988) The emergence of fungi as major pathogens. *J. Hosp. Inf.* **11** suppl. A: 411–26.

Burnett IA, Norman P (1990) *Streptococcus pyogenes*: an outbreak on a burns unit. *J. Hosp. Inf.* **15**(2): 173–6.

Burnie JP, Odds FC, Lee W *et al.* (1985) Outbreak of systemic *Candida albicans* in intensive care unit caused by cross infection. *Brit. Med. J.* **290**: 746–8.

Cancio-Bello TP, de Medina M, Shorey J *et al.* (1982) An institutional outbreak of Hepatitis B related to a human biting carrier. *J. Inf. Dis.* **146**(5): 652–6.

Cartmill TDI, Panigrahi H, Worsley MA *et al.*, (1994) Management and control of a large outbreak of diarrhoea due to *Clostridium difficile*. *J. Hosp. Inf.* **27**: 1–16.

Casewell MW, Desai N (1983) Survival of multiply-resistant *Klebsiella aerogenes* and other Gram-negative bacilli on finger-tips. *J. Hosp. Inf.* **18**(Suppl. B): 23–8.

Casewell MW, Phillips I (1977) Hands as a route of transmission for *Klebsiella* species. *Brit. Med. J.* **2**: 1315–7.

Cefai C, Richards J, Gould FK *et al.* (1990) An outbreak of *Acinetobacter* respiratory tract infection resulting from incomplete disinfection of ventilatory equipment. *J. Hosp. Inf.* **15**: 177–82.

Centers for Disease Control (1987) Recommendations for prevention of HIV transmission in health care settings. *MMWR* **36**(2S): 3S–18S.

Centers for Disease Control (1988a) Update: universal precautions for prevention of transmission of human immunodeficiency virus, hepatitis B virus and other blood-borne pathogens in health care settings. *MMWR* **37**(24): 377–88.

Centers for Disease Control (1988b) Update: acquired immunodeficiency syndrome and human immunodeficiency virus infection among healthcare workers. *MMWR* **37**: 229–34.

Centers for Disease Control (1991) Update: transmission of HIV infection during invasive dental procedures – Florida. *MMWR* **40**: 378–81.

Chadwick PR, McCann R (1994) Transmission of a small round structured virus by vomiting during a hospital outbreak of gastroenteritis. *J. Hosp. Inf.* **26**: 251–60.

Communicable Disease Report Weekly. (1994) AIDS and HIV Infection Worldwide. *CDR* **4**(20): 95–6.

Cradock-Watson JE (1990) Varicella-zoster virus infection during pregnancy. In *Current Topics in Clinical Virology* (Morgan-Capner, P., Ed.) pp. 1–28. Public Health Laboratory Service, London.

Crossley K, Landesman B, Zaske D (1979) An outbreak of infection caused by strains of *S. aureus* resistant to methicillin and aminoglycosides. *J. Inf. Dis.* **139**: 280–7.

Davies B, Blenkharn I (1987) On the right track. *Nursing Times* **83**(22): 64–8.

Day NE, Anderson RM, Darbyshire J *et al.* (1993) The incidence and prevalence of AIDS and other severe HIV disease in England and Wales for 1992–1997: projections using data to the end of June 1992. Report of a working group convened by the Director of the Public Health Laboratory Service. *CDR Suppl.* **3**(Suppl.1): S1–17.

De Louvois J (1993) *Salmonella* contamination of eggs. *Lancet* **342**: 367–8.

Denton M, Hawkey PM, Hoy CM *et al.* (1993) Co-existent cross-infection with *Streptococcus pneumoniae* and group B streptococci on an adult oncology unit. *J. Hosp. Inf.* **23**: 271–8.

Department of Health and Social Security (1984) *Management of patients with spongiform encephalopathy (Creutzfeldt–Jacob disease CJD). DHSS circular DA* **84**: 16.

Department of Health and Social Security (1986a) *The Report of the Committee of Inquiry into an Outbreak of Food Poisoning at Stanley Royd Hospital.* HMSO, London.

Department of Health and Social Security (1986b) *Memorandum on the Control of Viral Haemorrhagic Fevers.* HMSO, London.

Department of Health (1992a) *Immunisation Against Infectious Disease.* HMSO, London.

Department of Health (1992b) *Occupational Exposure to HIV and the Use of Zidovudine: a Statement from the Expert Advisory Group on AIDS* PL/CO(92). HMSO, London.

Department of Health (1993) *AIDS–HIV infected Health Care Workers: Guidance on the Management of Infected Health Care Workers* (Interim update). Expert Advisory Group on AIDS. HMSO, London.

Department of Health and Social Security (1989) *Listeriosis and Food.* PL/CMO(89)3. HMSO, London.

Efstratiou A (1989) Outbreaks of human infections caused by the pyogenic streptococci of Lancefields Group C and Group G. *J. Med. Micro.* **29**: 207–19.

European Collaborative Study (1991) Children born to women with HIV infection: natural history and risk of transmission. *Lancet* **337**: 253–60.

Evans BG, Gill ON, Gleave SR *et al.* (1991) HIV-2 in the United Kingdom – A Review. *CDR* **1** (2): R19–23.

Fekerty R, Kim KH, Brown D *et al.* (1981) Epidemiology of antibiotic associated colitis. *Am. J. Med.* **70**: 906–8.

French GL, Cheng AFB, Ling JML *et al.* (1990) Hong Kong strains of methicillin-resistant and sensitive *Staphylococcus aureus* have similar virulence. *J. Hosp. Inf.* **15**(2): 117–26.

George RH, Gully PR, Gill ON *et al.* (1986) An outbreak of tuberculosis in a childrens hospital. *J. Hosp. Inf.* **8**: 129–142.

Gormon LJ, Sanai L, Notman W *et al.* (1993) Cross-infection in an intensive care unit by *Klebsiella pneumoniae* from ventilator condensate *J Hosp. Inf.* **23**: 17–26.

Hamory BH, Parisi JT (1987) *Staphylococcus epidermidis*: a significant nosocomial pathogen. *J. Inf. Control.* **15**: 59–74.

Health and Safety Executive, Advisory Committee on Dangerous Pathogens (1990) *Statement on Cytomegalovirus and the Pregnant Woman.* HMSO, London.

Heptonstall J (1991) Outbreaks of hepatitis B virus infection associated with infected surgical staff. *CDR* **1**: R81–5.

Heptonstall J, Porter K, Gill N (1993a) *Occupational Transmission of HIV. Summary of Published Reports.* PHLS AIDS Centre, CDSC, London.

Heptonstall J, Gill ON, Porter K *et al.* (1993b) Health care workers and HIV: surveillance of occupationally acquired infection in the United Kingdom. *CDR Review* **3**(11): 147–153.

Hoffman PN (1993) *Clostridium difficile* and the hospital environment. *PHLS Microbiology Digest* **10**(2): 91–2.

Howard AJ (1991) Nosocomial spread of *H. influenzae. J. Hosp. Inf.* **19**(1): 1–4.

Humphries II, Johnson FM, Warnock DW *et al.* (1991) An outbreak of aspergillosis in a general ITU. *J. Hosp. Inf.* **18**(3): 167–78.

Hutchinson DN (1990) Nosocomial legionellosis. *Rev. Med. Micro.* **1**: 108–15.

Joint Tuberculosis Committee of the British Thoracic Society. (1990) An updated code of practice. *Brit. Med. J.* **30**: 995–1000.

Joint Tuberculosis Committee (sub-committee) of the British Thoracic Society (1992) Guidelines on the management of tuberculosis and HIV infection in the United Kingdom. *Brit. Med. J* **304**: 1231–3.

Jones D (1990) Foodborne listeriosis. *Lancet* **336**: 1171–4.

Joseph CA, Palmer SR (1989) Outbreaks of *Salmonella* infection in hospitals in England and Wales 1978–87. *Brit. Med. J.* **298**: 1161–4.

Kleemola M, Jokinen C. (1992) Outbreak of *Mycoplasma pneumoniae* infection amongst hospital personnel studied by a nucleic acid hybridisation test. *J. Hosp. Inf.* **21**(3): 213–22.

Kolmos HJ, Thuesen B, Nielsen SV *et al.* (1993) Outbreak of infection in a burns unit due to *Pseudomonas aeruginosa* originating from contaminated tubing used for irrigation of patients. *J. Hosp. Inf.* **24**: 11–21.

Korten V, Murray BE (1993) The nosocomial transmission of enterococci. *Curr. Opin. Inf. Dis.* **6**: 498–505.

Krishnan PU, Pereira B, Macaden R. (1991) Epidemiological study of an outbreak of *Serratia marcescens* in a haemodialysis unit. *J. Hosp. Inf.* **18**: 57–61.

Levin MH, Olsen B, Nathan C *et al.* (1984) *Pseudomonas* in the sinks of an intensive care unit: relation to patients. *J. Clin. Path.* **37**: 424–7.

Livornese LL, Dias S, Samuel C *et al.* (1992) Hospital-acquired infection with vancomycin-resistant *Enterococcus faecium* transmitted by electronic thermometers. *Ann. Int. Med.* **117**: 112–26.

Loomes S (1988) Is it safe to lie down in hospital? *Nursing Times* **84**(49): 63–5.

Madge P, Payton JY, McColl JH *et al.* (1992) Prospective controlled study of four infection control procedures to prevent nosocomial infection with respiratory syncytial virus. *Lancet* **340**: 1079–83.

Meers PD, Ayliffe GAJ, Emmerson AM *et al.* (1981) Report of the national survey of infection in hospitals – 1980. *J. Hosp. Inf.* **2**(Suppl.): 1–53.

Mitchell E, O'Mahoney M, McKeith I *et al.* (1989) An outbreak of viral gastro-enteritis in a psychiatric hospital. *J. Hosp. Inf.* **14**(1): 1–8.

Mok J (1993) Breast milk and HIV-1 transmission. *Lancet* **341**: 930–1.

Morgan D (Ed.) (1990) *A Code of Practice for the Safe Use and Disposal of Sharps.* British Medical Association, London.

Mortimer EA, Wolinsky E, Gonzaga AJ *et al.*, (1966) Role of airborne transmission in staphylococcal infections. *Brit. Med. J.* **1**: 319–22.

Musa EK, Desai N, Casewell *et al.* (1990) The survival of *Acinetobacter calcoaceticus* inoculated on fingertips and on formica. *J. Hosp. Inf.* **15**(3): 219–28.

NHS Estates (1993) The control of legionella in health care premises – a code of practice. Health Technical Memorandum 2040.

Newton L, Hall SM, Pelevin M *et al.* (1992) Listeriosis Surveillance: 1991. CDR Review **2**(12): R142–4.

Nowak R (1994) Flesh-eating bacteria: not new but still worrisome. *Science* **264**: 1665.

Nye FJ (1993) Clinical features and treatment of *Clostridium difficile* diarrhoea. *PHLS Micro. Digest* **10**(2): 77–8.

Olsen B, Weinstein RA, Nathan C *et al.* (1984) Epidemiology of endemic *Pseudomonas aeruginosa*: why infection control efforts have failed. *J. Inf. Dis.* **150**: 808–16.

Pallett AP, Strangeways JEM (1988) Penicillin-resistant pneumococci. *Lancet* **i**: 1452.

Piedra PA, Kasel JA, Norton JH *et al.* (1992) Description of an adenovirus type 8 outbreak in hospitalised neonates born prematurely *Paed. Inf. Dis J.* **11**(8): 460–5.

Polakoff S (1976) Hepatitis B in retreat from dialysis units in United Kingdom in 1973. *Brit. Med. J.* **i**: 1579–81.

Public Health Laboratory Service (1993) Unlinked anonymous monitoring of HIV prevalence in England and Wales: 1990–92. *CDR Review* **3**(1): R1–11.

Reid JA, Breckon D, Hunter PR (1990) Infection of staff during an outbreak of viral gastroenteritis in an elderly persons' home. *J. Hosp. Inf.* **16**: 81–5.

Ridgeway EJ, Allen KD, Galloway A *et al.* (1991) Penicillin-resistant pneumococci in a Merseyside hospital. *J. Hosp. Inf.* **17**: 15–23.

Report of a Working Group of the Royal College of Pathologists (RCP). (1992) *HIV Infection: Hazards of Transmission to Patients and Health Care Workers During Invasive Procedures.* Royal College of Pathologists, London.

Reybrouck G (1983) Role of hands in the spread of nosocomial infection: 1. *J. Hosp. Inf.* **4**: 103–10.

Sanderson PJ, Weissler S (1992) Recovery of coliforms from the hands of nurses and patients: activities leading to contamination. *J. Hosp. Inf.* **21**: 85–94.

Schlech WF (1991) Listeriosis: epidemiology, virulence and the significance of contaminated foodstuffs. *J. Hosp. Inf.* **19**(4): 211–24.

Shanson DC (1989) *Microbiology in Clinical Practice*, 2nd edn. Wright, London.

Skaliy P, Sciple GV, Savannah GA (1964) Survival of staphylococci on hospital surfaces. *Arch. Env. Health.* **8**: 636–41

Thomas CGA (1988) *Medical Microbiology*, 6th edn. Baillière Tindall, London.

Thornbury G (1988) TB or not TB. *Nursing Times.* Aug. 7: 43–4.

Tookey P, Peckham CS (1991) Does cytomegalovirus present an occupational risk? *Arch. Dis. Childhood* **66**: 1009–10.

UK Health Departments (1990) *Guidance for Clinical Health Care Workers: Protection Against Infection with HIV and Hepatitis Viruses.* HMSO, London.

UK Health Departments (1993) *Protecting Health Care Workers and Patients from Hepatitis B. Recommendations of the Advisory Group on Hepatitis.* HMSO, London.

Uttley AHC, Pozniak A (1993) Resurgence of tuberculosis. *J. Hosp. Inf.* **23**(4): 249–54.

Wade JJ, Desai N, Casewell MW (1991) Hygienic hand disinfection for the removal of epidemic vancomycin-resistant *Enterococcus faecium* and gentamicin-resistant *Enterobacter cloacae. J. Hosp. Inf.* **18**(3): 211–18.

Watson JM (1991) Tuberculosis in perspective. *CDR Review* **1**(12): R129–31.

Weems JJ (1993) Nosocomial outbreak of *Pseudomonus cepacia* associated with contamination of reusable electronic ventilator temperature probes. *Inf. Contr. Hosp. Epid.* **14**(10): 583–6.

World Health Organization (1993) *Global Programme on AIDS. The HIV/AIDS Pandemic: 1993 overview.* WHO, Geneva.

Worsley MA (1993) A major outbreak of antibiotic-associated diarrhoea. *PHLS Microbiology Digest* **10**(2): 97–99.

Further Reading

AIDS Briefing (1987) *New Scientist*, March 26, 36–59.

Breuer J, Jeffries DJ (1990) Control of viral infections in hospital. *J. Hosp. Inf.* **16**: 191–221.

Cameron S, Blakely A (1993) A protocol for the detection of *Chlamydia. Nursing Standard.* **8**(5): 25–27.

Carr P, Rothburn M (1989) Listeriosis in midwifery. *Nursing Times* **85**(18): 73–4.

Cartwright KAV, Stuart JM, Noah ND (1986) An outbreak of meningococcal disease in Gloucestershire. *Lancet* **ii**: 558–61.

Department of Health and Social Security (1988) *HIV Infection, Breast Feeding and Human Milk Banking.* PL/CMO(88)13. HMSO, London.

Fagan EA (1992) Hepatitis A to G and beyond. *Brit. J. Hosp. Med.* **47**(2): 127–31.

Greene WC (1993) AIDS and the immune system. *Scientific American* Sept.: 20–110.

King R (1992) Living safely with HBV. *Nursing* **5**(5): 28–31.

Oakley K (1992) Making sense of accidental exposure to blood and body fluids. *Nursing Times* **88**(23): 40–4.

Pratt R (1995) *AIDS: A Strategy for Nursing Care*, 4th edn. Edward Arnold, London.

Robinson P (1987) Ousting the Organism. Community Outlook. *Nursing Times* **83**(June Supp.): 20–22.

Sleigh JD and Timbury MC (1990) *Medical Bacteriology*, 3rd edn. Churchill Livingstone, Edinburgh.

Teo CG (1992) The virology and serology of hepatitis: an overview. *CDR* **2**(10): R109–113.

Terence Higgins Trust (1992) *HIV: How to Protect Yourself and Others*, London.

Terence Higgins Trust (1993) *Testing Issues. A Booklet for People Thinking of Having an HIV Test*, London.

4 The Immune System and the Immuno-compromised Patient

Introduction

The body possesses several different defence mechanisms for protection from invasion by micro-organisms or other foreign materials, known collectively as **antigens**. Some of these defences are non specific and act as general barriers to all types of micro-organisms. They include the skin, saliva, **lysozyme** in tears, mucus and **cilia** in the respiratory tract and acid and bile in the gastrointestinal tract (Fig. 4.1). If a micro-organism succeeds in invading the body the **inflammatory response** is initiated to limit its spread. White blood cells called **phagocytes** engulf the micro-organisms and destroy them. Phagocytes work more efficiently in the presence of **antibodies**, produced by special white blood cells called **lymphocytes**. The lymphocytes retain a 'memory' of micro-organisms or other antigens that have previously invaded so that when the same antigen enters the body again the correct antibodies can be produced very rapidly and the micro-organism will not be able to multiply and cause infection.

Fig. 4.1
*External defences to invasion
by micro-organisms.*

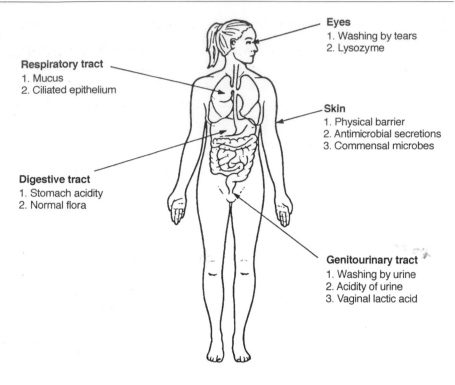

Respiratory tract
1. Mucus
2. Ciliated epithelium

Digestive tract
1. Stomach acidity
2. Normal flora

Eyes
1. Washing by tears
2. Lysozyme

Skin
1. Physical barrier
2. Antimicrobial secretions
3. Commensal microbes

Genitourinary tract
1. Washing by urine
2. Acidity of urine
3. Vaginal lactic acid

Non-specific Immune Response
External Defences

Skin

Intact skin provides the body with a tough outer layer that cannot be penetrated by microbes. Antibacterial substances are present in sweat and the secretions of sebaceous glands. The microbes which normally live on skin protect against invasion by **pathogens** through competition for nutrients. When patients are hospitalized this normal skin flora is often replaced by strains of hospital bacteria which are more resistant to **antibiotics** and which can cause serious infections if they enter the body during invasive procedures, for example methicillin-resistant *Staphylococcus aureus* (MRSA), *Klebsiella* and *Acinetobacter* species.

Cuts, abrasions or damaged skin (e.g. eczema) can be invaded by micro-organisms. Tetanus **spores** present in contaminated soil may be accidentally introduced through injured skin, HIV and hepatitis B by contact with infected blood or body fluids. Infection may also be introduced when skin is incised during surgical procedures or injured (e.g. stab wounds). Some **parasites** are injected through the skin by the bites of insects (e.g. malaria, typhus and yellow fever).

Ciliary Escalator System

The respiratory tract is protected from inhaled particles by hairs in the nose, which filter particles, and the cough reflex, which prevents aspiration. Particles that enter the airway are trapped in mucus, which is constantly moved by the cilia towards the mouth where it is swallowed.

Lysozyme

An enzyme present in tears and saliva breaks down bacterial cell walls, especially **Gram-positive** bacteria.

Gastrointestinal Tract

Acid in the stomach, at a pH of between 2 and 3, destroys most bacteria and is supplemented by the action of bile in the small intestine which also inhibits bacterial growth. The large intestine contains many bacteria which discourage the growth of pathogens by competing for nutrients and producing inhibitory substances.

Micro-organisms are prevented from adhering to the surface of the bladder and eyes by the constant flushing of urine and tears respectively.

Internal Defences

Inflammatory Response

When micro-organisms invade the body the first line of defence is the inflammatory response, which can be recognized by redness, heat, swelling and pain at the site of invasion. The aim of this response is to destroy as many of the invaders as possible and to limit their spread. It is a non-specific response initiated against any micro-organism or foreign substance.

The initial stages in the inflammatory response are illustrated in Table

Table 4.1
Stages in the inflammatory response

Response	Mediator	Effect	Visible sign
Dilation of blood vessels	Histamine from mast cells	Increases blood flow to area	Redness and heat
Blood vessels become more permeable	Prostaglandins	Plasma and white blood cells migrate into tissue	Swelling
Pressure on nerve endings	Swollen tissue	Discourages movement of affected part	Pain

Fig 4.2
Phagocytosis.

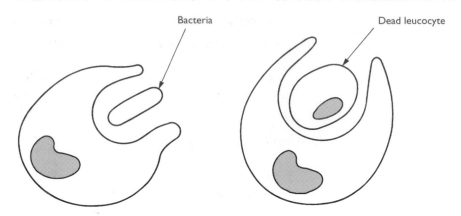

4.1. Once the blood flow to an area has been increased, chemicals released from the damaged tissue and from invading micro-organisms attract special white blood cells called phagocytes which engulf foreign substances by a process known as **phagocytosis** (Fig. 4.2). In humans there are two types of phagocytic cells; **polymorphonuclear neutrophil leucocytes (neutrophils)** and **mononuclear macrophages** (see Plate 4.1). Foreign cells or substances can be recognized and phagocytosed without assistance. However, the process is more effective when the cell has been marked or **opsonized** with proteins, such as **complement** or antibodies, so that the phagocytes can distinguish them from host cells.

The Complement System

The complement system is a series of structural **proteins** and **enzymes**, numbered C1 to C9, which circulate in the blood in an inactive form but when activated have several important effects, essential for phagocytosis to take place:

- promote vasodilation
- attract phagocytes
- increase the efficiency with which bacteria are engulfed by phagocytes (opsonization)
- destroy foreign cells by puncturing holes in their membranes

Complement is a non-specific immune response which is activated when the complement protein C3 binds on to microbial cell walls (the 'alternate pathway') or when the protein C1 binds to antibodies (the 'classic pathway'). The other complement proteins are then activated in an organized sequence (Fig. 4.3).

Clot Formation

A dense mesh of **fibrin** is formed around the site of invasion and prevents micro-organisms spreading away from the site. The **leucocytes,**

Fig. 4.3
The complement system.

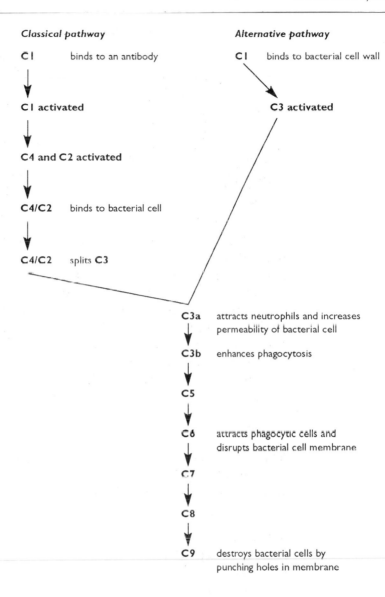

micro-organisms and damaged tissue are liquified by enzymes to form
pus. Pus can be absorbed or discharged through the skin, but if it forms
within the area walled off by the fibrin mesh, it cannot escape and an
abscess results.

This mechanism has no effect against bacterial **toxins** which travel in
the bloodstream to cause damage at sites distant to the site of infection,
for example diphtheria, in which the initial infection by *Corynebacterium
diphtheriae* occurs in the throat, but its toxin damages the heart, kidneys
and nerves.

Fever

The temperature of the body is maintained by a centre in the hypothalamus of the brain. Increased body temperature is a systemic effect of the inflammatory response. Fever is induced by pyrogens, proteins released by **white blood cells** and hormones such as **prostaglandins**. These substances stimulate the hypothalamus and cause a rise in body temperature. Aspirin inhibits prostaglandins and is used to reduce fever in adults.

Pyrexia is assumed to confer some advantage on the host, although the exact benefit is uncertain. High temperature increases the metabolic rate of the body and this may speed tissue repair and potentiate the immune response (Mackowiak, 1994). Most pathogenic microbes prefer a temperature of around 37°C and therefore an increase in body temperature may help the body to destroy them.

The effect of fever on the patient can be exhausting; the heart and respiratory rates increase and violent shivering or rigors may occur in severe fever. This increased activity may cause depletion of the glycogen energy reserves in the body and so protein may need to be broken down as a source of energy, the patient becomes debilitated and tissue repair is delayed. Children have immature temperature control and may experience febrile convulsions if the pyrexia develops rapidly. Although they are usually transient with no long-term effects they may lead to aspiration of secretions and asphyxia.

Evidence for the value of fever reduction is conflicting. The febrile patient is already responding as if to a cold environment and further cooling can increase discomfort. The use of antipyrexial drugs can disguise symptoms which may indicate a change in treatment is necessary, for example antibiotics (Styrt and Sugarman, 1990).

Guidelines for Practice

The Care of Pyrexial Patients

The nursing care should aim to reduce the discomfort associated with a raised body temperature, whilst replacing body fluids lost through sweating. Cooling the skin by sponging with warm water or with a fan may be of some benefit, but frequently causes greater discomfort and stress to the patient (Kinmouth *et al.*, 1992)

- Cover with one sheet, remove nightclothes if necessary
- Administer cool drinks frequently
- Offer frequent mouth care to counter the effects of dehydration
- Administer antipyrexial drugs if prescribed

The Specific Immune Response

Some microbes are not readily ingested by phagocytic cells and therefore other cells in the immune system, the lymphocytes, are required to destroy them. Unlike phagocytes, lymphocytes interact with specific antigens, they are able to remember a previous encounter with an antigen and provide a very rapid response the next time the same antigen invades.

There are two types of lymphocytes, B and T, both of which recognize and bind to receptors on specific antigens. **B lymphocytes** produce antibodies against the specific antigen, and are referred to as the **humoral immune system**. Humoral means 'of the body fluids' and is used to describe antibody production because they operate outside the cells in the blood and tissue fluids. **T lymphocytes** destroy abnormal or tumour cells and cells infected with viruses or other microbes. T lymphocytes are referred to as the cellular or **cell-mediated immune system**. The T lymphocytes also produce protein molecules which activate other lymphocytes and **macrophages**.

The lymphocytes do not operate independently, but act collectively to destroy the invading antigen. They interact with each other, with phagocytic cells and the complement system. The differentiation of blood cells into red cells, lymphocytes, leucocytes and macrophages is illustrated in Fig. 4.4.

Fig. 4.4
Differentiation of blood cells.

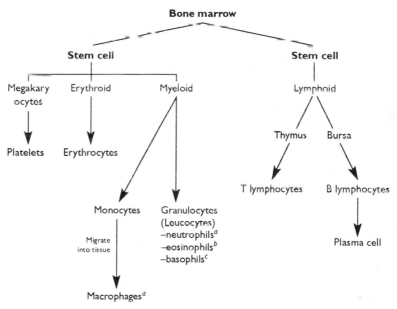

[a] Phagocytic cells
[b] Active against parasites, important in allergic reactions
[c] Unknown activity

B Lymphocytes

B lymphocytes originate from stem cells in the bone marrow. They are referred to as B cells because in birds they mature in a structure called the 'bursa of Fabricius'. B lymphocytes are responsible for the production of antibodies.

Structure of Antibodies

Antibodies are Y-shaped proteins called globulins, or **immunoglobulins.** The two arms of the Y vary in structure and are the parts of the molecule that enable the antibody to recognize or fit around different molecules on the surface of an antigen (Fig. 4.5). The stem of the Y activates complement and attaches to phagocytes, triggering them to engulf the invader. There are five different types of immunoglobulin distinguishable by their structure and number of amino acid chains (see Table 4.2)

Synthesis of Antibodies

Thousands of B lymphocytes are produced and circulate around the body. Each B lymphocyte has a different antibody on its surface. When

Fig. 4.5
The structure of immunoglobulin G. IgG is made of two long and two short peptide chains. The variable regions determine the specificity of the antibody.

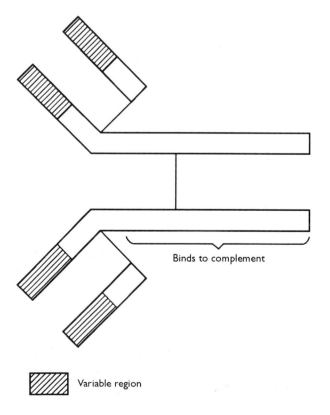

Binds to complement

Variable region

	Immunoglobulin	Activity
Table 4.2 *Different classes of immunoglobulin (antibody)*	IgG	The most abundant, diffuse from blood vessels into tissue fluids. Coat bacteria to facilitate phagocytosis and neutralize bacterial toxins. Cross the placenta in the last 3 months of pregnancy
	IgM	A large molecule made up of five short and five long chains of amino acids. Appear first in an attack against an antigen, but confined to blood. Assist phagocytosis by coating antigen, agglutinate bacteria and interact with complement
	IgA	Act as the early defence against microbial invasion of mucous membranes. Found in the secretions of reproductive, respiratory and gastrointestinal tract
	IgE	Mainly attached to mast cells where they influence the release of histamine. Secreted mainly in the respiratory and gastrointestinal tract, associated with allergic response
	IgD	Maximum levels are detected during childhood but function is unknown

a lymphocyte encounters an antigen that fits the antibody it is carrying, it binds to the antigen and is stimulated to divide repeatedly, generating a large number of identical cells, or **clones**, all of which carry the same antibody. These clones differentiate into **plasma cells**, which synthesize and release the antibody but die after a short time, and **memory cells**, special antibody-producing cells which persist in the blood for many years.

The division and maturation of plasma cells is controlled by T cells. The plasma cells produce IgM (see Table 4.2) for the first few days, the same cells are then instructed to produce IgG (see Table 4.2), which can be produced for up to a year.

If the same antigen invades the body again the memory cells circulating in the blood recognize it and begin the production of the appropriate plasma cells immediately. This very rapid response prevents the micro-organism becoming established in the host and is the mechanism that confers immunity after initial exposure to an infection (e.g. measles, mumps).

Effect of Antibodies

One micro-organism may have several receptor sites recognized by different antibodies. Once antibodies have bound to its surface the complement system and phagocytes are activated and the micro-organism is destroyed.

T Lymphocytes

These lymphocytes are formed in the bone marrow but mature in a gland at the base of the brain, the thymus. The thymus is prominent in children but atrophies with age.

T lymphocytes have two main roles: firstly, to provide a defence against micro-organisms which can enter and survive in host cells and secondly, to co-ordinate the immune response by helping to turn antibody production on and off and by enhancing the activity of phagocytic cells. They are particularly important for the control of intracellular parasites, for example mycobacteria, fungi, viruses, some bacteria and protozoa.

Antibodies can attack these microbes whilst they are in the blood or tissue fluid but not if they are inside the cell. Many micro-organisms can survive and multiply inside phagocytic cells which engulf them. When a microbe is engulfed by a macrophage, the macrophage displays (or presents) an antigen from the microbe on its surface. T lymphocytes, like B lymphocytes, have receptors specific to a large number of different antigens. These receptors recognize the antigens expressed on the surface of an infected cell, but only if they are adjacent to one of the host cell's own 'self markers', characteristic molecules present on the surface of every host cell. In this way the host cell is identified as infected and marked for destruction (Fig. 4.6).

When the helper or T4 lymphocyte binds to an invaded host cell it starts to divide and produce a range of **lymphokines**, of which the two most important are **interleukins** and **interferons**. Lymphokines play a very important role in co-ordinating and facilitating the immune response (Table 4.3).

Several types of T lymphocyte are produced and each has a different function (Fig. 4.7).

Cytotoxic cells recognize and destroy host cells which have been invaded by micro-organisms and other non-self cells (e.g. the rejection of grafted tissue or organs).

Memory cells keep a record of the antigen and enable rapid production of the appropriate T lymphocytes the next time the same antigen enters the body.

Suppressor cells or T8 lymphocytes inhibit the activity of the T4 or helper lymphocytes and are necessary to turn off the response when the infection has been successfully resisted.

Natural Killer Cells

These are lymphocytes which lyse both microbial and host cells. They are neither B or T cells and do not need to be activated by a specific antigen.

Table 4.3
The role of the lymphokines

- Attract macrophages and induce them to kill intracellular parasites
- Promote the production of B lymphocytes and control the manufacture of antibodies
- Induce the proliferation of T lymphocytes and stimulate their activity

Fig. 4.6
T cells recognize an antigen
on the surface of a
macrophage. The T cells
are the small spherical
objects, the macrophage
the larger, flat object.

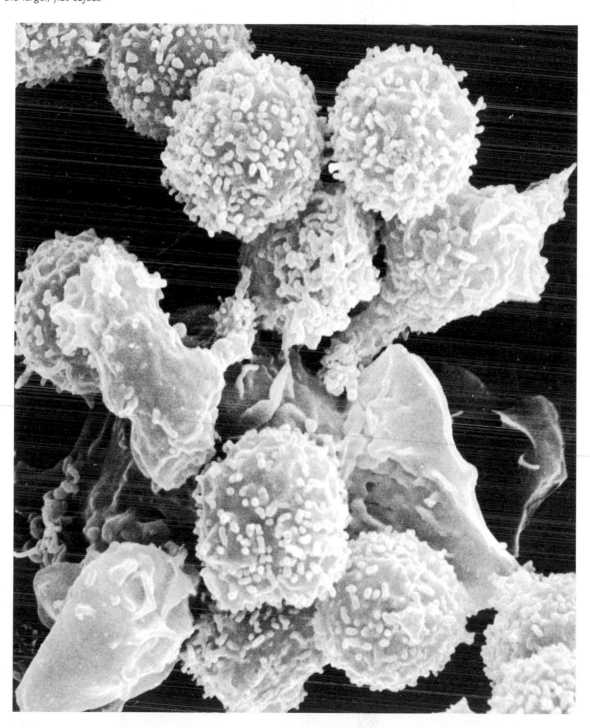

Fig. 4.7
*The specific immune
response. The B cells, T cells
and macrophages all
interact to fend off the
attack from invading
micro-organisms.*

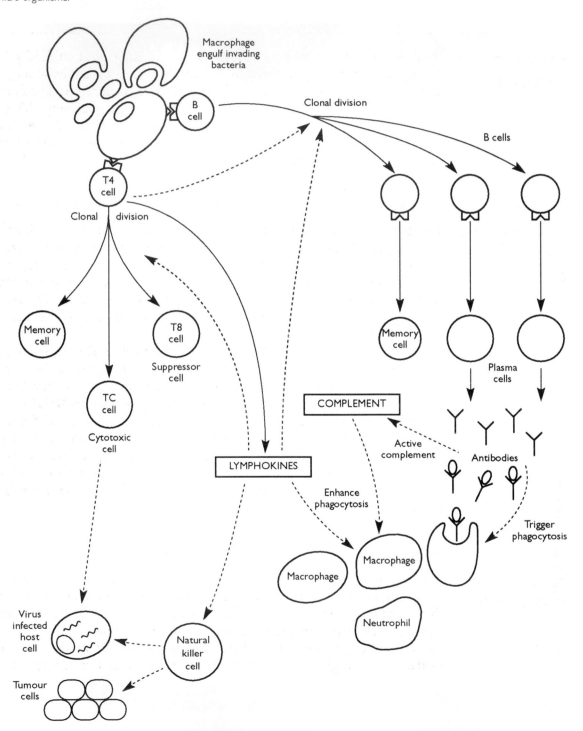

They probably have a role in controlling the differentiation of immune system cells and help prevent cancers, particularly leukemias. They also destroy cells invaded by **viruses**, aid in the rejection of grafted tissue and provide resistance against infection by some **fungi** and **protozoa**. The activity of killer cells is promoted by the lymphokine, interferon.

| Monoclonal Antibodies | A large amount of a single antibody can be manufactured artificially by fusing a cell producing specific antibodies with a cell from a B lymphocyte tumour. The fused cells survive and multiply indefinitely in tissue culture and produce many copies of the single specific antibody. These monoclonal antibodies are used in research on infectious diseases and the immune system and for the identification of some micro-organisms (e.g. *Legionella*, *Chlamydia*, viruses). |

The Recognition of Self and Non-self

Defence against an invader is only possible if the immune system is able to distinguish between the cells of the host (self) and those of the invader (non-self). At birth the immune system is immature and does not respond to self and non-self antigens that it encounters, possibly because neonatal macrophages are unable to present antigens or because all the self-reacting B and T lymphocytes are inactivated or because of the action of T-suppressor cells.

Each cell of the body also carries a distinct marker of selfness which not only differs between species but between individuals of the same species. The segment of **chromosome** that codes for these 'self marking' molecules is called the **human leucocyte antigen system (HLA)**.

The HLA markers enable the immune system to recognize and destroy tissue grafted into the body from another person. Grafted material is less likely to be attacked by the immune system if the HLA markers of the donated material are similar to those of the host. Tissue typing is used to find donors whose HLA markers are very similar to the intended recipient of the tissue.

Organs of the Immune System

The cells of the immune system originate in the bone marrow but settle in lymphoid tissue which then sustains them (Fig. 4.8). The spleen and liver contain lymphoid tissue and these organs filter and destroy foreign particles and micro-organisms from the blood. Lymphoid tissue is also found in the gut (Peyer's patches), the tonsils and adenoids. **Lymph nodes** are small glands scattered throughout the body but concentrated

Fig. 4.8
*The organs of the immune
response.*

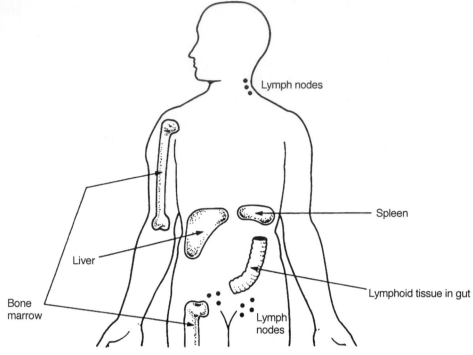

in areas of the body most likely to be invaded by pathogens; the mouth, eyes, nose, the gut and limbs. They are connected together by a network of small channels, called the **lymphatic system**. Lymph nodes contain many lymphocytes and macrophages and when an antigen enters a node the B lymphocytes are induced to produce antibody which is then released into the bloodstream. The nodes closest to the site of infection will mount the immune response and this is apparent when they become swollen and painful, for example an infection of the leg may cause lymph nodes in the groin to swell, whilst an infection of the upper respiratory tract causes nodes in the neck to swell.

Immunity to Infection

As already described, both B and T lymphocytes make memory cells after exposure to a particular infection. If the same microbe is encountered again, these memory cells are able to mount a very rapid response and prevent the invading organism from establishing infection. This enables the host to develop **immunity** to infections. Immunity can be conferred either naturally following an infection or artificially by the inoculation of an organism or its products into the body. Immunity can also be conferred by injecting antibody (IgG) against a specific micro-organism. This is called **passive immunity** because it does not cause the production of

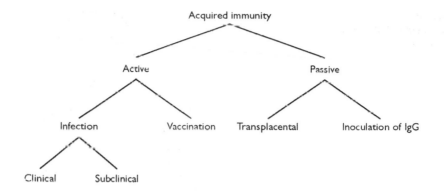

Fig. 4.9
*Acquired immunity to
infection.*

Fig. 4.9
*Acquired immunity to
infection.*

memory cells and protection is only conferred for the lifetime of the IgG. IgG crosses the placenta from mother to foetus so that the baby has some protection against infection for the first few months of life (Fig. 4.9).

Immunization

In the developed world, the ravages of **infectious** disease have declined dramatically in the last 100 years and immunization is one of several factors which have played a part in this decline (Table 4.4). The principles of immunization were developed in the early 1800s. They were pioneered by Edward Jenner, who in 1796 demonstrated that humans could be protected against smallpox by inoculation with a similar virus which caused cowpox in cows, this was the first use of a **vaccine** (Plate 4.2).

Vaccines

Most vaccines produce their protective effect by stimulating the production of antibodies, although Bacillus Calmette–Guérin (BCG) vaccine for tuberculosis, promotes cell-mediated immunity.

Table 4.5 illustrates the different types of vaccine that are used. They must be able to induce an immune response but without establishing infection and causing harm to the recipient. Some vaccines are made of dead micro-organisms. Others are made of live micro-organisms which

Table 4.4
*Factors that influence the
control of infectious disease*

- Improved living conditions
- Improved hygiene
- Clean water supply
- Sewage disposal
- Improved nutrition
- Understanding how to prevent the spread of disease
- Antibiotics
- Immunization

Table 4.5
Types of vaccine in routine
use

Live vaccines
  Attenuated
    e.g. polio, measles, mumps, rubella, BCG
Killed organisms
  Whole bacterial cells
    e.g. whooping cough, cholera, typhoid
  Inactivated toxin
    e.g. diphtheria, tetanus
  Capsule polysaccharide
    e.g. meningococcal, pneumococcal
Genetically engineered vaccines
  Antigen incorporated into yeast
    e.g. hepatitis B

have been altered to prevent them causing infection (**live-attenuated vaccines**). A few vaccines are made from bacterial products such as altered toxins.

Killed vaccines can be made of whole bacterial cells such as *Bordetella pertussis* used to immunize against whooping cough, or purified parts of the cell. The vaccines for *Haemophilus influenzae*, *Pneumococcus* and *Neisseria meningitidis* are derived from proteins in their **capsules** and the influenza vaccine is made from viral proteins.

Live-attenuated vaccines usually produce a stronger immunity and often confer protection with a single dose. This type of vaccine is used to immunize against poliomyelitis, measles, mumps and rubella. The BCG vaccine for tuberculosis is also a live-attenuated vaccine of a related organism, *Mycobacterium bovis*.

The vaccines for tetanus and diphtheria contain *toxoid*. These are toxins produced by the organisms but inactivated by treatment with formaldehyde. Although the toxoid induces an immune response, their toxic activity is destroyed.

More recently, genetic engineering techniques have been applied to vaccine production. The **genes** that code for specific microbial antigens (the part of the bacteria or virus, recognized by the immune system) are isolated and inserted into a piece of **DNA** which is transferred into a yeast and cultured in a very large fermenter. The yeast makes the antigen which is then recovered, purified and made into a vaccine. This method is used to make a vaccine for hepatitis B.

Some organisms present particular problems for vaccine production. The orthomyxoviruses, which cause influenza, undergo minor changes to the proteins on their surface (antigenic drift) and occasionally major changes (antigenic shift). Antibody made to the antigens on one strain of influenza may not recognize the antigens on the surface of the next season's strain. When an antigenic shift occurs, the population will have little immunity to the new strain and an **epidemic** of influenza may result. Influenza vaccine is made of several different viral strains and is prepared each year by identifying the strains most likely to be prevalent. It is mainly recommended for the elderly or those with heart and chest disease who are most vulnerable. The vaccine provides reasonable protection against the selected strains but protection only lasts for about 1 year (DOH, 1992).

The human immunodeficiency virus (HIV) presents similar problems because when it replicates the **genome** is frequently copied inaccurately. Copies of the virus vary slightly and make it difficult for the immune system to respond effectively.

Administration of Vaccines

Injection of a vaccine into an individual who has not been previously exposed to the infection induces a slow production of antibody, mostly IgM. The level rises to a peak within a few weeks and may then fall to undetectable levels. This is called the **primary response**. Further injections produce a more rapid response to a higher level, for longer; this is called the secondary response. The level of IgM produced is similar to the primary response but a much greater amount of IgG is produced (Fig. 4.10). After a full course of vaccine the level of antibody remains high for months or years. Another single dose of vaccine will increase the level of antibody rapidly because the immune system has been induced to make memory cells. Most immunizations require a course of at least three injections although some vaccines of live-attenuated micro-organisms, for example measles mumps rubella (MMR), produce a high level of antibody after one injection. In many cases, vaccination has been shown to confer protection for at least 15 years (e.g. rubella and BCG). Others may require a booster dose every few years (e.g. Hepatitis B, cholera).

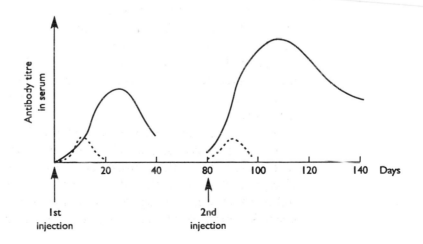

Fig. 4.10
Immunization – the primary and secondary response. A small amount of IgG (—) and IgM (- - -) are formed after the first injection but disappear fairly rapidly. After the second injection IgG reaches a higher level and persists in the serum for much longer.

Passive Immunization

The immunity conferred by active immunization with vaccine takes several weeks to establish as it depends on the production of specific antibodies or immunoglobulins. In certain situations, where an individual has been exposed to an infection and is known to have no immunity to it, a more rapid protection against infection is required. The specific antibodies or immunoglobulins made after exposure to particular micro-organisms can be collected from people recently infected or who have high levels of antibody following immunization. If inoculated into another person, these specific immunoglobulins will protect against infection, although the protection will only be temporary as they will gradually be lost from the body.

This type of **immunization** is used to protect against infection by hepatitis B following a needlestick injury and to protect **immunocompromised** individuals, who may develop serious illness, from chickenpox following exposure to the virus.

The Impact of Immunization Programmes

The aim of immunization can be the protection of the individual against a life-threatening or serious disease, the foetus (for example the immunization of women against rubella) or the community as a whole through the principle of 'herd immunity'. If sufficient numbers of a population are immune to the disease the micro-organism is unable to find susceptible hosts in which to cause infection. For herd immunity to be effective a minimum of 60% of the population must be immune and a higher level if the infection spreads rapidly and is highly **contagious**.

It is rare for an infection to be completely eradicated through immunization alone. The smallpox eradication programme was started in 1959 by the World Health Organization and not completed until the last case (outside of a laboratory) occurred in 1977. Its success depended on an effective vaccine, an easily identifiable disease with no animal or environmental reservoir and an intensive worldwide surveillance and immunization programme.

It is essential that high rates of immunization are maintained. In instances when diphtheria immunization has been relaxed, resurgence of the disease has occurred rapidly. Following fears in the mid-1970s about brain damage associated with the pertussis vaccine, the rate of immunization fell from over 80% to 30%. As a result the number of cases of whooping cough increased from around 2400 in 1973 to over 100 000 in 1977/79 (Fig. 4.11).

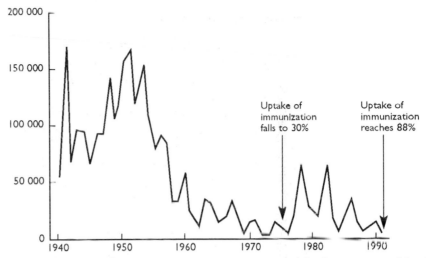

Fig. 4.11
*Pertussis notifications
(1940–1992).*

As with all medicines, vaccines carry some risk, but even with the pertussis vaccine, the risk is extremely small and less than that of the risk of serious complications from the disease itself

In the UK, the Department of Health recommends a schedule of immunization from early childhood and the primary health care services are responsible for its implementation (Table 4.6). Detailed information about all aspects of vaccines is available in the Department of Health publication *Immunisation against Infectious Disease* (DOH, 1992).

The Damaged Immune System

Individuals vary widely in their ability to resist infection and this depends on many factors, including age, general health, state of nutrition, previous exposure to infection and vaccination. Young children have an immature immune system and are more likely to succumb to infection until they

Table 4.6
*Schedule for routine
immunization*

Vaccine	Age	
Diphtheria, tetanus, pertussis polio, *Haemophilus influenzae* (HIB)	2 months 3 months 4 months	1st dose 2nd dose 3rd dose
Measles, mumps, rubella (MMR)	12–18 months	
Diphtheria, tetanus, polio, MMR (if not given previously)	4–5 years	Booster
Rubella	10–14 years	Girls only
BCG	10–14 years	
Tetanus, polio	15–18 years	Booster

have developed a range of specific memory cells. The elderly also have a diminished immune response, particularly by the T lymphocytes and are more susceptible to infection.

Physical or emotional stress, for example multiple traumatic injury or major surgery, can affect the immune response through the release of anti-inflammatory hormones such as **prostaglandin E** from damaged tissue and corticosteroids from the adrenal glands. In major burns, **immunosuppression** occurs through the loss of white blood cells and immunoglobulins and reduced phagocytic function. Poor nutrition impairs phagocytosis and reduces the production of white blood cells and antibodies (Conry, 1982).

These factors should be taken into account when assessing a patient's risk of acquiring an infection. The immune system of a patient who is malnourished or under stress will be less able to destroy bacteria which invade his/her wounds, intravenous cannula, etc. Planning the care of the patient towards improving the activity of his/her immune system is essential if infection is to be prevented. Risk assessment is discussed in more detail in Chapter 6.

Disease Associated with Immune Deficiency

Impairment of the immune response occurs as a result of a variety of genetic disorders, autoimmune disease, chemotherapy and certain viral infections, notably human immunodeficiency virus.

The most serious genetic disorder is severe combined immune deficiency disorder in which there is a failure of the bone marrow stem cells to differentiate into **B** and **T cells** and lymphocytes are not produced. It can be treated by bone marrow transplantation but the children often die of infection at a few months old, before the diagnosis has been made.

Autoimmune disorders occur as a result of a malfunction of the body's self-recognition mechanism. Antibodies are made against host tissue. The damage to the tissue or the deposition of antibody–antigen complexes in joints, blood vessels or kidney causes the symptoms of the disease (see Table 4.7).

In rheumatic fever, antibodies formed against *Streptococcus pyogenes* infection in the throat cross-react with tissue on the heart valves which

Table 4.7
Auto-immune diseases

Autoimmune disease	Self-antigen recognized
Pernicious anaemia	Gastric parietal cells
Juvenile insulin-dependent diabetes	Pancreatic islet cells
Multiple sclerosis	Central nervous system myelin
Lupus erythematosus	DNA, RBC, lymphocytes, platelets
Rheumatoid arthritis	IgG

has very similar receptors. The antibodies recognize the heart valves as an antigen, and the resulting damages is called endocarditis.

Chemotherapy can have profound immunosuppressive effects. Cytotoxic drugs interfere non-specifically in cell division but because bone marrow cells divide very frequently, about once every 12–30 h, the drugs have a major effect on bone marrow and the production of blood cells. Some antibiotics inhibit **cellular immunity** (e.g. chloramphenicol, tetracycline). Steroids have long-term effects on the production of immunoglobulins and interfere with the inflammatory response.

Leukemias are a group of malignant diseases affecting the white cell precursors in the bone marrow. Susceptibility to infection is increased through the overproduction of immature or abnormal white blood cells and the suppression of normal cell production.

Aplastic anaemia is a severe depression of the bone marrow which causes depletion of red blood cells, white blood cells and platelets. There are variety of causes of aplastic anaemia, including exposure to drugs (e.g. chloramphenicol), chemicals (e.g. benzene) or ionizing radiation.

Acquired Immune Deficiency Syndrome (AIDS)

The human immunodeficiency virus (HIV) attaches to and invades cells which carry particular protein called CD4. Several cells involved in the immune response carry CD4, including the T helper lymphocytes (T4 cells) and macrophages. HIV depletes circulating T4 cells sited in the lymph nodes and gradually damages the immune system. The lymph nodes appear to be the site of greatest viral replication and their eventual destruction has devastating effects on the immune response (Greene, 1993).

The main effect of T4 cell depletion is a diminished response to organisms which cause intracellular infection, for example tubercle bacilli and *Salmonella*, protozoa such as *Toxoplasma* and *Cryptosporidium* and viruses, in particular cytomegalovirus. Susceptibility to other organisms, which would not normally cause serious infection in an immune-competent host, is also increased (e.g. *Pneumocystis carinii*, Herpes simplex, *Candida albicans*. Certain malignant tumours which would normally be destroyed by T cells may also develop, for example B cell lymphomas and Kaposi's sarcoma (a cancer of endothelial cells).

Organ Transplants

It is now possible to treat many illnesses by replacing diseased organs or tissue with healthy tissue from another person, for example kidney, heart, lung and bone marrow. One of the major obstacles to successful organ transplantation is the rejection of the new or 'grafted' material by the recipients immune system. The surface markers on the foreign tissue cells are recognized as 'non-self' and the foreign material is gradually destroyed, primarily by the T lymphocytes of the cellular immune system. This response is called 'graft versus host disease' or GVHD. Successful transplantation therefore depends on tissue typing, the selection of donor material which is closely related to that of the recipient and less likely to be destroyed and the use of immunosuppressant drugs which interfere with the activity of T lymphocytes.

One of the most useful of these drugs was originally derived from a fungus and is called cyclosporin A. It blocks the production of lymphokines and therefore affects the immune response to new antigens but not the response by memory cells to previously encountered antigens. Another commonly used drug, azathioprine, inhibits the synthesis of **nucleic acids** and therefore prevents cell division. It has a preferential effect on T cells, but also affects cells in the bone marrow and intestine.

Preventing Infection in the Immuno-compromised Patient

Individuals who have a severely damaged immune system are at particular risk of life-threatening infection. This can be a problem whilst they are in hospital because they are more likely to be exposed to infection by contact with other patients, staff and through invasive procedures which bypass defences against microorganisms.

The Immunocompromised Host

The expression 'compromised host' is a vague term used to describe an individual who has a severely impaired immune system. Damage to the immune system renders these individuals particularly susceptible to infection, even by 'opportunists', micro-organisms which are not usually able to cause serious infection, for example *Pneumocystis carinii*, *Candida albicans*.

The types of infection associated with immunodeficiency depends on the part of the immune system that is affected. If the cellular or T cell response is reduced those microbes that cause **intracellular** infections predominate. Examples are *Salmonella*, *Listeria*, *Cryptococcus*, *Pneumocystis* and those viruses which persist in a latent form such as Herpes and Cytomegalovirus. If the humoral or B lymphocyte response is affected, protection against bacterial pathogens such as *Staphylococcus aureus* and *Pneumococcus* is reduced. The phagocytic cells or **granulocytes** are important for both the B and T lymphocyte responses, therefore a reduction in the number of these cells increases susceptibility to a wide range of infections, particularly **Gram-negative** bacteria, *Staphylococcus epidermidis* and *S. aureus*. Neutrophils account for the largest proportion of granulocytes and in immunocompromised patients, the number of neutrophils circulating in the blood is often used as an indicator of susceptibility to infection.

Protective isolation precautions are usually initiated when the level of neutrophils circulating in the blood falls below $0.5 \times 10^9/l$. A reduction to this level is associated with a significant increase in the risk of infection (Bodey *et al.*, 1966). Approximately half of the infections in these patients are caused by the patient's own microbial flora, the remainder are acquired from the hands of staff, equipment or food (Schimff *et al.*, 1972; Schimff, 1978; Remington and Schimff, 1981).

Many different systems of protecting these highly vulnerable patients from infection have been recommended, including the use of a plastic tent isolator (Trexler *et al.*, 1975), controlled airflow in a single room and standard care in a conventional hospital room.

Trexler Isolators

Trexler isolators consist of a plastic tent with built in 'suits' which enable staff to administer care from outside the tent. They provide an absolute barrier to micro-organisms from the environment and staff, but they are expensive, often of no benefit and now are rarely used.

Filtered Air

Two types of air filtration systems have been used to reduce the risk of airborne infection: plenum ventilation and laminar flow. In plenum ventilation, air is filtered, drawn into the room through vents in the ceiling and out of the room through vents in the walls. Laminar flow is a more efficient method of reducing the number of microbes in the air. Filtered air flows horizontally across the bed area and leaves on the opposite side of the room.

Infections acquired by the airborne route are a relatively uncommon problem in the immunocompromised patient. Outbreaks of life-threatening pneumonia caused by *Aspergillus* fungi have been reported and are usually associated with contaminated ventilation systems, fire-proofing materials or building works in the vicinity (Nauseef and Maki, 1981). Patients with severe burns may also be at increased risk of acquiring wound infection from bacteria which settle into the wound from dust particles. Filtered air is often recommended for rooms where dressings on extensive burns are changed (Ayliffe and Lilly, 1985).

Filtered air systems are expensive and although they may reduce the rate of infectious complications in patients with leukaemia, they do not appear to have a significant effect on the rate of survival from the disease (Schimff *et al.*, 1978). They may be justified in specialized bone marrow transplant units where patients have severely depleted T cells and outbreaks of airborne fungal infections may occur (Rogers and Barnes, 1988).

Simple Protective Isolation

Complex methods of protectively isolating an immunocompromised patient have been recommended, including the use of sterile equipment, masks, gowns, gloves and overshoes. However, such extensive precautions are expensive, increase the emotional deprivation of the patient and family and there is evidence that they are no more effective in preventing infections than more simple methods (Nauseef and Maki, 1981).

The following precautions are therefore recommended as an effective and practical method of minimizing the risk of infection in most severely immunocompromised patient:

Accommodation

An immunocompromised patient is probably as likely to acquire infection in a single room than in a ward with other patients (Nauseef and Maki, 1981). However, a single room acts as a reminder that special precautions are required. There is evidence that patients in **protective isolation** are able to cope better with the experience than those isolated because of an infectious disease. This may be because the immunocompromised are involved in the decision to isolate and prepared for the experience (Collins *et al.*, 1989). However, isolation can cause patients to become demanding and irritable and these behaviours should be recognized as a response to isolation (Denton, 1986). Psychosocial care of the patients is important to help them through the period of isolation but is frequently overlooked (Knowles, 1993) (Table 14.1). It should form part of the nursing care plan of all isolated patients.

Handwashing

Hands should be washed thoroughly with soap and water before contact with the patient to prevent the transfer of micro-organisms from other patients. Hands should also be washed immediately before direct contact with vulnerable sites on the patient such as intravenous cannulae, urethral catheters and wounds. An alcohol handrub is a useful, quick alternative to soap and water when hands are not visibly soiled (see Chapter 7). Handwashing is probably the most important method of protecting the immunocompromised patient.

Protective Clothing

Protective clothing should be used to prevent micro-organisms from other patients in the ward and from the patients own flora gaining access to vulnerable sites. Gloves and aprons should be used for contact with body fluids and changed before contact with wounds, cannulae, catheters or drains. Sterile protective clothing is probably unnecessary as it is unlikely to reduce the risk of infection. There is little evidence that masks provide protection against respiratory pathogens (Taylor, 1980; Nauseef and Maki, 1981). Staff with upper respiratory tract infections should be excluded from direct contact with these patients as this is a safer means of protecting the patient from respiratory pathogens than masks. The use of unnecessary protective clothing should be avoided as this may increase the patient's sense of isolation.

Visitors

Visitors with infections should be excluded but since they have minimal contact with the patient, there is no reason for them to wear protective clothing. They should be instructed to remove potential pathogens by washing their hands before seeing the patient.

Equipment

In general, there appears to be no reason to treat equipment differently. Low-risk equipment used only on intact skin should be processed in the usual way (e.g. linen, bedpans, crockery). However, some equipment is easily contaminated and not usually cleaned thoroughly (e.g. commodes, washbowls). It is therefore preferable to allocate one of these items for use only by the patient and clean each item thoroughly with detergent and water after each use. There is little value in autoclaving a wide range of items used by immunocompromised patients, especially newspapers, toys and books. The only equipment which needs to be sterile are those items used for invasive procedures.

Cleaning

Dust harbours micro-organisms and should be removed regularly from all horizontal surfaces where it collects. Disinfection of surfaces is of no value. Dry floors and surfaces are an unlikely source of infection and contamination is only removed temporarily by **disinfectants** (Ayliffe *et al.*, 1967).

Food

Food normally contains micro-organisms which are not harmful provided they are present in low numbers. Hospital food often contains Gram-negative bacilli (Shooter *et al.*, 1969; Remmington and Schimpff, 1981), which can cause serious infection in an immunocompromised host. Whilst it is impractical to sterilize food, particularly as the process may significantly alter the taste, every effort must be made to ensure that food is hygienically prepared and handled (see Chapter 12). Meat should be cooked thoroughly, fruit and vegetables should be washed and peeled before consumption and hospital-prepared salads should be avoided.

Fig. 4.12
An example of a simple protective isolation policy.

Indication

Protective isolation is necessary for patients with a severely compromised immune system

Aims

- To prevent the transmission of infection to an immunologically compromised patient
- To give psychological support and reassurance to the patient whilst in isolation
- To ensure all staff (including domestic staff) are aware of the correct precautions to take

Equipment

- A single room with a washbasin
- The room must be clean before the patient is isolated

Inside room: soap
paper towels
washbowl, sphygmomanometer
alcohol handrub
disposable clean gloves
plastic aprons

- Display a protective isolation card at the entrance to the room

Practice	Rationale
Patient – explain reason for isolation and give reassurance	To reduce anxiety and gain the patient's co-operation
Apron – put on a plastic apron before contact with the patient and between dirty and clean procedures	To prevent transmission of organisms from clothing to patient
Gloves – not necessary except for aseptic procedures and contact with blood and body fluids	To prevent contamination of vulnerable sites
Masks – not necessary	
Hands – always wash hands before entering the room. Repeat before handling cannula sites, etc.	To remove transient micro-organisms
Staff – exclude staff with infections. Staff who are nursing patients with infections should avoid nursing patients in protective isolation during the same span of duty	To minimize the risk of transferring micro-organisms
Equipment – clean thoroughly with detergent and water before use. Where possible reserve for the patient	To remove micro-organisms
Crockery – use normal utensils and wash in the normal way	The risk of cross-infection is minimal. Washing in hot water and detergent is sufficient
Visitors – instruct to wash hands on entering room, discourage those with infections	To remove potential pathogens

	Practice	Rationale
Fig. 4.12 *Continued*	*Other department* – should be notified in advance and where possible the patient seen on the ward	To enable appropriate arrangements to be made
	Cleaning – ensure that a high standard of cleaning is maintained. Explain the precautions to domestic staff	Dust may harbour micro-organisms. Regular cleaning will remove them
	Food – always wash hands and put on a plastic apron before handling food. Food must be served from the trolley without delay and meals must not be retained for reheating later	These patients are more susceptible to illness from pathogenic bacteria in food. Bacteria multiply in food unless stored at above 65°C or below 5°C
	If a microwave is used ensure that the instructions on the packet are followed precisely	To ensure the food reaches an even temperature throughout
	The following food should be avoided: salads, 'take-away' foods (including delicatessen), soft-boiled eggs, soft ripened cheeses (e.g. Brie)	Soft cheese and ready-to-eat meals may be contaminated with listeria
	Fruit should be washed and peeled	
	Fresh tap water and fresh pasteurized milk are permissible	

Cooked food, opened tins and jars should always be stored in the refrigerator and discarded after 24 h, before micro-organisms have the chance to multiply. Reheating of meals should be avoided, except 'ready-to-eat' meals which should be heated exactly as described by the manufacturers' instructions.

The main foods to avoid are soft cheeses, patés and freshly cut salads which may contain listeria, and cold meats, which are easily contaminated during handling (Lund *et al.*, 1989; Jones, 1990). Eggs are sometimes contaminated with *Salmonella* and should be thoroughly cooked before eating (De Louvois, 1993). Food which contains raw egg should be avoided (e.g. mayonnaise). Tap water from a drinking supply usually contains very few micro-organisms and is probably safe to drink provided it is fresh from the tap. Ice made in ice-making machines can be more hazardous because the water supplied to the machine may be contaminated, the ice may be present for considerable periods and ice in the machine may be contaminated by patients or staff using it. Outbreaks of infection caused by Gram-negative bacteria and *Cryptosporidium* have been associated with ice-making machines (Ravn *et al.*, 1991; Medical Services Directorate, 1993). Immunocompromised patients should not use ice from ice-making machines and where machines are in use they should be properly connected and maintained (Medical Services Directorate, 1993). Ice should not be removed by hand and vessels used to remove or store the ice should be washed with detergent and water after each use. Bottled water may contain large numbers of bacteria although probably no more than may be consumed on food. Bottled water should be stored in the refrigerator once opened and drunk within 3 days. It should not be drunk directly from the bottle as this may contaminate the water (Hunter, 1993).

Invasive Procedures

Probably the most important aspect of the care of the immunocompromised patient is rigorous attention to the care of intravenous cannulae. Nauseef and Maki (1981) suggest that a higher rate of **bacteraemia** observed when patients were isolated in a single room was related to the reduced attention to intravenous lines afforded to these patients. Total parenteral nutrition particularly increases the risk of infection associated with IV therapy. The recommended care for IV cannula and urethral catheters is outlined in Chapters 9 and 10. Fig. 4.12 illustrates a simple protective isolation policy which can be used to minimize the risk of introducing infection in an immunocompromised patient.

References

Ayliffe GAJ, Collins BJ, Lowbury EJL *et al.* (1967) Ward floors and other surfaces as reservoirs of hospital infection. *J. Hyg.* **65**: 515–36.

Ayliffe GAJ, Lilly HA (1985) Cross-infection and its prevention. *J. Hosp. Inf.* **6**(Suppl. B): 47–57.

Bodey GP, Buckley M, Sathe YS *et al.* (1966) Quantitative relationships between circulating leukocytes and infection in patients with acute leukaemia. *Ann. Int. Med.* **64**: 328–40.

Collins C, Upright C, Aleksich J. (1989) Reverse isolation: what patients perceive. *Onc. Nurs. Forum* **16**(5): 675–9.

Conry K (1982) Anergy: the hidden danger. *Heart Lung* **11**: 85.

Denton P (1986). Psychological and physiological effects of isolation. *Nursing* **3**(3): 88–91.

De Louvois J (1993) Salmonella contamination of eggs. *Lancet* **342**: 367–8.

Department of Health (1992) *Immunisation Against Infectious Disease.* HMSO, London.

Greene WC (1993) AIDS and the immune system. *Scientific American* **Sept**: 67–73.

Hunter P (1993) The microbiology of bottled natural mineral waters. *J. Appl. Bact.* **74**: 345–52.

Jones D (1990) Foodborne listeriosis. *Lancet* **336**: 1171–4.

Kinmouth AL, Fulton Y, Campbell MJ (1992) Management of feverish children at home. *Brit. Med. J.* **305**: 1134–6.

Knowles HE (1993) The experience of infectious patients in isolation. *Nursing Times* **89**(30): 53–6.

Lund BM, Knox MR, Cole MB (1989) Destruction of *Listeria monocytogenes* during microwave cooking. *Lancet* **i**: 218.

Mackowiak PA (1994) Fever: blessing or curse? A unifying hypothesis. *Ann. Int. Med.* **120**, 1037–40.

Medical Services Directorate (1993) Ice Cubes: Infection caused by *Xanthomonas maltophilia*. *Hazard* (**93**) 42.

Nauseef WM, Maki DG (1981) A study of the value of simple protective isolation in patients with granulocytopenia. *New Engl. J. Med.* **304**(8): 448–52.

Ravn P, Lundgren JD, Kjaeldgaard P *et al.* (1991) Nosocomial outbreak of cryptosporidiosis in AIDS patients. *Brit. Med. J.* **302**: 277–9.

Remington JS and Schimpff SC (1981) Please don't eat the salads. *New Engl. J. Med.* **304**: 433–5.

Rogers TR, Barnes RA (1988) Prevention of airborne fungal infection in immunocompromised patients. *J. Hosp. Inf.* **11**(Suppl. A): 15–20.

Schimpff SC (1981) Surveillance cultures. *J. Infect. Dis.* **144**: 81–4.

Schimpff SC, Young VM, Greene WH *et al.* (1972) Origin of infection in acute non-lymphocytic leukaemia: significance of hospital acquisition of potential pathogens. *Ann. Int. Med.* **77**: 707–14.

Schimff SC, Hahn DM, Brouillet MD *et al.* (1978) Comparison of basic infection prevention techniques with standard room reverse isolation or with reverse isolation plus added air filtration. *Leuk. Res.* **2**: 231–40.

Shooter RA, Cooke EM, Gaya H *et al.* (1969) Food and medicaments as possible sources of hospital strains of *Pseudomonas aeruginosa*. *Lancet* **1**: 1227–9.

Styrt B, Sugarman B. (1990) Antipyresis and fever *Arch. Int. Med.* **150**: 1589–97.

Taylor L (1980) Are face masks necessary in operating theatres and wards? *J. Hosp Inf.* **1**: 173–4.

Trexler PC, Spiers ASD, Gaya H. (1975) Plastic isolators for treatment of acute leukaemia patients under germ-free conditions. *Brit. Med. J.* **iv**: 549–52.

Further Reading

Bodey GP *et al.* (1989) Aspergillosis. *Eur. J. Clin. Micro. Inf. Dis.* **8**(5): 413–37.

Keithley J (1983) Infection and the malnourished patient. *Heart Lung* **12**: 23.

Lindgren PS (1983) The laminar air flow room – nursing practices and procedures. *Nurs. Clin. N. Am.* **18**(3): 553–61.

Mooney BR, Reeves SA, Larson E (1993) Infection control and bone marrow transplantation. *Am. J. Inf. Contr.* **21**: 131–8.

Roitt IM (1991). *Essential Immunology*, 7th edn. Blackwell Scientific, Oxford.

Scientific American (1993) September issue.

Selwyn S (1980) Protective isolation: what are our priorities? *J. Hosp. Inf.* **1**: 5–9.

Smith BJ (1983) The infection prone child – education and discipline. *Nursing Times* **July 13**: 62–4.

Weir DM, Stewart J (1993) *Immunology*. 7th edn. Churchill Livingstone, Edinburgh.

5

A Guide To Antimicrobial Chemotherapy

- **Introduction**
- **How Antibiotics Work**
- **Clinical Application of Antimicrobials**
- **Main Groups of Antibiotics**
- **Resistance to Antibiotics**
- **Antiviral Drugs**
- **Antifungal Drugs**
- **References and Further Reading**

Introduction

Effective treatment of infection involves the destruction of the invading micro-organism whilst, at the same time, not harming the cells of the host. Modern drugs used for antimicrobial chemotherapy affect characteristic features of the **procaryotic** cell which are not found in the **eucaryotic** cells of man.

The recognition of bacteria as the cause of fever and infection was soon followed by the search for substances that could destroy them. Chemicals such as carbolic acid and iodine, known to kill bacteria cultured in the laboratory, formed the basis of the antisepsis in surgery used by Lister in the late nineteenth century. Other chemicals which destroyed bacteria (e.g. mercury) were used to treat infection but invariably caused as much harm to the patient as to the microbe. Ehrlich first perceived that what was required was an agent which was selectively toxic to bacteria and he searched for such a substance amongst the azo dyes. Eventually, in the 1930s the dye prontosil was found to be a useful antimicrobial, although it was actually broken down in the body to form the effective compound, sulphonilamide. Other antimicrobial sulphonilamides were developed and widely used in the treatment of infection.

The ability to treat infections was revolutionized in the late 1930s with the discovery by Sir Alexander Fleming of the first naturally occurring antimicrobial substance. Plates of *Staphylococcus aureus* were inadvertently contaminated by a **fungus**, *Penicillium notatum*. Fleming noticed that the colonies of *Staphylococcus* close to the fungus were being lysed. He then grew the same fungus in a broth and found that the broth had marked inhibitory effect on many types of bacteria. The antibacterial substances were difficult to purify and unstable but after extensive work by Florey in the 1940s sufficient penicillin could be made for the treatment of patients. Commercial production of penicillin began during the Second World War and the search continued for new antimicrobials from a range of micro-organisms living in natural environments. In the 1940s streptomycin, chloramphenicol and tetracycline were isolated from soil organisms and cephalosporin from a fungus found in a sewage outlet. Erythromycin and rifampicin were discovered in the 1950s and gentamicin and fusidin in the 1960s, all from soil organisms.

The term **antibiotic** was used to describe these naturally occurring substances produced by one microbial species and capable of inhibiting the growth of another species. In the laboratory, small alterations to the chemical structure of naturally occurring antibiotics were found to alter the range of microbes against which the drug was effective, the absorption by the body and the duration of action. There are now over a hundred antimicrobial drugs available. Many are similar compounds but, with minor modifications, affect different species of bacteria.

Some people use the term antibiotic to refer only to the naturally occurring drugs made by bacteria or fungi, and the term antimicrobial agents to describe the whole range of antibacterial drugs now available, many of which are modifications of naturally occurring substances or are synthesized in the laboratory. Such a distinction is rather academic and for the purposes of this text the term antibiotic will be used for all drugs which are capable of destroying bacteria.

How Antibiotics Work

There are many species of bacteria and it is therefore to be expected that antibiotics affect each species differently. The effect may be **bactericidal**, that is cause the destruction of the bacterial cell; or **bacteriostatic**, that is prevent the cell replicating and enable them to be destroyed by the host's immune defences. Antibiotic activity depends on a number of different mechanisms.

Interfere With Cell Wall Synthesis

Bacteria differ from human cells in having a cell wall and this is a useful target for antibiotics. A number of different aspects of **cell wall** synthesis can be affected, for example penicillin binds to enzymes involved in making **peptidoglycan** whilst vancomycin prevents the cross-linkage process. The inhibition of cell wall synthesis causes the cells to lyse and destroy the bacteria. **Gram-negative** bacteria contain much less peptidoglycan in their cell walls and are therefore much less susceptible to penicillin than the **Gram-positive** bacteria.

Interfere With Protein Synthesis

Several antibiotics exert their effect by binding to bacterial **ribosomes** and are selective because they are unable to bind on to the much larger eucaryotic cell ribosomes. Protein synthesis either occurs abnormally or is completely prevented. Some substances do not bind permanently to the ribosome and their action is therefore bacteriostatic (e.g. tetracycline, chloramphenicol).

Inhibition of Nucleic Acid Synthesis

Nucleic acid synthesis can be affected in numerous ways. The sulphonamides and trimethoprim prevent the synthesis of folic acid, an important component in the production of **nucleotides**. Human cells also use folic acid but because they do not synthesize it but depend on a dietary source, they are not affected by these antibiotics. Bacteria which are able to use preformed folic acid are also resistant to these antibiotics.

Metronidazole inhibits an **enzyme** involved in nucleic acid production and rifampicin inhibits transcription of **DNA** into **RNA**.

Disruption of the Cell Membrane

Antibiotics such as amphotericin and nystatin disrupt membranes which contain cholesterol and cause the cell to lyse. Fungal cell membranes are particularly rich in cholesterol but because human cell membranes also contain some cholesterol many of these agents are toxic and can only be used topically.

Clinical Application of Anti-microbials

Considerable skill and knowledge is necessary to make the best use of the wide range of antibiotics that are available. In the UK, advice on antibiotic therapy is provided by a medical microbiologist, who is a doctor with a specialist knowledge and training in microbiology. Although the nurse is not responsible for the prescription of antimicrobial therapy, he/she does have an important role to play in administering and monitoring the drugs prescribed and discussing the treatment with the doctor when therapy seems unnecessary or unsuccessful.

These are some of the characteristics of antibiotics which need to be taken into account when choosing an antibiotic to treat an infection.

Spectrum

The term spectrum is used to describe the range of organisms against which an antibiotic is effective. Some antibiotics kill only a few different bacteria (e.g. only Gram-positive bacteria) and are said to have a narrow spectrum of activity. Penicillin is a narrow-spectrum antibiotic since it acts mainly on Gram-positive bacteria, the aminoglycosides are also narrow-spectrum because they are active mainly against Gram-negative bacteria, whilst metronidazole destroys only **anaerobic** bacteria and some **protozoa**.

Tetracycline, ampicillin and the modern cephalosporins are broad-spectrum antibiotics; that is, they are effective against a wide range of Gram-negative and Gram-positive bacteria. Broad-spectrum antibiotics are useful where the cause of the infection is unknown and action against a wide variety of organisms may be necessary. Unfortunately, they will also kill bacteria which make up the **normal flora** of the body as well as the infecting organism and other bacteria or fungi may multiply in the absence of this normal competition. This effect is called *superinfection*. *Clostridium difficile* is an organism which multiplies in the gut if other normal gut flora are destroyed by antibiotics. It causes a potentially serious, and sometimes life threatening, bowel infection called **pseudo-membranous colitis** (see Chapter 3).

Broad-spectrum antibiotics may also encourage the survival and multiplication of **strains** of bacteria that are resistant to antibiotics. When the cause of the infection is known, it is preferable to use an antibiotic that will destroy the **pathogen** only.

Combination of Antibiotics

Sometimes it is preferable to treat an infection with a combination of antibiotics, particularly where the cause of the infection is unknown. Some antibiotics (e.g. rifampicin) encourage the rapid emergence of strains resistant to the antibiotic and should be used with another drug to destroy resistant organisms. Some drug combinations enhance each other's activity (e.g. penicillin and gentamicin), others interfere with each other's activity (e.g. penicillin and tetracycline) or encourage the development of resistant strains (e.g. ampicillin and cloxacillin) (Shanson, 1989).

Pharmaco-dynamics

Pharmacodynamics of a drug relate to what happens to it in the body, whether it is absorbed from the intestine, how long it remains in the blood, what organs or tissues it reaches and how it is excreted. The distribution of an antibiotic through the body depends on how much it adheres to proteins, its solubility in lipids and whether it can pass through cell membranes. Chloramphenicol, which is highly lipid soluble, will spread widely, whereas gentamicin which is not very lipid soluble, tends to remain in the blood and in the fluid around cells. Most antibiotics do not readily pass through the blood–brain barrier, and although they may reach a higher concentration in the brain when the meninges are inflamed, many cannot be used to treat meningitis successfully.

Antibiotics that are not absorbed from the gut are given parenterally. Others are not absorbed properly if given before food as they are destroyed by gastric acid.

Antibiotics are eliminated from the body at different rates. Those that are eliminated fairly rapidly must be given in frequent doses, whilst others that are excreted slowly can be administered twice a day.

Duration of Therapy

Antibiotics should be given for long enough to ensure complete eradication of the bacteria, but not for too long since this may encourage the development of resistant strains. Usually treatment should be given for 7 days, but for serious or **systemic infection** prolonged therapy may be necessary.

Prophylaxis

Antibiotics can be used to prevent infection occurring. There are two situations in which prophylaxis is commonly used; at the time of an invasive procedure such as surgery or for intimate contacts of someone who has developed an infectious disease (e.g. meningococcal meningitis). The prophylactic antibiotic selected should be effective against the bacteria most likely to cause infection. For example, surgery on the large intestine will be most at risk from infection caused by **aerobic** coliforms and anaerobes of the gut flora. Prophylactic treatment should therefore include metronidazole to kill the anaerobes and gentamicin or a cephalosporin to kill the Gram-negative aerobes.

Antibiotic Policy

In some hospitals in the UK, the consultant medical microbiologist and pharmacy department have developed an antibiotic policy to discourage the indiscriminate use of antibiotics, minimize the development of antibiotic-resistant strains and reduce the costs of antibiotic prescribing. The policy provides guidelines on the use of a range of antibiotics and limits others unless advised by the microbiologist or infectious disease consultant.

Main Groups of Antibiotics
Penicillins

The penicillins cause bacterial cells to break apart by interfering with cell wall synthesis. The original, naturally occurring penicillins (e.g. benzyl-penicillin, penicillin V) have a narrow spectrum of activity and are mainly active against Gram-positive bacteria (e.g. streptococci). However, a large number of different penicillin antibiotics have been synthesized, which have the same basic β-lactam ring structure but, by modification of the side-chain molecules, are able to affect a wider range of bacterial species (see Fig. 5.1). Alterations to the side-chains can also influence the pharmacology of the drugs, for example benzylpenicillin is destroyed by gastric acid and so must be given intravenously whilst ampicillin is acid-stable and can therefore be given orally (see Table 5.1).

Penicillins are very useful antibiotics; they can infiltrate most sites of infection and they are usually used for initial treatment of infection until sensitivity testing indicates that an alternative drug is necessary. The penicillins are virtually non-toxic and can therefore be given in very high doses. Their main adverse effect is a **hypersensitivity** reaction which can range from minor rashes to severe **anaphylaxis**.

Resistance to penicillin was reported within a few years of its introduction and in certain species is widespread. For example, 90% of *Staphylococcus aureus* isolated in hospitals are resistant to penicillin. Resistant bacteria produce an enzyme, penicillinase (β-lactamase), which breaks open the β-lactam ring and destroys the activity of the antibiotic. Pharmaceutical manufacturers are constantly searching for side-chain modifications which prevent attack by β-lactamases. Flucloxacillin, a β-lactamase resistant antibiotic, was introduced in the 1960s and is the treatment of choice for many *S. aureus* infections.

Fig. 5.1
The structure of penicillin.

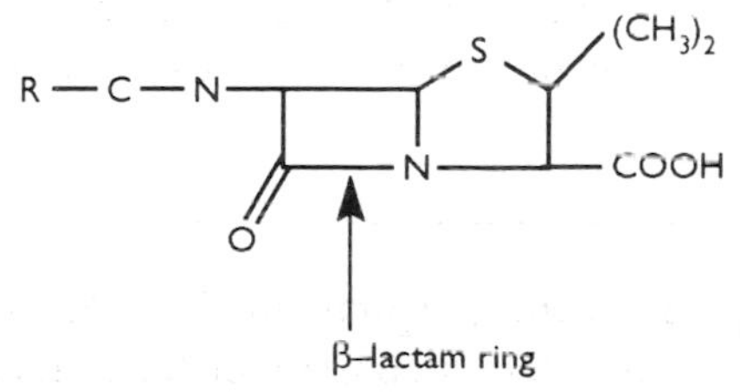

β-lactam ring

Table 5.1
Penicillins

Antibiotic	Spectrum of activity and principal uses
Natural penicillins	
Benzylpenicillin (Penicillin G)	Effective against Gram-positive bacteria and *Neisseria*. Used to treat a wide variety of infections by IM or IV route
Penicillin V	Same spectrum of activity as benzylpenicillin but used to treat mild tissue infections. Administered orally
Broad-spectrum penicillins	
Ampicillin	Effective against Gram-positive bacteria
Amoxycillin	*H. influenzae*, *Strep. faecalis*. Used to treat urinary and respiratory infections and some serious infections in combination with other drugs
Augmentin	A combination of amoxycillin and clavulanic acid. The clavulanic acid binds with penicillinases. Used for urinary tract, respiratory or soft tissue infections resistant to amoxycillin
Penicillinase-resistant penicillins	
Flucloxacillin	Same spectrum of activity as penicillin G and V, but also active against penicillinase producers such as *S. aureus*. Mainly used to treat staphylococcal infection
Methicillin	Methicillin is not used clinically
Anti-pseudomonal penicillins	
Mezlocillin Piperacillin Azlocillin	Derivatives of benzylpenicillin. Active against a range of Gram-negative and anaerobic bacteria. Used to treat urinary, respiratory and burns infections, especially those caused by *Pseudomonas aeruginosa*

Cephalosporins

The cephalosporins have a similar chemical structure to the penicillins, having a β-lactam ring, an additional side ring and different side–chains. They also cause bacterial cells to break open by interfering with cell wall synthesis.

Cephalosporins kill a wider range of bacteria and are less susceptible to β-lactamases than the penicillins, although some bacteria do produce cephalosporinase enzymes which break the β-lactam ring. The cephalosporins have been considerably modified since they were first introduced in the 1960s and are usually grouped according to their decade of development (see Table 5.2). The first generation cephalosporins were produced in the 1960s and many are still used today. The second generation cephalosporins are more potent and are active against a wider range of bacteria. They are used for prophylaxis in major surgery and in the treatment of penicillin-resistant strains of bacteria such as Gonococcus and Haemophilus. The third generation cephalosporins, introduced in the early 1980s, have greater effectivity against Gram-negative bacteria, but they are expensive and subject to widespread misuse in situations where a cheaper, narrower spectrum antibiotic would be more appropriate.

The main side-effect of cephalosporins is **hypersensitivity**. Twenty per cent of penicillin-allergic patients will have some cephalosporin allergy as well.

Table 5.2
Cephalosporins

Antibiotic	Spectrum of activity and principal uses
First generation Cephazolin Cephalexin Cefaclor	Active against a wide range of Gram-positive and -negative bacteria (although not *Ps. aeruginosa, Strep. faccalis, H. influenzae*) Not usually used as first choice of treatment for serious infections
Second generation Cefuroxime Cefamandole	Active against a wide range of Gram-positive and -negative bacteria (including *H. influenzae*) and resistant to action of β-lactamases. Used to treat severe systemic infection and for prophylaxis against infection
Third generation Cefotaxime Ceftazidime Cefsulodin	Similar spectrum of activity to 2nd generation cephalosporins but also active against *Ps. aeruginosa*. Used to treat serious sepsis, but prone to encourage superinfection by resistant organisms

Other β-Lactams

There are a variety of antibiotics that have a β-lactam ring as part of their structure. One group, the monobactams (e.g. Imipenem) are particularly useful as they are very potent and effective against a range of Gram-positive and Gram-negative bacteria.

Aminoglycosides

The aminoglycoside group of antibiotics interfere with protein synthesis by binding to bacterial ribosomes and preventing accurate reading of the **messenger RNA**. They are active against many Gram-negative, aerobic bacteria and some Gram-positive bacteria. They are often used in combination with another antibiotic to provide activity against a broad range of organisms. Aminoglycosides are not absorbed from the gut and so must be administered parenterally. The concentration of aminoglycosides in the blood must be closely monitored as they tend to accumulate in the tissues where they can cause damage, particularly the kidney and ear. Some bacteria acquire resistance to aminoglycosides by producing enzymes which can modify the molecule.

The main aminoglycoside antibiotics are illustrated in Table 5.3.

Table 5.3
Aminoglycosides

Antibiotic	Spectrum of activity and principal uses
Gentamicin Tobramycin Amikacin	Broad spectrum of activity against a range of Gram-negative and Gram-positive bacilli. Potent antibiotics used to treat serious infection, especially Gram-negatives. Must be given IM or IV. Blood levels should be checked regularly to avoid ototoxicity or nephrotoxicity
Neomycin	Only for topical use, toxic if absorbed. Used to treat otitis externa
Streptomycin	Used to be used more widely but largely replaced by gentamicin. Important drug for treatment of tuberculosis in combination with other drugs

Tetracyclines

The name tetracyclines is derived from their structure of four rings fused together. They bind to bacterial ribosomes and block protein synthesis by preventing **transfer RNA** attaching to **messenger RNA**. The attachment to the ribosomes is reversible and their effect is therefore bacteriostatic rather than bactericidal. Tetracyclines also inhibit protein synthesis in human cells to some extent and this may account for their main side-effects; gastrointestinal upset, staining of teeth and bone development in children.

Tetracyclines are effective against a broad range of Gram-positive and Gram-negative bacteria and are useful for unusual infections such as brucellosis and *Chlamydia*. They should not be given intramuscularly as this causes considerable pain.

Bacteria that acquire resistance to tetracycline are able to prevent the drug entering the cell. Tetracyclines have decreased in use because of the incidence of resistant bacteria and the availability of more effective broad-spectrum antibiotics.

Erythromycin

Erythromycin inhibits bacterial protein synthesis by binding to the ribosome. It is bacteriostatic as the attachment to the ribosome is reversible. It has broad activity against Gram-positive and Gram-negative bacteria and is one of the safest antibiotics available. Side-effects of gastrointestinal upset occur rarely. It is commonly prescribed for patients who are allergic to penicillin.

Quinolones

Ciprofloxacin and norfloxacin are derivatives of a bactericidal antibiotic, naladixic acid. Naladixic acid is excreted in high levels in the urine and active against most Gram-negative pathogens of the urinary tract but resistance to it develops very rapidly. The quinolones are also highly effective against Gram-positive bacteria. These antibiotics interfere with DNA replication by preventing the two strands unwinding prior to **transcription** and should not be given to pregnant women and children.

Chloramphenicol

Chloramphenicol prevents protein synthesis by binding to bacterial ribosomes. It is active against a wide range of bacteria including unusual ones such as *Rickettsia*, spirochaetes, *Chlamydia* and *Mycoplasma*. Its most important side effect is bone marrow suppression and on rare occasions can cause aplastic anaemia. It is therefore not used systemically except for

Table 5.4
Other antibiotics

Antibiotic	Spectrum of activity and principal uses
Erythromycin	Effective against a similar range of bacteria as penicillin but also some others e.g. *H. influenzae, Listeria pneumophilia, Chlamydia*. Used for respiratory infections (including whooping cough and legionella), non-specific urethritis and instead of penicillin for patients who are penicillin-allergic
Tetracycline	Effective against a wide range of both Gram-positive and -negative bacteria, although some are now commonly resistant. Used to treat exacerbations of chronic bronchitis, atypical pneumonia and non-specific urethritis
Naladixic acid	Effective against Gram-negative bacteria but not *Ps. aeruginosa*. Prone to resistance and only used to treat urinary tract infection.
Ciprofloxacin	Much wider range activity against Gram-positive and Gram-negative bacteria, including *Ps. aeruginosa*, but not anaerobes
Norfloxacin	Used to treat infection due to *Ps. aeruginosa*, chronic urinary tract infection and enteric infection
Chloramphenicol	Has potent, broad-spectrum activity but association with aplastic anaemia has restricted its use. Used to treat meningitis, typhoid fever. Eye infections (topically)
Sulphonomides	Although they work slowly, are active against a wide range of Gram-positive and -negative bacteria. Resistance develops readily and now rarely used on their own, except for urinary tract infection
Trimethoprim	Active against most common pathogens, resistance frequently reported. Used for urinary and respiratory tract infection
Cotrimoxizole	Combination of sulphamethoxazole and trimethoprim. Active against both Gram-positive and -negative bacteria. Widely used for urinary and respimtory infection
Metronidazole	Active only against anaerobic bacteria and protozoa e.g. *Giardia, Entamoeba*. Used to treat any anaerobic infection e.g. abdominal, gynaecological wound infection, abscesses, peritoneal infection and as prophylaxis for colonic surgery. Can be administered orally, IV and rectally
Vancomycin	Effective against staphylococci, streptococci and *Clostridia*. Used to treat serious infection e.g. endocarditis, septicaemia, especially *S. epidermidis* and MRSA. Given orally for pseudomembranous colitis. Blood levels should be monitored because of oto- and nephrotoxicity
Rifampicin	Mostly used for the treatment of tuberculosis and as prophylaxis for meningococcal meningitis. Turns urine, sputum and tears red during therapy

life-threatening infections. It can be used safely as a topical preparation for eye infections.

Sulphonamides

The sulphonamides were the first antimicrobials found to be effective against bacteria whilst not harming the patient. Introduced in the 1930s, they are still available today although resistance and toxicity now restrict their use. The sulphonamides prevent the synthesis of folic acid, an essential ingredient for the production of nucleic acids.

Trimethoprim

Trimethoprim also affects folic acid synthesis and, as it enhances the activity of sulphonamides, is often used in the combined form of cotrimoxazole. Cotrimoxazole is a useful treatment for urinary tract infection as the drug is excreted in the urine.

Metronidazole

Metronidazole was originally introduced as a drug for protozoal infections such as *Trichomonas* and *Giardia*. These are anaerobes and depend on specialized enzymes for energy production; these enzymes convert the drug into toxic substances which then destroy the cell. Anaerobic bacteria use the same enzymes and metronidazole has now become the main treatment for anaerobic bacterial infections.

Metronidazole is distributed throughout the tissues and adverse reactions and resistance are rare.

Glycopeptides

Vancomycin and teicoplanin are large glycopeptide molecules which interfere with cell wall synthesis and affect the permeability of the cell membrane. Vancomycin is effective against Gram-positive but not Gram-negative bacteria. It is used to treat infections caused by strains of *S. aureus* resistant to flucloxacillin (**MRSA**), infections caused by *S. epidermidis* which is naturally resistant to penicillin antibiotics, and pseudomembranous colitis caused by *Clostridium difficile*. Resistance to vancomycin is so far very rare. Although the modern, purified drug has fewer side-effects, vancomycin can cause damage to the kidney and ears. Levels in the blood should be closely monitored and it should be administered in a slow intravenous infusion.

Teicoplanin has greater activity against Gram-positive bacteria, is less toxic, and can be given by intramuscular injection.

Antituberculosis Therapy

Tuberculosis is a difficult infection to treat because the mycobacteria may be multiplying in cavities in the lungs and be dormant in closed cavities and macrophages. A combination of antibiotics must be used to kill both multiplying and intracellular mycobacteria and to prevent resistant bacteria emerging. The main drugs used are isoniazid, rifampicin, ethambutol and pyrazinamide. Prolonged therapy is given, three drugs together for the first 8–10 weeks, followed by two drugs for about 4 months.

The prolonged nature of therapy affects compliance with the treatment regime. Recently, shorter courses of therapy, with doses given once or twice a week under supervision, have been developed to address these problems. The emergence of resistance is encouraged by incomplete courses of treatment. Although resistance to antituberculous drugs is very rare in the UK, rates as high as 30% resistance to one or more drugs has been reported in other parts of the world (Uttley and Pozniak, 1993).

Patients with acquired immune deficiency syndrome are particularly susceptible to an atypical mycobacterium, *Mycobacterium avium-intracellulare*. These bacteria are usually highly resistant to antituberculosis drugs and treatment of the infection can be extremely difficult (Lewis, 1989).

Resistance To Antibiotics

Micro-organisms are not all intrinsically sensitive to all antibiotics. The terms sensitive and resistant to antibiotics are used to distinguish between those antibiotics which will or will not destroy a micro-organism. A bacteria is *sensitive* to a particular antibiotic if its growth is inhibited or it is killed by a concentration of the drug which could be achieved by the usual dose regimen. *Resistant* bacteria are not inhibited or killed by this concentration of the drug.

Bacteria may have a *natural resistance* to certain antibiotics because the drug cannot penetrate their cells or because they do not possess the protein to which the drug attaches. Some bacteria are naturally resistant to several commonly prescribed antibiotics (e.g. *Pseudomonas aeruginosa, S. epidermidis*.

Resistance by selection occurs when one or two cells in a population of bacteria are naturally resistant to the antibiotic. These cells are able to survive and multiply and eventually the sensitive cells are replaced by resistant ones. This type of resistance develops rapidly when sulphonamides are used and is also a problem with antituberculosis drugs.

Previously sensitive bacteria can *acquire resistance* to antibiotics for one of three reasons:

- the permeability of the cell membrane changes so that the drug cannot enter the cell (e.g. resistance to tetracycline)
- the site with which the drug reacts is altered and the drug is unable to affect the cell (e.g. resistance to trimethoprim)
- the bacteria produces enzymes that inactivate the antibiotic (e.g. β-lactamases which destroy penicillins, cephalosporins)

Acquired resistance to antibiotics has been evident since antibiotics were first widely used. It occurs by the transfer of genetic information between bacterial cells and even between different bacterial species. These 'resistance' genes are often carried on **plasmids**, circular pieces

Table 5.5
Practices that encourage the development of antibiotic resistant micro-organisms

- Inappropriate use of antibiotics
- Use of antibiotics in animal feeds
- Uncontrolled sale of antibiotics without prescription
- Indiscriminate use of antibiotics (especially broad-spectrum)

of DNA independent of the **chromosome**, which can be replicated and transferred into another bacterium. *Multiple drug resistance* is a term used to describe bacteria that have developed resistance to several, unrelated antibiotics, for example Gram-negative bacilli that are resistant to both streptomycin and the sulphonamides. These multiresistant bacteria often have one plasmid that carries several genes conferring resistance to several antibiotics.

Preventing the emergence of drug resistance depends on controlling the indiscriminate use of antibiotics (see Table 5.5) and can be detected by surveillance of laboratory results (WHO, 1983). In the UK, antibiotic use is fairly well controlled and drugs cannot be obtained without a prescription. This is not the case in other parts of the world and antibiotic-resistant strains are often prevalent in those areas. Patients from countries without reasonable controls on antibiotic consumption are more likely to be infected or colonized by antibiotic-resistant bacteria.

Clinical Problems Associated with Antibiotic-Resistant Bacteria

Resistance is a problem because it limits the choice of antibiotics that can be used to treat infection and can mean that a more toxic or expensive drug must be used instead. This is a particular problem in hospitals, where antibiotic treatment is used frequently. Resistant organisms often emerge and spread by cross-infection through lapses in infection control procedures such as handwashing.

The microbiology laboratory routinely test **pathogenic** bacteria isolated from specimens for their sensitivity to a range of antibiotics. This provides the clinician with useful information about which drugs could be effectively used against the infection. The medical microbiologist provides expert advice about the best drug to use.

Most pathogenic bacteria are not sensitive to all antibiotics. The laboratory looks out for bacteria that are resistant to more antibiotics than usual and would be particularly concerned if they were resistant to the drug normally used to kill them. For example, *Pseudomonas aeruginosa* is naturally resistant to many antibiotics and infections would normally be treated with an aminoglycoside such as gentamicin. A *Ps. aeruginosa* resistant to gentamicin is unusual and could make treatment difficult. Other antibiotics would be tested to find one to which it is sensitive and the patient isolated to prevent the spread of the organism to other patients.

The most common examples of unusually resistant bacteria encountered in hospitals are methicillin-resistant *Staphylococcus aureus* (MRSA), *Enterococcus* and various Gram-negative bacilli (e.g. *Klebsiella*, *Serratia*, *Acinetobacter*, *Pseudomonas* and *Enterobacter*), which can cause serious outbreaks of infection. The intensive care unit provides a particularly fertile ground for the emergence of resistant strains; the usage of antibiotics is high, the patients have many skin sites susceptible to **colonization** and they may have a compromised immune system. Such patients are susceptible to infection by **opportunistic pathogens** that may be highly resistant to antibiotics, and which may then spread easily to other patients on equipment and the hands of staff (Casewell and Desai, 1983; Wade *et al.*, 1991).

Methicillin-resistant *Staphylococcus aureus* (MRSA)

Staphylococci have a remarkable capacity to adapt to the presence of antibiotics in their environment by developing resistance (see Table 5.6). β-Lactamase producing strains of *S. aureus*, resistant to penicillin appeared very soon after the antibiotic came into use. Now approximately 90% of strains in hospitals and about 50% of strains in the community are resistant to penicillin.

Modifications to the β-lactam ring were made to prevent attack by β-lactamases and in 1960 methicillin, a penicillin resistant to β-lactamases, was introduced. It could only be administered **parenterally** and was therefore replaced by flucloxacillin, which could also be given orally. Flucloxacillin soon became established as the drug of choice for the treatment of staphylococcal infection, since resistance to other penicillins was widespread. Methicillin is now only used in the laboratory for sensitivity testing.

Soon after the introduction of methicillin, resistant strains of *S. aureus* (MRSA) were reported. The incidence of MRSA increased until the 1970s and caused many serious outbreaks of infection in hospitals. During the 1970s outbreaks of MRSA diminished but unfortunately, this was not the end of the problem; in the early 1980s, the third generation cephalosporins and new penicillin derivatives were introduced and

Table 5.6
The development of antibiotic resistance in Staphylococcus aureus

1960	Methicillin introduced
1961	Methicillin-resistant *S. aureus* first reported
1970	5% of *S. aureus* isolates methicillin-resistant
1976	*S. aureus* resistant to gentamicin and methicillin reported
1980	New penicillins and cephalosporins introduced. Epidemic strain of MRSA reported in London
	Incidence of MRSA increases
1990	MRSA affecting most parts of the UK. Many different strains identified

this coincided with increased reports of MRSA. Epidemics of MRSA first occurred in London in the mid-1980s. Sporadic outbreaks of MRSA have continued to be reported throughout the country and several distinct strains have been identified (Marples and Reith, 1992). MRSA occurs worldwide and the importation of strains of MRSA from other countries remains a problem.

Virulence

S. aureus causes a variety of infections ranging from mild infection of the skin, boils and abscesses, to serious systemic infection, **septicaemia**, **pneumonia** and major wound infection. *S. aureus* also accounts for about one-third of all wound infections (Meers *et al.*, 1981). MRSA causes the same type of infection as sensitive strains of *S. aureus* and most studies suggest that it has equal pathogenicity (French *et al.*, 1990). In addition to causing infection, *S. aureus* is a part of the normal flora of the skin, especially in axillae, groins, perineum and nose. Some people are heavily colonized with *S. aureus* and areas of damaged skin are especially prone to colonization (e.g. wounds, cannula sites). MRSA may replace sensitive strains of *S. aureus* on the skin, which it will colonize without causing infection but provide a reservoir from which it may spread to other patients or staff (Muder *et al.*, 1991).

MRSA is usually found in hospitals where extensive use of antibiotics encourages the survival of bacteria that are resistant to antibiotics, such as MRSA. Patients discharged into the community may lose the strain as resistance to antibiotics is of no advantage in the home environment.

Treatment of Infections

Strains of *S. aureus* resistant to methicillin are also resistant to many other antibiotics and treatment of serious infection with MRSA presents particular problems. Usually the only drug that the organism is reliably sensitive to is vancomycin, which is expensive and potentially toxic.

Treatment of Colonization

Colonized patients provide a reservoir from which resistant bacteria can be spread to other patients. *S. aureus* can be removed from colonized sites by topical treatment with antistaphylococcal solutions and creams. The most effective of these is mupirocin applied to skin lesions or to the nose, for 1 week, three times a day and this is usually sufficient to eliminate MRSA. Unfortunately, resistance to mupirocin has already been reported although, so far, infrequently (Cookson, 1990). Antiseptic skin disinfectant solutions (e.g. Chlorhexidine handwash) also remove *S. aureus* and daily washing with these solutions will help to remove MRSA from colonized skin.

Spread

Although many strains of MRSA do not spread from person to person easily, a number of strains do have a particular propensity to transmit and are often referred to as **epidemic** strains. It is not unusual for such epidemic strains of MRSA to colonize and infect several patients on one ward and may spread throughout a hospital if left unchecked. The more patients that are colonized with MRSA, the greater the chance of serious infection occurring among them which may be extremely difficult to treat.

MRSA is spread in the same way as sensitive strains of *S. aureus*. The most important route of transmission is on the hands of staff who acquire the organism through direct contact with infected or colonized skin and if **carriage** is not removed by handwashing, will deposit it on patients (Mortimer *et al.*, 1966). Heavily contaminated uniforms, equipment or surfaces could potentially transmit infection. Airborne spread is theoretically possible and commonly cited but there is little direct evidence that it occurs (Boyce, 1991; Haley, 1991). It is probably not a significant route of transmission unless patients are shedding excessive amounts of skin scales or the standard of cleaning is very low.

Colonization of Staff

Staff may acquire MRSA in the nose and on skin, particularly if damaged and, once colonized, may contribute to the spread of the organism. However, the probability of staff becoming colonized is low and usually related to the extent of contact with infected or colonized patients. More importantly, carriage is usually transient and the organism will generally disappear after a few hours (Cookson *et al.*, 1989). None the less, the screening of staff for MRSA colonization during outbreaks may be necessary to help control the spread. Colonized staff may require treatment to eliminate the organism and this is usually arranged by the occupational health department.

Controlling the Spread of MRSA

A variety of measures are recommended to prevent the spread of MRSA (Hospital Infection Society, 1990; Keane *et al.*, 1991). A simple and practical approach to the problem is summarized in Table 5.7. The key to successful control is good isolation techniques, especially rigorous attention to handwashing by all members of staff who have contact with the **infected** or colonized patient. The aim should be to treat the infection or colonization as rapidly as possible and ensure the patient's period of isolation is kept to a minimum.

Table 5.7
The control of methicillin resistant Staphylococcus aureus *(MRSA)*

Recommended practice	Rationale
Isolation of infected/ colonized patients	To help prevent the spread to other patients. Standard isolation until approximately 3 sets of screening swabs do not grow MRSA.
Isolation of several infected patients in one room or bay	One or two nurses responsible for the care of the patients can help to ensure compliance with isolation precautions and prevent spread.
Treatment of infected/ colonized patients	7 days of antistaphylococcal cream applied to lesions, antiseptic soap solution used to wash skin and hair will usually remove MRSA. Swabs to check if treatment successful should not be taken until 24 h after last application. 3 sets of swabs are required to confirm eradication
Discharge home of infected/colonized patients	Antibiotic-resistant strains are often lost outside hospital. Removes from contact with vulnerable patients
Labelling medical notes of previously infected/colonized patients	Some patients will continue to carry MRSA for prolonged periods, particularly in chronic wounds. Indicating previous colonization on the front of the medical notes enables early detection and prompt isolation of these patients
Screening patient contacts	Other patients who have contact with an infected or colonized patient may need to have nose and skin lesions swabbed for MRSA, especially if transferred to other wards
Screening staff contacts	If there is evidence of spread of MRSA, staff who have had direct contact with infected or colonized patients may need to have nose and skin lesions swabbed for MRSA
Ward closure	If several patients on one ward are found to be infected/colonized with MRSA or if MRSA has spread extensively on a ward or unit, particularly if the ability to isolate patients effectively is compromised. Closure of part or all of the ward may be recommended
Screening patients transferred from other hospitals	Patients admitted from other hospitals in the UK or abroad may be colonized with MRSA. Early detection can enable prompt isolation and treatment

The infection control team will co-ordinate the management of outbreaks of MRSA among hospital patients and will work closely with the occupational health department to monitor and treat colonized staff.

Antiviral Drugs

Conventional antibiotics are not effective against **viruses** because the virus has none of the structures, such as cell walls or ribosomes, against which antibiotics are active. Viral infections are difficult to treat because the virus invades the cell and antiviral agents must enter the cell and destroy the virus without harming the host cell. Many viral infections are relatively mild and resolve spontaneously after a few days. Treatment is therefore confined to the control of symptoms during the acute phase of the illness.

Recently, antiviral compounds that interfere with viral replication and are mostly active against Herpes viruses have been developed. The most important of these is acyclovir, which is used to treat systemic Herpes infection (e.g. **encephalitis**). A close relative of acyclovir, gancyclovir is much more active against cytomegalovirus but is also more toxic and is only used for life-threatening infection. Zidovudine inhibits the activity of an enzyme called **reverse transcriptase** which is essential for the replication of retroviruses. It slows the replication of the human immunodeficiency virus, the cause of AIDS, although it is also associated with toxic side-effects.

Antifungal Drugs

Fungi may cause a variety of infections ranging from superficial infections of the skin, nails, hair or mucous membranes (e.g. thrush) to serious systemic infection, which may be fatal, usually associated with **immunosuppression** (e.g. aspergillosis). Since fungi are eucaryotic cells, conventional antibiotics have no effect on them and special antifungal agents must be used. These agents are associated with considerable toxicity as they affect human cells as well as the fungi. Superficial infections are therefore treated topically to avoid the toxic side-effects. Nystatin and clotrimazole are used to treat *Candida* infections. The latter belongs to a large group of antifungals called imadazoles which inhibit the production of sterols in fungal cell membranes. Griseofulvin produced by a species of *Penicillium* is concentrated in the skin and widely used to treat chronic fungal infections of the skin and nails. Amphotericin is active against most fungi and yeasts and, although highly toxic, is the most important drug for systemic use. Its side-effects range from pyrexia to severe malaise and renal damage (White, 1991).

References

Boyce JM (1991) Should we vigorously try to contain and control methicillin resistant *Staphylococcus aureus*? *Inf. Control Hosp. Epid.* **12**: 46–54.

Casewell MW, Desai N (1983) Survival of multiply-resistant *Klebsiella aerogenes* and other Gram-negative bacilli on finger-tips. *J. Hosp. Inf.* **18**(Suppl. B): 23–8.

Cookson BD. (1990) Mupirocin resistance in staphylococci *J. Antimicro. Chemo.* **25**: 497–503.

Cookson BD, Peters B, Webster M *et al.* (1989) Staff carriage of epidemic methicillin resistant *Staphylococcus aureus. J. Clin. Micro.* **27**(7): 1471–6.

French GL, Cheng AFB, Ling JML *et al.* (1990). Hong Kong strains of methicillin-resistant and sensitive *Staphylococcus aureus* have similar virulence. *J. Hosp. Inf.* **15**(2): 117–26.

Haley RW (1991) Methicillin resistant *Staphylococcus aureus* do we just have to live with it? *Ann. Int. Med.* **114**(2): 162–4.

Hospital Infection Society (1990). *Revised Guidelines for the Control of Epidemic Methicillin-resistant* Staphylococcus aureus. Working Party Report. *J. Hosp. Inf.* **16**: 351–77.

Keane CT, Coleman DC, Caffertey MT. (1991) Methicillin-resistant *Staphylococcus aureus* – a reappraisal. *J. Hosp. Inf.* **19**: 147–52.

Lewis MJ. (1989) Mycobacterial disease. In *Antimicrobial Chemotherapy* (D Greenwood, Ed.), pp. 279–88 Oxford Medical Publications, Oxford.

Livornese LL, Dias S, Samel C *et al.* (1992) Hospital-acquired infection with Vancomycin-resistant *Enterococcus faecium* transmitted by electronic thermometers. *Ann. Int. Med.* **117**: 112–26.

Marples RR, Reith S (1992). Methicillin-resistant *Staphylococcus aureus* in England and Wales. *CDR* **2** (Review 3): R25–9.

Meers PD, Ayliffe GAJ, Emmerson AM *et al.* (1981) Report of the national survey of infection in hospitals – 1980. *J. Hosp. Inf.* **2**(Suppl.): 1–53.

Mortimer EA, Wolinsky E, Gonzaga AJ *et al.* (1966) Role of airborne transmission in staphylococcal infections *Brit. Med. J.* **1**: 319–22.

Muder RR, Bennan C, Wagner MN *et al* (1991). Methicillin-resistant staphylococcal infection colonisation and infection in a long-term care facility. *Ann. Int. Med.* **114**: 107–12.

Shanson DC (1989) *Microbiology in Clinical Practice*, 2nd edn. Wright, Bristol.

Uttley AHC, Pozniak A (1993) Resurgence of tuberculosis. *J. Hosp. Inf.* **23**(4): 249–54.

Wade JJ, Desai N, Casewell MW (1991) Hygienic hand disinfection for the removal of epidemic vancomycin-resistant *Enterococcus faecium* and gentamicin-resistant *Enterobacter cloacae. J. Hosp. Inf.* **18**: 211–18.

White G (1991) Management of fungal infections *Nurs. Stand.* **6**(9): 38–40.

World Health Organization (1983) Control of antibiotic resistant bacteria. *Bull WHO* **61**: 423–33.

Further Reading

Ayliffe GAJ, Lowbury EJL, Geddes AM, Williams JD. (1992) *Control of Hospital Infection, A Practical Handbook*, 3rd edn. Chapman & Hall, London.

Brown EH, Spencer RC, Brown JMC (1990) The emergence of bacterial resistance in hospitals – a need for continuous surveillance. *J. Hosp. Inf.* **15**(Suppl. A): 35–9.

Burgen ASV, Mitchell JF (1986) *Gaddums Pharmacology*, 9th edn. Oxford University Press, Oxford.

Finch RG (1989) Viral infections. In *Antimicrobial Chemotherapy.* (D Greenwood, Ed.), pp. 302–9 Oxford Medical Publications, Oxford.

Greenwood D (Ed.) (1989) *Antimicrobial Chemotherapy.* Oxford Medical Publications, Oxford.

Marples RR (1988). Methicillin-resistant *Staphylococcus aureus. Curr. Opin. Inf. Dis.* **1**: 722–6.

Rose NR, Barron AL (Eds) (1983) *Microbiology – Basic Principles and Clinical Applications.* Macmillan, New York.

Sleigh JD, Timbury MC (1990) *Medical Bacteriology,* 3rd edn. Churchill Livingstone, Edinburgh.

Stucke VA. (1993) *Microbiology for Nurses – Applications to Patient Care,* 7th edn. Baillière Tindall, London.

Walters J (1988) How antibiotics work. *Prof. Nurse* **3**(7): 251–4.

Walters J (1989) How antibiotics work: the cell membrane. *Prof. Nurse* **4**(10): 508–10.

Walters J (1990) How antibiotics work. nucleic acid synthesis. *Prof. Nurse* **5**(12): 641–3.

Wood MJ, Geddes AM (1987) Antiviral therapy. *Lancet* **ii**: 1189–92.

6 The Epidemiology of Infection

- Introduction
- Sources and Reservoirs of Micro-organisms
- Routes of Microbial Transmission
- Epidemic and Endemic Infection
- Infection Acquired in the Community
- Infection Acquired in Hospital
- References and Further Reading

Introduction

The term **epidemiology,** derived from the Greek, means the study of things that happen to people. Historically, it has referred to the study of disease and particularly to the occurrence and distribution of infection.

The interaction between man and microbes has changed considerably through history. The microbes responsible for the great **epidemics** of the past have largely been controlled through improvements in living conditions, **immunization** and chemotherapy. However, many parts of the world have yet to benefit from our ability to understand and control **infectious** disease, whilst the re-emergence of old diseases like tuberculosis and the appearance of new diseases like acquired immune deficiency syndrome (AIDS) present new challenges. At the same time, rapid improvements in medical technology and changes in the way care is delivered have increased the risk of infection associated with hospitalization and this affects the costs of health care.

A knowledge of potential sources of micro-organisms and an understanding of how they spread enables us to take appropriate measures to prevent transmission and infection associated with health care. This chapter reviews the epidemiology of infection, it outlines how micro-organisms are spread from person to person and discusses the significance of infections acquired in the community and in hospital.

Sources and Reservoirs of Micro-organisms

Micro-organsims have a **reservoir** where they live. For some, particularly viruses which cannot replicate outside living cells, the human body is the reservoir and they survive by passing from person to person. The human body is also the reservoir for bacteria and fungi which colonize the bowel, skin and respiratory tract.

Animals provide a reservoir for some microbes which do not cause disease in the animal but establish infection when passed to man; for example, *Salmonella* which colonizes the intestine of chickens causes gastrointestinal infections in man.

Other micro-organisms, for example *Clostridium* and *Legionella*, normally inhabit the environment in soil, dust or water.

A **source** is the place from which an organism causing a particular infection originates. Not all microbial reservoirs are necessarily sources of infection. Vases of flowers probably contain a variety of potentially **pathogenic Gram-negative** bacteria but since these bacteria are unlikely to find a way out of the vase and into the patient the vase is an improbable source of infection. Similarly, washbasins are a major reservoir for Gram-negative bacilli and other environmental organisms but are also an improbable source of infection. (Levin *et al.*, 1984).

If the micro-organisms causing an infection are acquired from another person or the environment this is described as an **exogenous** source and the transmission is referred to as **cross-infection**. For example, *Streptococcus* infecting a leg ulcer may be transferred by the hands of staff to the wound of another patient. **Endogenous** or **self-infection** occurs when a micro-organism **colonizing** a site on the host enters another site and establishes infection. For example, the Gram-negative bacilli of the intestine are a common cause of wound infection following abdominal surgery or of urinary tract infections in catheterized patients. In practice, it can often be very difficult to distinguish between endogenous and exogenous infections.

Identification of the source of a micro-organism can be important during the investigation and control of outbreaks of infection. Once a source has been found, action can be taken to prevent further transmission (see 'A lesson to be Learnt').

Routes of Microbial Transmission

To cause disease a **pathogen** must have a way to enter the body – a portal of entry. To transmit to another host it must be able to leave the body via a portal of exit. The route of entry and exit may be different, for example enteric infections enter the mouth and leave in the faeces, or they may be the same; for example respiratory tract infections (see Fig. 6.1).

Micro-organisms use a range of different routes to find new hosts and

A Lesson to be Learnt How Routinely Used Equipment Became an Infection Hazard	The problem was first noticed when three patients on the same ward developed wound infections caused by an antibiotic-resistant strain of *Klebsiella*. Despite strict isolation, new cases of the same infection occurred in other wards. A wide range of ward equipment, including ventilators, humidifiers and suction equipment was investigated to identify the source of the organism. The resistant *Klebsiella* was found on a portable electric suction pump and immediately all other portable pumps were removed and examined in the laboratory. The organism was found in the collection bottles, internal tubing, filters, oil reservoirs and exhaust outlet of six of the seven pumps.

The suction pumps had been used for draining wound cavities and had been shared between several wards. Of the 66 patients affected by this organism, 80% had been nursed in areas where the portable suction had been used. The suction pumps became contaminated because drainage fluids were allowed to overfill the collection bottles and because filters designed to prevent contamination were not replaced regularly.

The equipment was sterilized, improved airfilters and overflow prevention devices were introduced and no further cases of infection were reported.

Davies and Blenkharn (1987)

one microbe may be able to spread by using more than one method. A broad distinction can be made between transmission through direct physical contact with an infected individual and transmission indirectly on other vehicles, objects and equipment.

Transmission by Direct Contact

Micro-organisms may spread through direct contact with the body fluids of an infected individual. Some examples of this type of transmission are sexually transmitted diseases such as *Neissera gonorrhoeae*, glandular fever which is transmitted by kissing and rubella transmitted from mother to baby *in utero*.

Transmission by Indirect Contact

Some micro-organisms depend on people, animals or inanimate objects for transfer from their reservoir to a new host.

Fig. 6.1
Routes of microbial invasion.

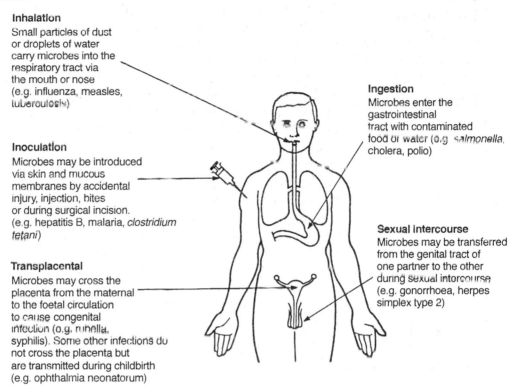

Inhalation
Small particles of dust
or droplets of water
carry microbes into the
respiratory tract via
the mouth or nose
(e.g. influenza, measles,
tuberculosis)

Ingestion
Microbes enter the
gastrointestinal
tract with contaminated
food or water (e.g. *salmonella*,
cholera, polio)

Inoculation
Microbes may be introduced
via skin and mucous
membranes by accidental
injury, injection, bites
or during surgical incision.
(e.g. hepatitis B, malaria, *clostridium
tetani*)

Sexual intercourse
Microbes may be transferred
from the genital tract of
one partner to the other
during sexual intercourse
(e.g. gonorrhoea, herpes
simplex type 2)

Transplacental
Microbes may cross the
placenta from the maternal
to the foetal circulation
to cause congenital
infection (e.g. rubella,
syphilis). Some other infections do
not cross the placenta but
are transmitted during childbirth
(e.g. ophthalmia neonatorum)

Hands

The first clear indication of the important role that hands play in the transmission of infection emanated from the work of Semmelweiss in the 1850s. He demonstrated a remarkable reduction in deaths from **puerperal fever** in the obstetric hospital by instructing doctors to wash their hand in chlorinated lime between contact with cadavers and women in labour. Previous to this practice *Strep. pyogenes*, which causes puerperal fever, was acquired on the hands of doctors as they performed post-mortems on patients who had died from the infection (Newsom, 1993).

Unfortunately, until the late 1960s, the significance of hands as vectors of hospital-acquired infection was not fully appreciated and airborne transmission was considered more important. This view was changed by a study published in 1966 (Mortimer *et al.*, 1966) where babies in the same nursery were divided into two groups attended by different staff. Although both groups occupied the same room, transmission of staphylococci occurred mostly between babies in the same group. When hands were not washed after handling the babies the rate of transmission was even greater. The results strongly implicated hands as the main vector of infection whilst illustrating that air was not a significant route of transmission.

Microbes acquired on hands through contact with excretions, secretions or infected lesions are readily transferred to another host by touch (Mackintosh and Hoffman, 1984). This type of contact is probably responsible for the transmission of a large number of infections, particularly among hospital patients where health care workers have frequent and intimate contact with secretions and excretions of patients (Reybrouck, 1983). Most micro-organisms acquired on the hands are not able to survive for long and are usually transferred rapidly to the next object or patient that is touched. Some species, including antibiotic-resistant strains of *Klebsiella* and *Acinetobacter* have been found to survive for several hours (Casewell and Desai, 1983; Musa *et al.*, 1990), providing plenty of opportunity for them to be transferred to another patient.

Food or Water

Bacteria, **viruses** and some **protozoa** use food or water as a vehicle in what is described as a faecal–oral route of transmission (Fig. 6.2). The microbe is ingested, causes gastrointestinal infection and is excreted in

Fig. 6.2
Faecal–oral spread of infection.

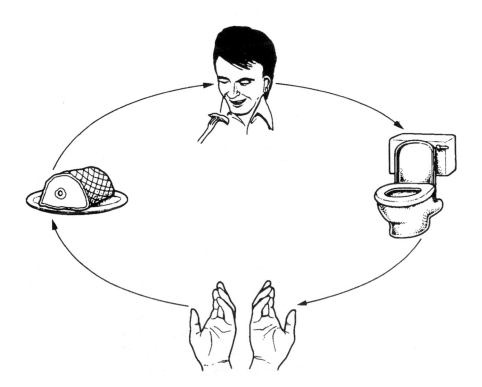

faeces. Transmission to another host occurs when the infected person contaminates his or her hands with faeces and the hands transfer the organism to food which is then ingested by someone else. Food that is cooked after handling is less likely to transmit infection since the organisms will be destroyed unless the **inoculum** is extremely large and the food not cooked thoroughly. Similarly, food that is cooked and then eaten cold, such as cold meats, desserts, sandwiches, salads, etc. may be easily contaminated by an errant food handler with poor hand hygiene and could more easily transmit infection as the organism will not be destroyed by further cooking.

Water contaminated by animal or human faeces is responsible for the transmission of a number of micro-organisms, in particular the bacterium which causes cholera, *Vibrio cholerae* and the protozoa *Cryptosporidium* and *Giardia*. Norwalk viruses can contaminate shellfish grown near to sewage outlets.

Airborne Particles

Contrary to popular belief microbes cannot travel through the air on their own but are carried on airborne particles.

Dust

The major source of micro-organisms in the air are skin squames, flat flakes of dead skin about 10–20 μm in diameter, which are shed from the surface of the skin into the air at a rate of about 300 million per day. A proportion of these squames carry bacteria and together with fibres from clothing and other fabrics are components of dust. The larger particles of dust settle within a few minutes on to exposed horizontal surfaces such as the floor, furniture and equipment. Small particles may remain airborne for several hours and microbes carried on them may be inhaled into the respiratory tract or settle into wounds. Most micro-organisms die rapidly in the absence of water and nutrients and cannot survive in the air for more than a few minutes or hours (Rhame, 1986). Some bacteria form spores which enable them to survive for many months. The spores of *Clostridium difficile* are released from the faeces of infected patients who have diarrhoea. If allowed to accumulate in dust, the environment may act as a source of infection (Hoffman, 1993).

The main significance of airborne dust particles is in the operating department where there is a strong correlation between the numbers of airborne particles and the number of personnel in the operating room. **Pathogens** carried on these particles may settle into the wound or on to surgical instruments and subsequently cause wound infection (Whyte *et al.*, 1982; Howarth, 1985). In wards, activities such as bedmaking can increase the number of bacteria carried in the air, although they settle rapidly on to surfaces (Overton, 1988).

Respiratory Droplets

Droplets are expelled from the respiratory tract by coughing, sneezing and talking. These droplets are composed mostly of saliva but may contain a small number of pathogenic organisms from the respiratory tract. The large droplets (more than 0.1 mm diameter) fall to the ground within a few seconds and are not inhaled. Small droplets (less than 0.1 mm in diameter) evaporate rapidly to a size of between 1 and 10 μm diameter. These very small particles can remain airborne in this form for hours and be inhaled in the same way as small dust particles.

Although some infections are transmitted by respiratory particles in the air, most notably *Mycobacterium tuberculosis* (Riley *et al.*, 1959), the probability of inhaling particles carrying pathogenic organisms is quite low. Many respiratory infections are more commonly transmitted through contact with respiratory secretions, for example on tissues, handkerchiefs and hands (Ansari *et al.*, 1991). Pathogens in droplets expelled onto the hand that covers the sneezer's mouth will be readily passed on to others unless they are removed by handwashing!

Water

Environmental water sources may also transmit infection. The bacterium, *Legionella pneumophilia*, commonly colonizes static water and is responsible for the respiratory infection, legionnaire's disease. Infection is acquired through inhalation of aerosols generated from contaminated water sources such as whirlpools or air-conditioning systems (Bartlett *et al.*, 1986).

Inanimate Objects and Equipment

Inanimate objects which become contaminated with pathogenic bacteria and then spread infection to others are often referred to as **fomites**. These objects include beds, curtains, bedclothes, toys, bedpans and sphygomanometers. Most micro-organisms are not able to survive in the absence of moisture, warmth and nutrients. Provided that such equipment is kept clean and dry bacteria will not be able to multiply and their presence on surfaces will be transitory. Occasionally, outbreaks of infection associated with inadequate decontamination have been reported (Barrie *et al.*, 1994). Bacteria or viruses on inanimate objects can be transferred by touch, with hands then acting as vectors of infection (Ansari *et al.*, 1991). Hands have been found to readily acquire micro-organisms during bed-making or through handling used linen or equipment in the sluice (Sanderson and Weissler, 1992).

Wet environments present a much greater hazard. Some bacteria, particularly *Pseudomonas*, *Acinetobacter* and other Gram-negative bacilli, are able to survive and multiply easily in moisture which may become a source of infection. Equipment that is filled with fluid, for example humidifiers, bowls of disinfectant or wash bowls, is particularly prone to contamination (Greaves, 1985; Gormon *et al.*, 1993). Again it is important to distinguish between sources and reservoirs. Many bacteria may be found in a washbasin but are unlikely to be transferred to a patient, whilst bacteria contaminating a nebulizer chamber are highly likely to be inhaled into the respiratory tract of the patient (see 'The Problem with Mattresses. . .')

Most outbreaks of infection associated with inanimate objects are caused by items that should be sterile but have been inadequately decontaminated. Instruments that enter sterile parts of the body or are in close contact with mucous membranes present particular cross-infection hazards. Infection can also be transmitted by accidental injuries such as the transmission of blood-borne viruses following a needle-stick injuries (Heptonstall *et al.*, 1993).

Animal and Insect Vectors

Other micro-organisms are spread by animal or insect vectors. Cockroaches, ants, rats or mice are often blamed for transmission of infection by carrying pathogens on the surface of their bodies, but there is little evidence to substantiate such claims. The main significance of these pests is in food preparation areas where severe infestation may result in the contamination of food with enteric pathogens.

The Problem With Mattresses. . .

Despite strict isolation precautions, infections caused by an antibiotic-resistant strain of *Acinetobacter* continued to colonize and infect patients on the burns and intensive care units. Whilst investigating the source of this organism, it was noticed that one patient's bed linen was wet, yet she was not incontinent or perspiring and there was no leakage from her burns. When the linen was removed a badly stained mattress cover was revealed and inside it the mattress was found to be wet. Further investigation found 23 mattresses with stained covers and all stained parts were no longer impermeable to fluid. Bacteria were isolated from inside 15 mattresses and the resistant strain of *Acinetobacter* was found in nine. The damage to the mattress covers may have been related to the use of phenolic disinfectants to clean the mattress cover and silver nitrate applied to burns. No further cases of the resistant *Acinetobacter* occurred once the stained mattresses were replaced, a regular system of mattress inspection implemented, and the use of phenolic to clean mattresses discontinued.
Loomes (1988)

Other animals and insects act a reservoir for human pathogens and transmit disease by bites. For example, *Rickettsia* which causes typhus is carried by lice (human and rat lice) and transmitted by their bites. Malaria (a protozoa) and yellow fever (a virus) are transmitted by the bite of mosquitos.

Fig. 6.3
Epidemic curves. (a) Classic epidemic curve. (b) Seasonal epidemic. (c) Single point epidemic of food poisoning with secondary spread by cross-infection.

(a)

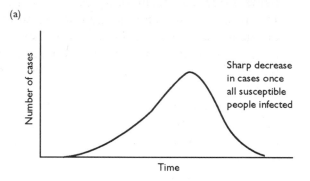

(b)

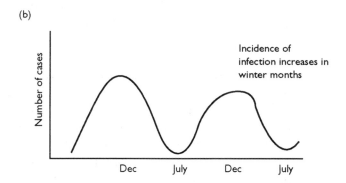

(c)

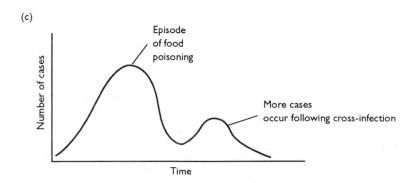

Epidemic and Endemic Infection

Within a population a disease can be *endemic* that (i.e. it is always present at a static level) or *epidemic*, (i.e. a definite increase in the incidence of the disease above its normal or **endemic** level).

A typical epidemic curve shows a gradual increase in the number of infections until all the susceptible individuals have become infected, followed by a fairly rapid decline in new cases of infection (Fig. 6.3a). Some epidemics occur every few years, for example whooping cough and measles. Children who are not **immune** through previous exposure or **vaccination** acquire the infection. When all susceptible children have been infected the number of new cases falls. Three to five years later there will be another increase in infections among the new population of non-immune children.

Other infections are associated with seasonal epidemics, for example influenza, rotavirus and chickenpox (Fig. 6.3b). Infections which induce long-term **immunity** usually cause epidemics amongst the very young or elderly who have either not been previously exposed or have a diminished immunity.

Epidemics of infection associated with a single exposure to infection (e.g. food poisoning) present with a sudden rise in the number of infections followed by a rapid fall. If the infection can be transmitted to others from infected individuals during the incubation period, then a second epidemic due to cross-infection may follow shortly after the first (Fig. 6.3c).

Two methods are commonly used to determine the occurrence of a disease within a population. A **prevalence** rate measures the number of infections present in a particular population at a particular time; for example 'the number of patients who have an infection on ward A on Saturday', expressed as a percentage of the total number of patients on the ward on that day. An **incidence** rate measures the number of new infections that occur in a particular population over a specified period of time; for example the number of patients who develop surgical wound infections during the year, expressed as a percentage of the total number of operations performed.

Infection Acquired in the Community

The principles of epidemiology were first recognized in the time of Hippocrates, 300 years BC. In Britain, the first form of record keeping began in the early sixteenth century with the introduction of 'Bills of Mortality' which provided information on deaths and disease. Epidemics of disease such as plague, typhus, smallpox and syphilis were commonplace in the Middle Ages and although some attempts to control spread through quarantine were employed, the widespread belief that diseases were punishment from God prevailed for hundreds of years.

Giralano Fracastoro, who published De Contagione in 1546, realized that diseases could be transmitted by contact with sick people, their bedding and excreta or through the air. The connection between **contagious** disease and the bacteria first seen under van Leeuwenhoeks' microscope, was not universally accepted until Louis Pasteur and Robert Koch began the study of micro-organisms in the late nineteenth century. These two scientists had to overturn the widespread and strongly held belief in evil humours released by decomposing matter and dirt as the cause of disease.

Pasteur was able to prove that **fermentation** was initiated by microbes and that cultures of anthrax *Bacillus* would cause the disease in sheep. Koch demonstrated that microbes were responsible for anthrax and tuberculosis. He isolated the microbes from infected tissue, cultured them outside the body, re-infected another animal with the culture and finally recovered the same microbes from the animal. Once the link between micro-organisms and human disease was established, other workers studied immunization as a method of protection against infection and the use of antimicrobial drugs to kill microbes without harming the host.

The Public Health Reform Acts

The progress made in the understanding of microbiology had an enormous affect on the control of infectious disease, but of parallel importance was the revolution in public health that took place in the second half of the nineteenth century. The Industrial Revolution of the 1800s brought with it rapid development of towns, which were built with no provision for water supply or sewage drainage. These newly industrialized towns, with overcrowded, squalid conditions and sewage and rotting carcasses filling the streets, were associated with frequent epidemics of disease, particularly typhus, typhoid fever, cholera, smallpox, scarlet fever and measles. Infant mortality of 200 deaths per 1000 births was recorded in some places.

The cholera epidemic of 1831, which killed 60 000 people, mostly in poor and densely populated areas, resulted in demands for action to improve the living conditions of the poor. Poor Law commissioners were appointed and Edwin Chadwick, Secretary to the Commissioners, compiled a report on the 'Sanitary condition of the labouring population of Great Britain (1842)'. This report highlighted the problems of inadequate sewage disposal, pointed to contaminated water as a cause of disease and suggested that a network of earthenware pipes, flushed with running water, should be used to drain sewage away. In response, the Act for Promoting Public Health was passed in 1848, which established the role of district Medical Officers responsible for initiating sanitary improvements and inspectors to monitor their implementation.

Unfortunately, the provisions in this first Public Health Act were not obligatory and it was not until Gladstone became Prime Minister in 1868 that a national Public Health Service was created by parliamentary acts in 1872 and 1875. These Acts resulted in the appointment of Medical Officers for Health (MOH) in each Local Authority. The MOH was responsible for all aspects of public health including sewage disposal, water supply, food hygiene, infectious disease control, child welfare, maternity and venereal disease clinics, the school medical service and, until the formation of the National Health Service in 1948, the Municipal hospitals.

Between 1840 and 1900, the death rate in Britain fell from 25 to 15 per 1000 and life expectancy increased from 40 to 50 years. By the end of the nineteenth century the combined effects of improved standards of hygiene, nutrition, drinking water supply and sewage control virtually eliminated the threat of epidemic disease in developed countries. Today, vaccination is widely used to control the spread of many infectious diseases, but different challenges in disease control develop as a result of changes in life styles. For example, the increase in sexual freedom has been associated with a rise in sexually transmitted diseases and the emergence of the human immunodeficiency virus.

The Public Health Service of Today

In the 1970s, the National Health Service was restructured and many of the community health services previously under the control of the Local Authority moved to the newly formed District Health Authorities (DHA). Monitoring of environmental services such as water and sewage supply, food hygiene and housing remained with the Local Authorities within Environmental Health Departments. The old Public Health Inspectors became Environmental Health Officers (EHO). The EHOs also retained responsibility for the control of communicable disease and food poisoning within the community. The office of MOH was abolished and replaced by a Medical Officer for Environmental Health (MOEH) employed by the Health Authorities. The medical specialty of community medicine was established to train doctors in all aspects of public health and the planning of health services.

Since 1988, the monitoring of disease and the investigation of outbreaks of infection are the responsibility of the DHA. Each DHA appoints a Director of Public Health (DPH) to advise the DHA, Local Authority (LA) and the general public on issues related to public health. The DPH also monitors progress towards the 'Health of the Nation' targets determined by the Department of Health. The Consultant in Communicable Disease Control (CCDC) works for the DPH and is responsible for the prevention and control of outbreaks of infection which occur in the community. The CCDC co-ordinates the activities of the LA and DHA and is designated as the 'Proper Officer' to whom cases of infectious disease must be notified. (NHSME, 1993).

Notification of Infectious Disease

A system of recording cases of infectious disease was recognized as an essential part of the control of epidemics in the early 1900s. Local Authorities have a statutory responsibility to control infectious diseases within their boundaries and to facilitate this some diseases must be notified to the Proper Officer, usually by the doctor who makes the diagnosis. Table 6.1 shows the infectious diseases that are notifiable in England and Wales.

There are several reasons why notifications of infectious disease are necessary. Firstly, close family or other contacts may have been exposed to the infection and require treatment or monitoring for signs of infection (e.g. tuberculosis, meningococcal meningitis). Secondly, the infection may have been acquired from contaminated food or water and require

Table 6.1
Notifiable diseases

Public Health (Control of Diseases) Act 1984
  Cholera
  Food poisoning
  Plague
  Relapsing fever
  Smallpox
  Typhus

Public Health (Infectious Diseases) Regulations 1988

Acute encephalitis	Ophthalmia neonatorum
Acute poliomyelitis	Paratyphoid fever
Anthrax	Rabies
Diphtheria	Rubella
Dysentery	Scarlet fever
Leprosy	Tetanus
Leptospirosis	Tuberculosis
Malaria	Typhoid fever
Measles	Viral haemorrhagic fever
Meningitis	Viral hepatitis
Meningococcal septicaemia	Whooping cough
Mumps	Yellow fever

Local Authorities have the power to prevent the spread of infectious diseases by adding to or subtracting from this list. AIDS is not a notifiable disease but doctors are asked to report cases to a voluntary, confidential scheme at CDSC. Sexually transmitted diseases are reported anonymously by Genitourinary clinics to the Department of Health investigation to identify the source of infection (e.g. food poisoning). Finally, the information is analysed and used at both a local and national level to monitor fluctuations in the levels of infection and the effect of vaccination programmes, detection of epidemics at an early stage and planning preventative programmes.

Public Health Laboratory Service

A network of laboratories providing microbiological services to local public health departments was established during the Second World War. There are now 52 of these laboratories, many on the sites of hospitals, which are able to culture specimens and assist in the diagnosis and control of infectious disease in the community

The Communicable Disease Surveillance Centre (CDSC)

CDSC is based at the headquarters of the PHLS in Colindale, London. It receives data on a voluntary basis from laboratories and CCDCs through out England and Wales. Data on the incidence of infectious diseases are published weekly in the Communicable Disease Report. CDSC also provides advice and information about infectious diseases to Public Health departments and LAs. A similar department in Scotland, the Communicable Disease Surveillance Unit, provides the same service for Scotland.

Infection Acquired in Hospital

A **nosocomial** or **hospital-acquired infection** (HAI) is any infection that develops as a result of hospital treatment from which the patient was not suffering or incubating at the time of admission to hospital. The infections acquired by patients in hospital are usually quite different from those acquired at home. Most HAIs are caused by **opportunistic pathogens** which are introduced to susceptible sites as a result of invasive procedures. Occasionally, epidemics of HAI occur associated with spread of infection from an infectious patient or a breakdown in infection control procedures.

Historical Perspective of HAI

Hospitals for the sick existed in the civilized world as early as 5000 BC, in particular in Asia, Egypt, Palestine and Greece. The standards of hygiene in these early hospitals were based on religious rituals and were far superior to those found in the hospitals of later centuries. Patients were generally housed in separate beds or rooms, good ventilation was considered essential and many of the rudiments of infection control were practised such as not touching wounds, isolation of infected patients and use of cleaning and hot ovens to 'sterilize' instruments.

Unfortunately, after the fall of the Roman empire, standards deteriorated because of the influence of Christianity, which was associated with an aversion to washing and an absence of laws on hygiene. Severe overcrowding, with several patients sharing one bed, and poor ventilation were features of hospitals until the late nineteenth century and it is therefore not surprising that the mortality due to infection was extremely high and death rates from postoperative infection of more than 50% were frequently reported.

John Simpson, Professor of Medicine and Midwifery at Edinburgh University and an early advocate of infection control measures, made a detailed study of the epidemiology and prevention of 'surgical fever'. He observed a significantly higher rate of infection amongst patients operated on in hospital than those operated on by a country surgeon (Simpson, 1869).

Various attempts over the centuries to implement simple infection control measures met with considerable opposition. Many doctors recommended cleanliness of clothes, hands and dressings, but surgeons preferred to blame 'intrinsic defects' in the patient or the 'atmosphere'. An increasing understanding of bacteria, asepsis and transmission of disease, combined with improvements in hospital conditions introduced by Florence Nightingale, finally brought hospital acquired infection under some control by the end of the nineteenth century. In the 1940s, further reductions in the incidence of HAI were associated with the emergence of antimicrobial drugs as effective treatments for infection.

In the early twentieth century, *Streptococcus* was the main problem of cross-infection. Later, in the 1950s, this was replaced by staphylococci, already resistant to a number of antibiotics. The HAI problems of today reflect the nature of the hospital population; highly susceptible patients who in the past would have died from their illness and extensive invasive procedures – each with an attendant risk of infection.

The Infection Control Advisory Service

The development of an organized structure within hospitals to prevent and control infection in hospital began in the 1940s with appointment of part-time Control of Infection Officers and the formation of Infection Control Committees. In 1959 the first Infection Control Nurse was appointed to provide a full-time infection control service. The increasingly complexity of medical care, the cost of HAI and the effects of several outbreaks of HAI (Fig. 6.4) have established infection control as an essential hospital service (DOH, 1995). Most hospitals in the UK appoint key personnel responsible to an infection control team (ICT) who are responsible for ensuring that standards of infection control are maintained:

The Infection Control Doctor (ICD)

The ICD is usually a microbiologist and should have training and a special interest in infection control. He or she is responsible for identifying potential infection control problems, providing advice on the prevention of infection and the management of outbreaks of infection.

The Infection Control Nurse (ICN)

The ICN is usually the only full-time member of the infection control department. The ICN acts as a specialist resource for all health care workers, providing advice on the prevention and control of infection, educating staff, identifying infection hazards, monitoring infection control procedures, developing and implementing infection control policies, managing outbreaks of infection and collecting data on infection rates.

Fig. 6.4
Outbreaks of hospital-acquired infection can cause considerable alarm.

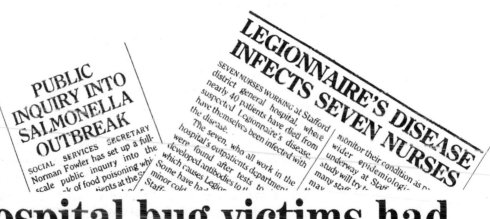

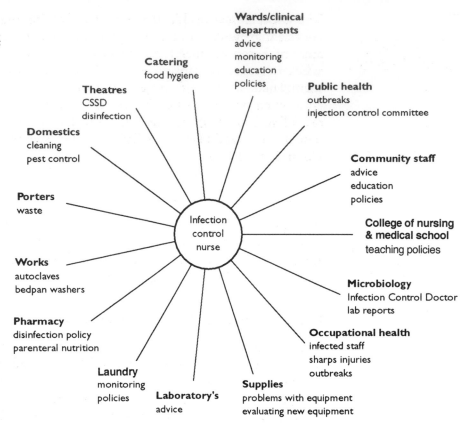

The ICN plays a crucial role in motivating all health care workers to take the prevention and control of infection seriously and in educating where there is misunderstanding or lack of knowledge (Fig. 6.5).

Specialist training in infection control is available for ICNs in the form of a certificate, diploma or degree in Infection Control Nursing.

The Infection Control Committee

The priorities and strategy for infection control should be developed by an hospital infection control committee. This committee should include the members of the ICT and have representatives from medical and nursing staff, pharmacy, central sterile supply, occupational health, environmental health, public health department and the chief executive. If an outbreak of infection occurs in the hospital an emergency meeting of the infection control committee may be convened to co-ordinate control of the outbreak.

The ICT has close links with the Consultant in Communicable Disease Control in the DHA, particularly when outbreaks of infection occur.

The Occupational Health Advisory Service

The occupational health department has an important role in infection control and works closely with the infection control team. The main areas of liaison are health surveillance for infectious diseases which may affect fitness to work (e.g. tuberculosis, gastroenteritis); health surveillance where staff are exposed to hazards such as glutaraldehyde; controlling hazards to health (e.g. management of sharps injuries); and providing advice on the use of protective equipment and ergonomic design of workplaces (RCN, 1991; Health Services Advisory Committee, 1993).

Factors that Affect the Risk of Acquiring Infection in Hospital

A hospital constantly exposes the patient to microbiological risks which he or she would not encounter in his/her own home. From the time of admission to hospital the patient's risk of acquiring infection is strongly influenced by the following factors:

Breach of Natural Defence Mechanisms

The natural defence of the body, which protect us against invasion by micro-organisms, is frequently damaged or breached as a result of hospital treatment. The integrity of the skin may be broken by surgery, intravenous device or decubitous ulceration. The activity of cilia in the upper respiratory tract may be bypassed by intubation or respiratory ventilation and normally sterile organs may be exposed to contamination by invasive procedures.

Contact With Other People

Any place where many people are in close proximity with each other encourages the spread of disease. However, the problem is exacerbated in hospitals because of the regular and intimate contact that occurs between patient and health care workers and which enables micro-organisms to transfer from person to person. A patient may have contact with many different health care workers: nurses, doctors, physiotherapists, occupational therapists, social workers, porters, pharmacists, etc.

Hospital Pathogens

In the 1950s and 60s *Staphylococcus aureus* was the most important hospital pathogen. However, in the last decade Gram-negative bacilli have become a major cause of hospital-acquired infection (Fig. 6.6). Their emergence has coincided with the increase in the proportion of elderly

Fig. 6.6
Common causes of hospital-acquired infection. Compiled using data from Meers et al. (1981).

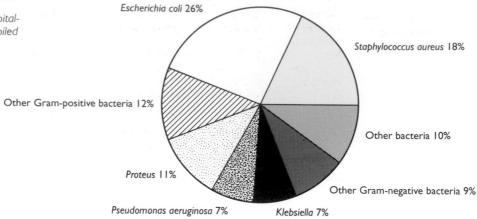

Escherichia coli 26%

Staphylococcus aureus 18%

Other bacteria 10%

Other Gram-positive bacteria 12%

Other Gram-negative bacteria 9%

Proteus 11%

Pseudomonas aeruginosa 7%

Klebsiella 7%

people in the population and advances in medical care. Patients who in the past would have died, now survive. Critically ill patients admitted to a neonatal or intensive care unit, rapidly change their normal bacterial flora, acquiring Gram-negative hospital pathogens (Noone *et al.*, 1983).

Antibiotic therapy is an extremely common part of hospital care. Antibiotic-resistant bacteria survive in favour of antibiotic-sensitive strains and may be carried by patients or staff or may colonize the environment in dust or on equipment. Many strains have a particular ability to spread between patients (Casewell and Desai, 1983; Wade *et al.*, 1991). Over 90% of strains of *S. aureus* isolated from hospital patients are resistant to penicillin, compared with approximately 50% of *Staphylococcus* strains isolated from patients in the community. The degree of antibiotic resistance encountered in a particular hospital tends to reflect antibiotic usage and can often be controlled by the use of an effective antibiotic policy (see Chapter 5).

Susceptibility of the Host

Each individual has a different resistance to infection but those admitted to hospital are often particularly susceptible. Bowell (1992) has suggested a scoring system to identify patients who are particularly at risk. The score takes into account invasive procedures, underlying diseases, drugs and other general factors which increase an individual's susceptibility to infection (Table 6.2). Once the risks have been recognized, actions required to manage or prevent them can be incorporated into the patient's care plan (Kingsley, 1992); for example, the safe management of an intravenous infusion or urinary catheter, improving the patient's nutrition or hydration.

	General factors	Local factors	Invasive procedures	Drugs	Diseases
Table 6.2 *Identifying patients at risk of infection. From Bowell (1992) with permission.*	*Age* Very young Very old	*Oedema* Pulmonary Ascites	*Cannulation* Peripheral Central Parenteral	Cytotoxics	Carcinoma
	Nutrition Emaciated Thin Obese Dehydrated	*Ischaemia* Thrombus Embolus Necrosis	*Surgery* Anaesthesia Wound Wound drainage Wound/colostomy Implant	Antibiotics	Leukaemia
	Mobility Limited Immobile Temporary Permanent	*Skin lesions* Trauma Burns Ulceration	*Intubation* Endobronchial suction Humidification Ventilation	Steroids	Aplastic anaemia
	Mental state Confused Depressed Senile	*Foreign body* Accidental Planned	*Catheterization* Intermittent Closed drainage Irrigation		Diabetes mellitus
	Incontinence Urine Faeces Temporary Permanent				Liver disease
	General health Weak Debilitated				Renal disease
	General hygiene Dependence Mouth/teeth Skin				AIDS

Each factor listed in this table increases the risk of a patient acquiring infection. An infection risk assessment can be made by counting the risk factors for an individual patient. The higher the number counted, the greater the risk that the patient will develop an infection.

The Size of the Problem

The number of infections that are acquired in hospital is very difficult to measure. The presence of infection is often not accurately recorded in medical or nursing records and very few hospitals have systems in place to collect and analyse information about infections. Outbreaks of infection are fortunately quite rare and probably only account for about 2–3% of all HAI (Haley *et al.*, 1985a). Endemic infection of wounds, urinary tract and respiratory tract, presents a much greater problem. The most comprehensive study of HAI in the UK was a prevalence survey by Meers and colleagues in 1980. This study found that on the day of the survey more than nine out of every 100 patients had a hospital-acquired infection (Meers *et al.*, 1981). This survey method tends to overestimate the true level of infection because patients who develop an infection are more likely to stay in hospital for longer and will therefore account for a disproportionate number of hospital in-patients at a single point in time. A more accurate measure is provided by incidence studies which suggest that around 6% of patients admitted to hospital acquire an infection. There is also evidence that the rate of infection is increasing by approximately 0.5% every 5 years, probably related to the increasing complexity of medical care (Haley *et al.*, 1985b).

Types of Hospital-acquired Infection

The most common types of infection acquired in hospital are illustrated in Fig. 6.7.

Surgical Wound Infection

This accounts for approximately 20% of all HAI and occurs mostly as a result of microbial contamination of the wound during surgery. Bacteria may be derived from the **normal flora** of the patient, for example during surgery on the bowel, from instruments or from the skin of the surgeons or their assistants. The factors that influence the acquisition of wound infection and methods of prevention are discussed in more detail in Chapter 8.

Fig. 6.7
The frequency of different types of hospital-acquired infection. Compiled using data from Meers et al. (1981).

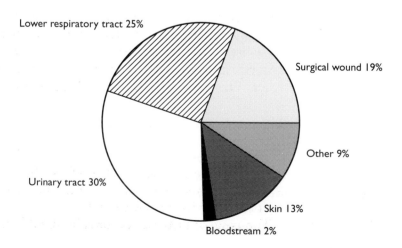

Lower respiratory tract 25%

Surgical wound 19%

Other 9%

Skin 13%

Bloodstream 2%

Urinary tract 30%

Skin Infections

Many breaks in the integrity of the skin caused by pressure sore
and burns sustain a population of colonizing micro-organisms that
no harm. Occasionally, the organisms invade causing infection but
addition they are a potential source for cross-infection. Preventing
infection associated with these wounds is discussed in Chapter 8.

Bloodstream Infections

These account for only 1–2% of HAI but can be very serious and are
associated with a considerable mortality. Up to 40% of patients who
develop bloodstream infection (**septicaemia**) do not survive, and if the
infection is caused by *Pseudomonas* or *Candida* up to 60% may die (Maki,
1981). Approximately 20% of bloodstream infections are caused by
bacteria from an infection at another site in the body invading the
bloodstream (e.g. urinary tract, respiratory tract or wound infections).
Of the remaining 80% most originate from intravenous devices (Maki
1981). The prevention of infection associated with intravenous devices is
discussed in Chapter 9.

Urinary Tract Infection (UTI)

UTI are the most common HAI, although associated with fewer serious
complications that other infections. Nearly all UTI acquired in hospital
occur in patients who have an indwelling urethral catheter or have
undergone a urological procedure (Stamm, 1986). The prevention of
UTI associated with urinary catheters is discussed in Chapter 10.

Lower Respiratory Tract Infection (LRTI)

LRTI accounts for approximately 20% of infections acquired in hospital
but is the leading cause of death associated with HAI (Gross *et al.*, 1980).
Most are caused by bacteria and are related to respiratory therapy or
surgery, although outbreaks of respiratory infections especially by viruses,
occur. The prevention of LRTI is discussed in Chapter 11.

Costs of Hospital-acquired Infection

There have been many studies which have attempted to quantify the
costs of HAI but most have not addressed the total costs to the hospital,
the health service or the patient.

The costs of HAI can be broadly divided into:

to the Patients

may range from a few extra days' absence from work, to consider-
ain and immobility. Loss of earnings, loss of productivity and social
y payments may also be attributable to HAI but are extremely
lt to quantify.

ths attributable to HAI are also difficult to quantify because the
in may be one of several factors contributing to the death of a
y ill patient. Studies in the USA suggest that 1% of patients die
as a direct result of the HAI and they are a significant contributory
factor in a further 3% (Hughes *et al.*, 1983).

Cost of Treatment

Prolonged treatment with intravenous drugs can be very expensive. In
addition, some patients may require further surgery, intensive care or
increased nursing costs such as wound dressings.

Cost of Extra Days Spent in Hospital

Estimates of the effect that infection has on the period of stay in hospital
suggest an average increase of between 4 and 10 days, depending on the
type of infection (Table 6.3). Additional days spent in hospital increase the
cost of care and prevent the admission of another patient into the bed.

In England and Wales, 4.75 million patients are treated as in-patients
every year. If 5% of these patients acquire an infection and stay an average
of 4 days longer in hospital as a result, then the total cost to the health
service will be in the region of 100 million pounds. If the infection rate
could be reduced by just 1% then 22 million pounds would be saved each
year (Ayliffe *et al.*, 1990).

Reducing Hospital-acquired Infection Rates

Prevention of HAI is therefore of enormous importance, not only to the
individual, affected patients but also to the finances of the health service
as a whole.

Meers *et al.* (1981) estimated that as much as 50% of HAI could be

Table 6.3
Days added to hospital stay by nosocomial infection. From Haley, 1985.

Type of infection	Average added hospital days
Surgical wound	7
Bloodstream	7
Pneumonia	6
Urinary tract	1
Other	5
All types	**4**

avoided and the Study on the Efficacy of Nosocomial Infection Control (Haley *et al.*, 1985) found that as many as 32% of HAI could be avoided by the implementation of an effective infection control programme. This included effective monitoring or surveillance of the occurrence of infection, combined with control activities by the infection control team, such as education of staff and development of infection control policies (Haley, 1985).

Providing staff with data about the incidence of infection in their clinical area can be an effective tool in improving practice. For example, if the rate of bacteraemia in an intensive care unit is found to be high, attention can be focused on the way that intravenous infusions are managed and changes in practice implemented to try and reduce the number of infections.

References

Ansari SA, Springthorpe S, Sattar SA *et al.* (1991) Potential role of hands in the spread of respiratory infections : studies with human parainfluenza virus 3 and rhinovirus 14. *J. Clin. Micro.* **29**: 2115–9.

Ayliffe GAJ, Collins BJ, Taylor LJ (1990) *Hospital-acquired Infection. Principles and Prevention*, 2nd edn. Butterworth, London.

Barrie D, Hoffman PN, Wilson JA, Kramer JM (1994) Contamination of hospital linen by *Bacillus cereus*. *Epid. Infect.* **113**: 297–306.

Bartlett CLR, Macrae AD, Macfarlane JD (1986) *Legionella Infections.* Edward Arnold, London.

Bowell B (1992) Protecting the patient at risk. *Nursing Times.* **88**(3): 32–5.

Casewell MW, Desai N (1983) Survival of multiply-resistant *Klebsiella aerogenes* and other Gram-negative bacilli on fingertips. *J. Hosp. Inf.* **4**: 350–60.

Davies B, Blenkharn I (1987) On the right track. *Nursing Times* **83**(22): 64–8.

Department of Health (1995) *Hospital Infection Control – Guidance on the Control of Infection in Hospitals*. Prepared by the DH/PHLS/Hospital Infection working party. HMSO, London.

Greaves A (1985) We'll just freshen you up, dear. *Nursing Times* **Mar 6** (Suppl). : 3–8.

Gormon LJ, Sanai L, Notman W *et al.* (1993) Cross-infection in an intensive care unit by *Klebsiella pneumoniae* from ventilator condensate. *J. Hosp. Inf.* **23**: 17–26.

Gross PA, Neu HC, Aswa PO *et al.* (1980) Deaths from nosocomial infection: experience in a university hospital and community hospital. *Am. J. Med.* **68**: 219.

Haley RW (1985) Surveillance-by-objectives: a new priority-directed approach to the control of nosocomial infections. *Am. J. Inf. Control* **13**: 78–89.

Haley RW, Tenney JH, Lindsay JO *et al.* (1985a) How frequent are outbreaks of nosocomial infection in community hospitals? *Infection Control* **6**: 233–6.

Haley RW, Culver DH, White JW *et al.* (1985b) The efficacy of infection surveillance and control programs in preventing nosocomial infections in US hospitals (SENIC Study). *Am. J. Epid.* **121**: 182–205.

Heptonstall J, Porter K, Gill N (1993) *Occupational Transmission of HIV. Summary of Published Reports*. PHLS AIDS Centre, London.

Hoffman PN (1993) *Clostridium difficile* and the hospital environment. PHLS *Micro. Digest* **10**(3): 91–2.

Health Services Advisory Committee (1993) *The Management of Occupational Health Services for Healthcare Staff*. HMSO, London.

Howarth FH (1985) Prevention of airborne infection during surgery. *Lancet* **i**; 386–8.

Hughes HM, Culver DH, White JW *et al.* (1983) Nosocomial infections surveillance, 1980–1982. *MMWR* **32**: 1SS.

Kingsley A (1992) First step towards a desired outcome. Preventing infection by risk recognition. *Prof. Nurse* **7**(11): 725–9.

Levin MH, Olsen B, Nathan C *et al.* (1984) *Pseudomonas* in the sinks of an intensive care unit: relation to patients. *J. Clin. Path.* **37**: 424–7.

Loomes S (1988) Is it safe to lie down in hospital? *Nursing Times* **84**(49): 63–5.

Mackintosh CA, Hoffman PN (1984) An extended model for the transfer of microorganisms via the hands: differences between organisms and the effect of alcohol disinfection. *J. Hyg.* **92**: 345–55.

Maki DG (1981) Nosocomial bacteraemia. An epidemiological overview. *Am. J. Med.* **70**: 719–31.

Meers PD, Ayliffe GAJ, Emmerson AM *et al.* (1981) Report of the National Survey of Infection in Hospital. *J. Hosp. Inf.* **2**(Suppl.): 1–51.

Mortimer EA, Wolinsky E, Gonzaga AJ *et al.* (1966) Role of hands in the transmission of staphylococcal infections. *Brit. Med. J.* **1**: 319–22.

Musa FK, Desai N, Casewell MW *et al.* (1990) The survival of *Acinetobacter calcoaceticus* inoculated on fingertips and formica. *J. Hosp. Inf.* **15**: 219–228.

Newsom SWB (1993) Ignaz Philip Semmelweiss. *J. Hosp.I nf.* **23**: 175–88.

NHS Management Executive (1993) *Public Health: Responsibilities of the NHS and the Roles of Others*. HSG (93)56. HMSO, London.

Noone MR, Pitt TL, Bedder M *et al.* (1983) *Pseudomonas aeruginosa* in an intensive therapy unit: role of cross infection and host factors. *Brit. Med. J.* **286**: 341–4.

Overton E (1988) Bed making and bacteria. *Nursing Times* **84**(9): 69–71.

Reybrouck G (1983) Role of hands in the spread of nosocomial infections 1. *J. Hosp. Inf.* **4**: 103–10.

Rhame F (1986) In *Hospital Infections* (JV Bennett, PS Brackman, Eds), pp. 223–50. Little Brown, Boston.

Riley RL, Mills CC, Nyka W *et al.* (1959) Aerial dissemination of pulmonary tuberculosis: a two year study of contagion in a tuberculosis ward. *Am. J. Hyg.* **70**: 185.

Royal College of Nursing (1991) A guide to an Occupational Health Nursing Service. A handbook for employers and nurses. Scutari, London.

Sanderson PJ, Weissler S (1992) Recovery of coliforms from the hands of nurses and patients: activities leading to contamination. *J. Hosp. Inf.* **21**: 85–93.

Simpson JY (1869) Some propositions on hospitalism. *Lancet* **Oct 16**: 535–8.

Stamm WE (1986) In *Hospital Infections* (JV Bennett, PS Brackman, Eds), pp. 375–84. Little Brown, Boston.

UK Health Departments (1992) *Immunization Against Infectious Disease*. HMSO, London.

Wade JJ, Desai N, Casewell MW (1991) Hygienic hand disinfection for the removal of epidemic vancomycin-resistant *Enterococcus faecium* and gentamicin-resistant *Enterobacter cloacae*. *J. Hosp. Inf.* **18**: 211–18.

Whyte W, Hodgson R, Tinkler J (1982) The importance of airborne bacterial contamination of wounds. *J. Hosp. Inf.* **3**: 123–35.

Further Reading Currie E, Maynard A (1989) *The economics of hospital-acquired infection.* Centre for Health Economics Consortium. Discussion paper 56. Centre for Health Economics, University of York, York.

Department of Health (1988) *Public Health in England.* Report of the committee of enquiry into the future development of public health function. HMSO, London.

Haley RW (1986) *Managing Hospital Infection Control for Cost Effectiveness.* A strategy for reducing infectious complications. American Hospital Publishing, USA.

McCormick A (1993) The notification of infectious diseases in England and Wales. *CDR* **3**(2): R19–24.

Morgan D (Ed.) (1989) *Infection Control.* The British Medical Association Guide. Edward Arnold, London.

Parker L (1990) From pestilence to asepsis. *Nursing Times* **86**(49): 63–7.

Selwyn S (1991) Hospital Infection the first 2500 years. *J. Hosp. Inf.* **18**(Suppl A): 5–65.

Ward K (1988) The role of the infection control nurse. *Nursing* **3**(30): 5–8.

The Central Principles of Infection Control

- **Introduction**
- **What are Infection Control Precautions?**
- **Routine Infection Control Practice**
- **Education and Training**
- **References and Further Reading**

Introduction

Infection is a common, but largely avoidable complication of hospitalization. In Chapter 6 we considered the impact that **hospital-acquired infection** has on the patient and the health service. In this chapter we will look at the use of simple infection control precautions to minimize the spread of infection both from one patient to another and between patient and health care worker.

A small proportion of patients admitted to hospital will have or be incubating an **infectious** disease and precautions are necessary to prevent transmission to other patients or staff. In addition, approximately 5% of patients admitted to hospital will acquire an infection during their stay and it has been estimated that around one-third of these infections could be prevented by improved infection control practice (Haley *et al.*, 1985).

Health care workers are healthy and less susceptible to infection than their patients. Infections commonly acquired by health care workers include skin infections caused by streptococci, staphylococci, Herpes simplex and fungi (Greaves *et al.*, 1980); respiratory infections such as chickenpox, respiratory syncitial virus and *Mycobacterium tuberculosis* (Hall, 1981; George *et al.*, 1986) and enteric infections, particularly viral gastro-enteritis (Reid *et al.*, 1990). Health care workers are also at risk of acquiring blood-borne viruses such as hepatitis B and C (West, 1984). At least 64 health care workers worldwide have acquired human immunodeficiency virus occupationally since it was first recognized as the cause of AIDS in the 1980s (Heptonstall *et al.*, 1993).

Health care workers infected with blood-borne viruses may transmit infection to their patients, although the main risk of transmission is associated with invasive procedures in which injury to the health care worker could result in blood entering the patient's open tissues (UK Health Departments, 1991; Ciesielski *et al.*, 1992; DOH, 1993).

What are Infection Control Precautions?

Infection control precautions are used routinely to prevent the transmission of micro-organism between patients, from patient to staff and vice versa. Special isolation precautions are used for those patients who are known or suspected to have a particular infectious disease (Fig. 7.1).

Routine infection control practices are used in the care of all patients and include the key procedures which minimize the transmission of micro-organisms such as handwashing, use of protective clothing and disposal of body fluids. The basic principles are covered in more detail in this chapter. Chapters 8, 9, 10 and 11 examine the more specific precautions required to prevent infection associated with invasive devices such as urinary catheters, intravenous devices and respiratory therapy and wounds. Chapter 12 describes the principles of sterilization and disinfection of equipment.

Isolation precautions were originally developed to prevent the spread of infectious disease amongst vulnerable hospital patients and are used to prevent or control outbreaks or **epidemics** of infection in hospital, for example of antibiotic-resistant bacteria. They are initiated when an infectious disease is diagnosed in a particular patient, include the isolation of the patient and use of protective clothing to handle infectious body material. They are discussed in more detail in Chapter 14.

Patients may be infectious before the clinical illness becomes apparent, for example patients with chickenpox are infectious for 2–3 days before

Fig. 7.1
The role of infection control precautions.

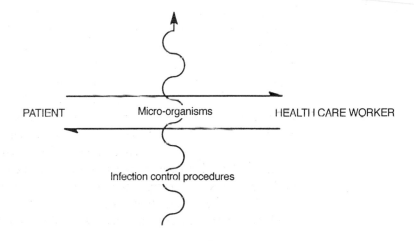

PATIENT   Micro-organisms   HEALTH CARE WORKER

Infection control procedures

the rash appears. This is particularly the case with HIV and hepatitis B, both of which are associated with prolonged asymtomatic **carriage** of which even the patient may be unaware. The implementation of special precautions on diagnosis of infection may not prevent cross-infection prior to the diagnosis being made.

Universal Blood and Body Fluid Precautions

The problem of identifying infected patients was acknowledged by the Centers for Disease Control in the USA in their advice to health care workers on preventing the transmission of blood-borne pathogens. The precautions necessary to minimize this risk required the health care worker to use appropriate protective clothing to prevent exposure of skin and mucous membranes to blood or body fluids and to use these precautions with all patients because infected patients could not be reliably identified (CDC, 1987).

Universal precautions were originally applied to all body fluids but it became clear that blood-borne viruses were not transmitted by all body fluids (e.g. faeces, urine, sputum), and a recommendation to exclude those fluids from universal precautions, unless they contained visible blood, was made later (CDC, 1988).

In the UK the Department of Health advised similar measures to protect clinical health care workers against infection with blood-borne viruses (UK Health Departments, 1990) and endorsed the use of the same level of precaution with all patients. The concept has caused some controversy and it has been suggested that where the prevalence of blood-borne viruses is low the precautions are unnecessary and should only be used with individuals known or suspected to be infected (Speller *et al.* 1990). Unfortunately, it is often difficult to identify infected individuals and patients who practice high risk behaviours are frequently not detected.

Since body fluids frequently contain large numbers of micro-organisms, they are a major source of pathogens which cause hospital-acquired infection. Many workers have therefore recognized that universal blood and body fluid precautions, as well as protecting health care workers from infection with blood-borne viruses, could prevent the transmission of many other pathogens and make a major contibution to the reduction of

Table 7.1
Transmission of blood-borne viruses to health care workers

Infected body fluids:
- inoculated through skin
- contaminate damaged skin
- contaminate mucous membranes
  (eyes or mouth)

hospital-acquired infection (Lynch *et al.*, 1987; Leclair *et al.*, 1987; Wilson and Breedon, 1990; UK Health Departments, 1990). Others have suggested that it is difficult to maintain the routine use of precautions with all patients and question the benefit of the increased costs of protective clothing (Garner and Hierholzer, 1993).

A further advantage of universal blood and body fluid precautions is the simplification of the traditional approach to isolation of infectious patients (Jackson and Lynch, 1985). If the same precautions are taken with all body fluids there is no need to identify different levels of protection for many infectious diseases. For example, *Salmonella* is transmitted by contact with faeces but if protective clothing is always used for contact with faeces, additional precautions may not be necessary for patients known to be infected with *Salmonella*.

Routine Infection Control Practice

The infection control practices outlined below incorporate the principles of universal blood and body fluid precautions and represent a standard of care that should be used routinely with all patients to minimize the spread of potential pathogens including blood borne viruses between patients and staff.

Handwashing

The hands of staff are the most common vehicle by which micro-organisms are transmitted between patients and hands are frequently implicated as the route of transmission in outbreaks of infection (Reybrouck 1983, Casewell and Phillips, 1977; Ansari *et al.*, 1991).

Transient Skin Flora

Microbes acquired on the surface of the skin through contact with other people, objects or the environment are known as *transient skin flora*. They are particularly easily acquired on the hands when the object touched is moist (Marples and Towers, 1979). The composition of this transient flora varies but reflects the extent of contact with patients or their environment and the prevalent micro-organisms. For example, **methicillin-resistant *Staphylococcus aureus* (MRSA)** is frequently found on the skin of nurses who are caring for patients infected with the organism (Cookson *et al.*, 1989). The antibacterial properties of skin prevent the survival of these transient micro-organisms for more than a few hours (Reybrouck, 1983) but within this time the organisms are readily transferred to other people or objects (Mackintosh and Hoffman, 1984).

Hands and the Spread of Infection

Over a period of one month the same type of *Klebsiella pneumoniae* was isolated from the respiratory secretions of six patients on an intensive care unit. Four patients developed infections caused by the organism. During the investigation to identify the source of the organism it was noticed that the water traps collecting condensate from ventilator tubing were emptied into foil dishes. These remained by the bedside until full when they were emptied into the sink. Although hands were washed after contact with tracheal secretions, hands were not washed after handling the condensate.

The *Klebsiella* was found in samples of the condensate and in the foil bowls and was also recovered from the hands of staff. No further cases of infection occurred once staff had been alerted to the potential hazard of the condensate and handwashing after contact with ventilator tubing and traps had been instituted.

Gorman *et al.*, (1993)

The potential extent of transmission has been demonstrated by experiments using a fluorescent powder, visible only under ultraviolet light, to represent micro-organisms. This study demonstrated that 2 h after the powder was applied to a baby, traces of it were found on the hands of all the nurses responsible for the care of the baby, the hands of at least one other nurse and in the environment (Scanlon and Leikkanen, 1973).

Pathogens are likely to be acquired on the hands in greatest number when handling moist, heavily contaminated substances such as body fluids. However, Casewell and Phillips (1977) showed that even during routine procedures such as touching, lifting or washing a patient, transient bacteria are easily acquired on the hands. They are also acquired simply by touching the buttocks of a baby, even if the nappy is not soiled (Sprunt *et al.*, 1973) and have been recovered from hands after bed-making, handling curtains or using the sluice (Sanderson and Weissler, 1992). Pathogens present on the skin surrounding an infected wound are readily transferred to the hands even if forceps are used to dress the wound (Tomlinson, 1987). Viruses are also easily acquired, for example during nappy changing (Samadi *et al.*, 1983) and hands are commonly contaminated by respiratory viruses (Ansari *et al.*, 1991).

Removal of Transient Micro-Organisms: Handwashing with Soap and Water

Fortunately, the majority of micro-organisms acquired in this way are easily removed mechanically by washing with soap and water, even by a brief, 10-s wash (Sprunt *et al.*, 1973) (Plate 7.1). Hands should be washed to remove these transient organisms before and after any patient contact but especially in the situations described in Table 7.2.

Table 7.2 *Indications for handwashing*	Hands should be washed with soap and water before any direct contact with patients and especially:

- before and after handling invasive devices
- before and after dressing wounds
- before and after contact with immunocompromised patients
- before and after handling food
- after handling equipment contaminated with body fluid
- after contact with blood or body fluid
- after removing gloves
- after using the toilet
- before leaving the clinical area

Resident Skin Flora

The skin also supports the growth of a wide variety of microbes known as the resident or **normal flora**. These organisms live in deep crevices in the skin, in hair follicles and sebaceous glands. The type and distribution of organisms varies according to humidity, temperature, body site and the person's general health. The bacteria present in largest number include staphylococci, micrococci, streptococci, corynebacteria and to a lesser extent *Neisseria* and *Candida*. Although not conventionally considered part of the resident flora, many **Gram-negative bacilli** appear able to withstand the desiccation and antibacterial effects of skin, are often present in large numbers, especially on humid parts of the body such as the axilla, and may consitute a **reservoir** for **infection** (Knittle *et al.*, 1975). Gram-negative bacilli have been recovered from skin at ring sites but the clinical significance of these organisms is unknown (Hoffman *et al.*, 1985).

Removal of Resident Flora – Antiseptic Soap Solutions

The resident microbial flora are not easily removed by the mechanical action of washing with soap, but their numbers can be reduced by the combination of a detergent and a **microbicide**, such as chlorhexidine or povidone-iodine. Both these agents supress the skin's resident flora if used repeatedly (Lowbury and Lilley, 1973).

Removal of resident skin flora during routine clinical care is usually not necessary as they are not readily transferred to other people or surfaces and most are of low pathogenicity. However, some resident bacteria could cause infection if introduced during invasive procedures into normally sterile body sites, or to sites on particularly vulnerable individuals (e.g. neonates, intensive care).

These detergent microbicides are designed to be used by surgeons a few times a day. If used in ward situations where staff wash their hands much more frequently they have been associated with damage to skin and increased levels of bacteria on the hands (Ojajärvi *et al.*, 1977).

Their use is therefore best restricted to operating theatres, prior to invasive procedures and occasionally for the control of outbreaks of infection. Gram-negative bacilli, especially antibiotic-resistant strains, are often difficult to remove by the mechanical action of soap and water and microbicide detergents may be necessary to prevent their spread (Wade *et al.*, 1991).

Handwashing Technique

Hands must be washed properly to remove micro-organisms. Taylor (1978) observed that nurses washed their hands for an average time of 20 s and that large areas of the skin was frequently left unwashed. Micro-organisms may remain on parts of the hands not exposed to soap and water and would still be available for transfer to other patients.

Hands should be washed by systematically rubbing all parts of the hands and wrists with soap and water, being particularly careful to include the areas that are most frequently missed (Fig. 7.2). Similarly, the efficacy of antiseptic soap solutions depends on the adequacy of the handwash; micro-organisms will only be removed by these solutions if all parts of the hands are reached. None the less, even a brief 10-s handwash appears to remove transient micro-organisms effectively (Sprunt *et al.*, 1973).

Thorough drying afterwards is also an important part of the procedure. More bacteria are probably removed by the towel or hot-air drier (Ansari *et al.*, 1991) and moisture remaining on the skin may cause it to become dry and cracked.

Unfortunately, research has shown that hands are frequently not washed at all after contact with patients and even after dirty procedures (Gould, 1993). Medical staff have been found to be especially unlikely to wash their hands (Albert and Condie, 1981). Williams and Buckles (1988) demonstrated that even though handwashing frequency increased significantly after an extensive promotional campaign, 6 months later the rate of handwashing had decreased to the previous level (Fig. 7.3).

Alcohol Handrub Solutions

Although a single hand wash and dry takes about 1 min to perform properly, a considerable amount of time is spent on repeated hand washing, more if there is some distance between the patient and the nearest sink. An inadequate supply of handwashing facilities can adversely affect the frequency of handwashing (Kaplan and McGuckin, 1986).

One means of encouraging effective and frequent handwashing is by using alcohol handrubs. These can be applied more quickly (15–20 s)

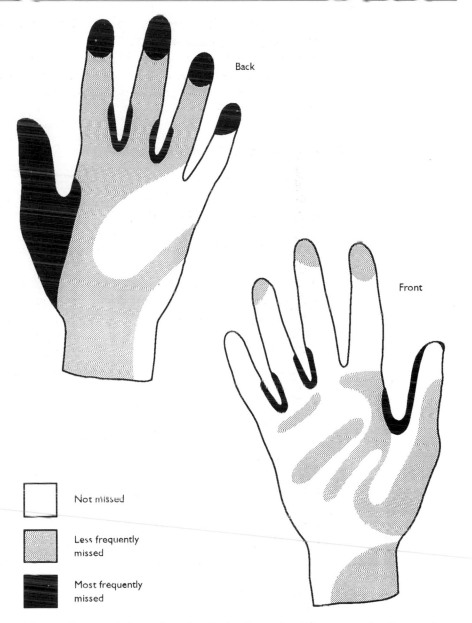

Fig 7.2
Parts of the hands most frequently missed during handwashing.

Back

Front

☐ Not missed

▨ Less frequently missed

▧ Most frequently missed

without the need for a handwash basin and will remove both transient organisms and resident bacteria. In most situations they can be used instead of soap and water but should not be used if hands are visibly soiled (Mackintosh and Hoffman, 1984). Handrubs are particularly useful during aseptic techniques, outside isolation rooms, in intensive care settings where hands may need washing frequently and in the patient's home where access to handwashing facilities may be difficult. Although not popular, they are a suitable alternative to surgical scrubs and are associated with less skin damage (Ojajärvi *et al.*, 1977; Lilley *et al.*, 1979).

Fig. 7.3

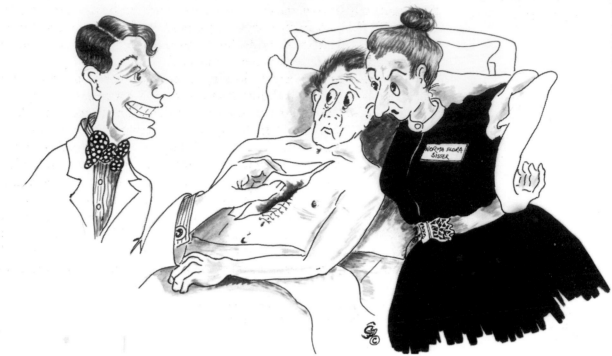

"NOW WASH YOUR HANDS- OR, DON'T PEEK!"

Handcreams

Frequent handwashing, especially with antiseptic soap solutions or if hands are not properly dried, can cause damage to skin. Cracked skin may harbour more bacteria and increase the risk of cross-infection (Larson *et al.*, 1986). Regular use of hand creams may help to prevent skin damage but communally used creams can become a potential source of infection (Morse and Schonbek, 1968).

Covering Cuts

Intact skin protects tissue from invasion by micro-organisms. Damaged skin may become infected superficially by bacteria or fungi to cause a local abcess and blood-borne viruses may enter the body through damaged skin. Whilst at work health care workers should therefore always protect any damaged skin, particularly on the hands and fore-arms, with a waterproof dressing.

Protective Clothing

Many excretions and secretions of the body are a major source of **pathogenic micro-organisms** associated with hospital-acquired infection (Table 7.3). Protective clothing should therefore be worn for any direct contact with these body fluids, to interrupt the transmission of micro-organsims between patients and staff.

The choice of protective clothing selected depends on the anticipated risk of exposure to body fluid during the particular activity. This strategy is called **risk assessment** and is a common approach to Health and Safety (COSHH, 1988). Many clinical activities involve no direct contact with body fluid and do not require the use of protective clothing, for example washing a patient or taking a pulse, blood pressure or temperature. Other procedures may result in contamination of the hands or clothing and require the use of gloves and a plastic apron, for example assisting a patient with a commode or handling of specimens. Procedures which involve a risk of blood or body fluid splashing require protection of the mouth and eyes, therefore a mask, eye protection and water-resistant gown will be necessary. Figure 7.4

Table 7.3
Potentially infectious body fluids

Body fluids which may contain blood-borne viruses:
  Blood
  Blood-stained body fluids
  Semen
  Vaginal secretions
  Tissues
  Cerebrospinal fluid
  Amniotic fluid, synovial fluid, pleural fluid, etc.

Body fluids which may contain other pathogens:
  Faeces
  Urine
  Vomit
  Sputum
  Saliva

Fig. 7.4
The selection of protective clothing. The risk of exposure to blood or body fluids should be assessed before commencing the procedure.

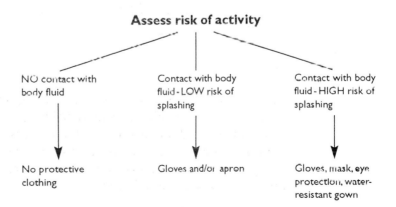

Assess risk of activity

NO contact with body fluid → No protective clothing

Contact with body fluid - LOW risk of splashing → Gloves and/or apron

Contact with body fluid - HIGH risk of splashing → Gloves, mask, eye protection, water-resistant gown illustrates the principles of risk assessment in the selection of protective clothing.

These same principles should be applied in all situations, with all patients and in all areas of clinical practice.

Gloves

The contribution that the hands of staff make to the transmission of infection in health care settings has already been demonstrated. Disposable gloves for direct contact with body fluids and moist body sites provide a reliable method of reducing the acquisition on hands of micro-organisms from these sources. Some studies have demonstrated a reduction in the incidence of infection where gloves are routinely used for handling body fluids, although they must be used appropriately (Leclair *et al.*, 1987; Gerding *et al.*, 1988; Lynch *et al.*, 1990). Gloves will also protect the health care worker from infection if cuts and abrasions are present on the hands.

Gloves should be worn for any activity where body fluid may contaminate the hands but hands should be washed after removal because gloves may be punctured and hands are easily contaminated as the gloves are taken off (Olsen *et al.*, 1993). To prevent transmission of infection gloves must be discarded after each procedure (Patterson *et al.*, 1991). Washing gloves between patients is not recommended; the gloves may be damaged by the soap solution and if punctured unknowingly, may cause body fluid to remain in direct contact with skin for prolonged periods (Adams *et al.*, 1992).

Gloves should also be worn for procedures involving direct contact with mucous membranes, for example mouth care and vaginal examination. Micro-organsims **colonizing** or infecting mucous membranes may be easily transmitted on hands and infect another person. For example: papilloma virus or *Candida* in the vagina, Herpes simplex virus or *Candida* in the mouth (Burnie *et al.*, 1985).

If gloves are to be used appropriately they must be readily available in all clinical areas. The gloves used should not split or tear easily, be disposable and do not need to be sterile unless used in sterile body sites (e.g. surgical procedures, lumbar puncture, central line cannulation). Latex gloves conform to the hands and are suitable for procedures requiring a fine degree of dexterity, although sensitization to latex has been reported by some staff (Booth, 1994). Vinyl gloves are looser fitting but not usually associated with adverse skin reactions.

Disposable gloves will not prevent needlestick injuries (Palmer and Rickett, 1992). There is some evidence that needlestick injury is less likely to occur if two pairs of gloves are worn, although the loss of sensitivity may impede the user (Matta *et al.*, 1988). In one study involving orthopaedic surgery the incidence of glove puncture was 14% when one pair was worn and when two pairs were worn, 19% for the outer glove and 6% for the inner glove (McCleod, 1989). Double gloving should be considered for activities associated with a high risk of skin puncture, for example surgery, especially orthopaedic or dental surgery where sharp pieces of bone or teeth are most likely to cause injury.

Considerable controversy surrounds the use of gloves for venepuncture. The UK Health Departments (1990) recommend that gloves should be worn when the venepuncturist is inexperienced, has cuts or abrasions on their hands which cannot be covered by a dressing, the patient is restless or is known to be infected with blood-borne virus. However, staff will probably find the procedure more difficult if they are not used to wearing gloves. A more logical approach is to train staff from the beginning to use gloves for taking blood. Experience with phlebotomists who always use gloves demonstrates that gloves can be successfully worn for venepuncture.

Eye Protection and Masks

In the past, nurses wore masks with the intention of protecting vulnerable sites on the patients such as wounds, from contamination by micro-organisms expelled from the respiratory tract of the nurse. It is now recognized that a healthy member of staff expels few micro-organisms from the respiratory tract and that masks are not necessary for most procedures (Ayliffe, 1991)

Unlike intact skin, micro-organisms can pass through mucous membranes to cause infection. In two reported incidents, health care workers have acquired HIV as a result of blood splashing into the face (Heptonstall *et al.*, 1993). Masks and eye protection are therefore important to protect health care workers from splashes of body fluid.

Eye protection and a mask should be worn for any activity where there is a risk of body fluid splashing into the face (Fig. 7.5). Such activities are not commonly encountered in ward settings, the main risks are associated with respiratory suction where excessive secretions are present, scrubbing of instruments, endoscopy, management of women in labour and some surgical procedures, particularly orthopaedic and cardiac surgery.

In common with people in other occupations whose work involves a risk of damage to the eyes, health care workers are often reluctant to protect their eyes properly. Masks and eye protection must be readily available in any clinical area where such procedures are performed. In the past, eye protection has been cumbersome to wear, but now a variety of types are available and some look like ordinary spectacles.

Fig. 7.5
Eye protection. Mask and eye protection should be worn for procedures where there is risk of splashing of blood or body fluids.

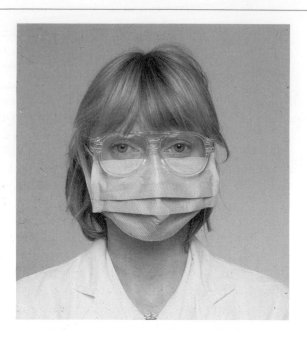

Water-repellant Aprons or Gowns

Water-repellent protection should be worn for procedures anticipated to cause significant contamination of skin or clothing with blood or body fluid. This will protect the skin of the health care worker from contamination by potentially infected body fluid and reduce the risk of **cross-infection** of micro-organisms to other patients on the clothing.

Since the front of the body is the part most frequently contaminated by body fluid, plastic, disposable aprons provide adequate protection in most circumstances (e.g. dealing with body fluid spills, handling bedpans, dressing wounds). Plastic aprons should be readily available in all clinical areas.

Exposure to body fluid during surgical procedures varies; minor surgery such as biopsy, lump removal or laparoscopy, involves little exposure to body fluid. Some orthopaedic, abdominal and cardiac procedures may result in considerable contamination with blood or body fluid and then a water-repellant gown should be worn.

Water-repellant gowns may be disposable or re-usable and made of specially woven or treated cotton. The most impervious have a plastic layer but are expensive.

Safe Handling of Sharp Instruments

Sharp instruments frequently cause injury to health care workers and are a major cause of transmission of blood-borne viruses (Heptonstall *et al.*, 1993).

Sharps include needles, scalpels, broken glass or other item that may cause a laceration or puncture. The risk of acquiring hepatitis B from a single sharps injury involving blood from a hepatitis B carrier can be extremely high and the inoculation of a minute quantity of blood is sufficient to transfer infection. Approximately one in four such injuries involving blood from a highly infectious **carrier** will result in the health care worker acquiring hepatitis B. HIV is not so easily transmitted with less than 1% of health care workers acquiring infection following a single injury involving HIV-infected blood (Royal College of Pathologists, 1992; Heptonstall *et al.*, 1993).

Strategies aimed at reducing the risk of needlestick injury have been described but are unlikely to work unless a clear written policy informs employees what is expected of them. Containers used for sharps should conform to the British Standard for sharps containers which is summarized in Table 7.4. Small, portable sharps bins are available for use in community settings. Disposal of used sharps in inappropriate places may present a considerable risk to other employees and every health care worker has a responsibility to ensure proper disposal of the sharps that they have used.

Research into the frequency and causes of sharps injuries has been hampered by under reporting of injuries (Jagger *et al.*, 1988). Injury due to used needles often happens after use but before disposal, for example during resheathing or whilst being carried to a sharps container (Eisenstein and Smith, 1992). Resheathing of needles is particularly

Table 7.4
Summary of contents of the British Standard for sharps containers

Containers intended to hold sharps should:

- have a handle
- have a closure device which remains closed when the container is carried or dropped
- be resistant to penetration
- not leak or break open when dropped
- be yellow
- be marked with the words:
    Danger
    Contaminated sharps only
    Destroy by incineration
- be marked to indicate when 70–80% full

dangerous because if the needle misses the sheath it will puncture the hand holding it. In one study resheathing was responsible for 33% of injuries (Jagger *et al.*, 1988).

Other factors commonly responsible for causing needlestick injuries include; insufficient sharps containers, leaving used sharps on trolleys or beds after use, leaving lancets for blood glucose testing on lockertops, discarding sharps into plastic waste bags and careless assembly or closure of sharps bins, which subsequently break open during transport (Saghafi *et al.*, 1992).

Particular care should be taken during procedures where sharp instruments are passed between two people, for example during surgery. The risk of injury can be reduced by the use of a receiver to pick up and deposit instruments rather than placing into the hand. In the future, sharps instruments may be increasingly replaced by self-sheathing needles, laser surgery, blunt suture needles and electrocautery (Davies, 1994).

Table 7.5 outlines the principles of good practice for the safe management of sharp instruments.

Vacuum Blood Collection Systems

These systems are now widely used for venepuncture and are generally considered safer than taking blood with a needle and syringe, as blood is drawn directly into the specimen bottle and not injected in after collection.

Some vacuum collection systems incorporate a re-usable barrel from which the needle has to be unscrewed, but this can only be done safely if the needle is resheathed in a resheathing device (Fig. 7.6). Ideally, the barrel and needle should be discarded as one unit. If a re-sheathing device is not available the sheath should be placed on a flat surface to receive the needle and not held by hand.

Table 7.5
The safe handling of used sharp instruments

Used sharps should be handled as little as possible to minimize the risk of injury:

- needles must not be resheathed. If a needle and syringe needs to be disassembled then it should first be resheathed using a single handed technique or a resheathing device (Fig. 7.6).
- sharps must be discarded *immediately* after use into a designated sharps container
- sharps must never be carried in the hand to the point of disposal, but either carried in a tray or a sharps container brought to the point of use
- they should not be passed by hand between staff
- needles should not be removed from syringes but discarded as a single unit
- sharps bins must be of adequate capacity, conform to the British Standard and placed out of the reach of children. In the community, small portable bins should be available
- the bins must *never* be more than 3/4 filled, sharps protruding from the aperture of a sharps bin present a major hazard to other users
- bins must be securely closed and labelled with the date and point of origin before being sent for disposal

Fig. 7.6
A resheathing device. If it essential to resheathe a needle than a resheathing device should be used.

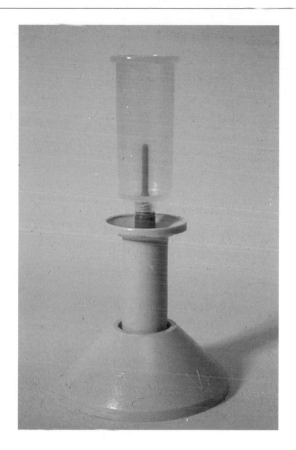

Treatment of Sharps Injuries

Exposure to blood or body fluid, from a sharps injury, bite or from splashing into the eyes, mouth or broken skin, must always be properly followed up because of the risk of infection from blood-borne viruses (Fig. 7.7).

The occupational health department assesses whether any action is necessary to prevent infection with hepatitis B or HIV. The recipient of the injury needs a blood test to establish whether he/she has immunity to hepatitis B virus. If the source of the blood/body fluid is known then the patient can be tested, with their informed consent, for hepatitis B infection. Specific **immunoglobulin** can be administered to the recipient if not immune and the source is a carrier of hepatitis or cannot be identified. This will prevent or moderate the infection by hepatitis B virus provided that it is adminstered quickly, preferably within 48 h of the injury. If the health care worker is not immune, a full course of hepatitis B **vaccination** should be commenced, whether or not hepatitis B immunoglobulin has been given.

At present, there is no vaccination or specific immunoglobulin

Fig 7.7
*Management of sharps injuries
or exposure to blood or body
fluid.*

**SHARPS INJURIES OR
EXPOSURE TO BLOOD AND BODY FLUID**

In case of an injury with a used needle or other sharp or if blood/body fluid is splashed into mouth, eyes or onto broken skin, carry out the following procedure.

1. **Needlepricks, cuts, bites or scratches.**

a) Encourage bleeding by squeezing

b) Wash thoroughly with soap and water.

c) Cover with a waterproof dressing.

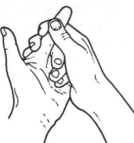 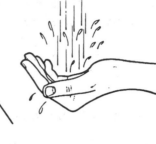 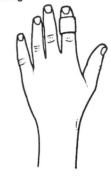

2. **Splashes to mouth or eyes.**
Rinse thoroughly with plenty of running water.

3. **Inform your manager immediately.**

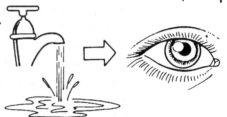

4. **Complete the Accident/Incident Form.**
If known, include the name of the patient from whom the sharp/body fluid came.

5. **Report to the Occupational Health Department immediately.**

6. **If the Occupational Health Department is closed,** attend the Accident and Emergency department for further advice.

**It is the responsibility of the member of staff involved and their
manager to see that this procedure is carried out.**

available for HIV. The occupational health department can offer counselling and arrange, with his/her consent, for the health care worker to be tested for HIV infection (including repeat testing 3, 6 and 12 months following the exposure). Storage of a baseline sample of the health care worker's blood is recommended for subsequent testing if the health care worker acquires HIV to demonstrate that **seroconversion** occurred as a result of the incident.

The use of prophylactic Zidovudine has been recommended when an exposure involves known HIV-infected blood and either a large volume of blood has been inoculated or the needlestick injury was deep (DOH, 1992a). However, it must be administered within 1 h of the injury and there is no clear evidence that it is effective in preventing infection (Jeffries 1991). Each hospital should have a policy specifying the action to be taken in the event of exposure to HIV-infected blood (DOH, 1992a, UK Health Departments, 1993).

There is a legal requirement for employers to keep records of accidents to staff and the records provide a important method of identifying hazardous procedures or inadequate equipment. Accurate records of the time of the injury are essential if compensation is to be awarded. Health care workers who acquire HIV or hepatitis B at work are considered eligible for industrial injury compensation.

Hepatitis B Vaccination

A safe and effective **vaccine** against hepatitis B is available and recommended for immunization of health care workers who have direct contact with blood, blood-stained body fluids or tissues; for staff and clients in residential homes; for people with learning difficulties, where there is known to be a high prevalence of hepatitis B carriage and where behavioural problems increase the risk to staff. **Immunization** should also be considered for other staff who may not directly handle blood but who are at risk from injury by blood contaminated sharps (Department of Health, 1992b; UK Health Departments, 1993).

The Safe Disposal of Waste

Waste from hospitals, clinics, surgeries, veterinary practices or pharmacies which may be toxic, hazardous or infectious, is described as **clinical waste**. The responsibilities of those who produce waste are described in the Environmental Protection Act 1990.

To control infection, waste material contaminated with blood or body fluid must be discarded carefully to prevent exposure or injury to others, particularly those who handle it, and incineration is recommended (HSE, 1992). A colour coding system for waste bags has been adopted nationally (Table 7.6). Potentially infectious waste should be discarded into yellow bags and kept separate for ultimate incineration. If leakage of body fluids is likely, a second bag or a special, impervious container should be used. This particularly applies to the disposal of human tissue, which should not be mixed with other waste.

When approximately three-quarters full waste bags must be properly sealed as if over-filled they tend to break open during removal. They

Table 7.6
Colour coding for clinical waste. Health Services Advisory Committee of the Health and Safety Executive (1992)

Colour of bag	Type of waste	Method of disposal
Black	Uncontaminated paper and other household waste	Landfill
Yellow	Material contaminated with blood or body fluid, human or animal tissue	Incineration
Yellow sharps bin	Syringes, needles, broken glass and any other sharp items	Incineration

should be labelled with the point of origin so that any problem that arises during disposal can be investigated. Bags should only be handled by the neck to minimize the risk of injury from protruding items. A procedure for dealing with spills from a bag should be available.

Clinical waste is often stored for considerable periods prior to collection. The storage area must be dry, the area secure, particularly from children and animals, and free from rodents and insects. Different coloured bags should be separated.

Staff involved in the disposal of clinical waste should be trained in how to handle the waste and what protective clothing is necessary.

Disposal of Clinical Waste in the Home

The situation in the home is different as much smaller amounts of clinical waste are generated and householders are exempt from the 'Duty of Care' for their own household waste. Waste produced and handled only by the patient or his or her family can usually be discarded with the normal household waste where, because it is mixed with large amounts of ordinary waste, it does not present a hazard. Contaminated needles, such as those used by insulin-dependent diabetics, could be hazardous and should if possible be discarded into sharps containers. Some local authorities collect sharps bins from diabetics by arranging for their collection from chemists. If sharps bins are not available then some other form of rigid container, such as a bottle or can should be used to contain the needles, or the needle blunted using needle-clippers.

Health care workers who produce clinical waste in the home, for example community nurses or dialysis technicians, are obliged under the Health and Safety at Work Act to transport and dispose of the clinical waste safely. Small amounts of waste can be discarded into sharps bins, larger quantities (e.g. dressings) present a problem and employers have a responsibility to make arrangements for its disposal (Environmental Protection Act 1990).

Local Authorities have a legal obligation to provide a collection service for infectious waste if requested, but this usually only applies to waste from dialysis patients or those known to be infected with blood-borne viruses. This in itself presents difficulties to the client who may fear possible loss of anonymity if an infected waste collection service is arranged for them. They may prefer to make their own arrangements to take waste to a health centre or GP surgery.

Linen

Laundry staff sort linen by hand into batches of sheets, pillow cases, towels, etc. before washing and may be exposed to potential pathogens on soiled linen, particularly where instruments or 'sharps' are carelessly discarded with linen (Fig. 7.8). The risks can be minimized by the use of protective clothing and the segregation of particularly hazardous linen for disinfection by washing prior to sorting, for example linen from patients infected with enteric pathogens or heavily blood-stained linen (Table 7.7). This infected linen should be sealed in a water-soluble or soluble stitched bag and distinguished from other linen by placing it in a red outer bag. The water-soluble bag can then be removed from the outer bag and placed directly into the washing machine without opening (DOH, 1987).

The micro-organisms are physically removed from linen by the detergent and water and most are destroyed by the high temperature in the wash. Some micro-organisms which remain after washing are destroyed by tumble drying and ironing. Some fabrics are damaged by high wash temperatures and must be decontaminated by the addition of a chemical disinfectant to the rinse cycle instead. Bed linen made of these types of fabrics should be avoided because these chemicals damage the fire-retardancy of the fabric.

Fig 7.8
Sharps found in laundry bags. These sharps present a considerable hazard to the laundry staff.

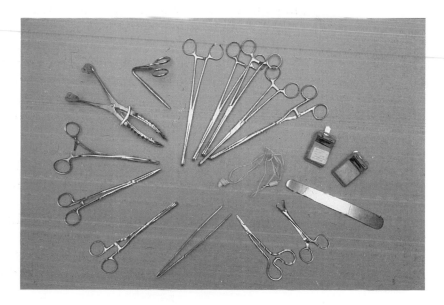

Category	Description	Recommended process
Soiled	Used and fouled linen	Send to laundry in white bags. Thermally disinfect by washing at 65°C for 10 min or 71°C for 3 min
Infected	Linen from patients with enteric infection, open TB, notifiable diseases and other infections specified by Infection Control Doctor	Send to laundry in water-soluble bag and outer red bag Do not sort prior to washing. Thermally disinfect by washing at 65°C for 10 min or 71°C for 3 min
	Heavily blood-stained linen may be included in this category	
Heat-labile	Fabrics damaged by thermal disinfection e.g. wool, synthetics	Send to laundry in bags with orange stripe Wash at 40°C, add hypochlorite to penultimate rinse

Table 7.7
Categorization of hospital linen

Some wards use domestic washing machines to wash patient's clothing. Whilst satisfactory for this purpose, they should not be used to wash bedlinen or other items that will be used by different patients. The normal wash temperatures of 40 or 60°C may not acheive satisfactory heat disinfection and the items are difficult to dry quickly and thoroughly.

Increasingly, duvets are used in clinical areas. Fabric duvets must withstand a wash temperature of 71°C and comply with Department of Health standards of fire retardancy. The duvet cover should be washed between patients and when soiled. The duvet should be washed when soiled and at least once evey 3 months (Webster *et al.*, 1986). PVC-coated duvets should be cleaned with detergent and water between patients in the same way as mattresses.

Excreta

Excreta and other body fluids can contain considerable numbers of potential pathogens and must be discarded safely to minimize the risk of transmission of infection to others. Excreta should be discarded directly into the bedpan washer, macerator or toilet. There is no advantage in adding disinfectant to excreta prior to disposal as it is unlikely to penetrate the organic material. Pathogens are constantly introduced to the drainage system from infected people in the community and it is therefore not worth attempting to remove those from the relatively small amounts entering the system from hospitals.

The risk of transmission of infection between patients on bedpans can be minimized by the use of a bedpan washer with a heat–disinfection cycle, where the bedpan is flushed with water at a temperature of 80°C for a few minutes after washing. Faults in these machines must be reported promptly.

Bedpan macerators should have an effective seal around the door to prevent the escape of aerosols which may contain pathogenic bacteria or viruses.

Decontamination of Equipment

There are numerous examples of infection transmitted between patients on inadequately decontaminated equipment and concerns about the transmission of HIV have highlighted the need to ensure equipment used for invasive procedures is properly decontaminated after every patient, not only those known to be infected.

The method selected should be sufficient to prevent transmission of blood-borne viruses and it should not be necessary to use a higher level of decontamination after use on patients known to be infected by a blood-borne virus.

In some instances it is possible to reduce exposure to equipment contaminated by body fluid by changing practice. For example, swabs used during operations present a considerable hazard to staff who handle and count them on to a swab rack. This risk can be reduced if such swabs are counted directly into clear plastic bags and the contamination of the swab rack can be avoided.

Departments such as intensive care and theatres, which use suction frequently, may choose a disposable suction system to avoid the need to decontaminate suction jars.

Any equipment contaminated by body fluid which required servicing or repair must be decontaminated before it is given to the engineer or returned to the manufacturer (NHS Management Executive, 1993). The principles of decontamination are discussed in more detail in Chapter 13.

Treatment of Spills of Blood or Body Fluid

Dealing with spills of blood or body fluid may expose the health care worker to blood-borne viruses or other pathogens. The task can be carried out more safely if any pathogens in the spillage are first destroyed by a disinfectant.

High concentration chlorine-releasing compounds provide the most economical and effective method of treating body fluid spills (Table 7.8). Chlorine-releasing granules have the advantage of containing the spill rather than adding to it, they have a longer shelf life than hypochlorite

Table 7.8
Methods of treating body fluid spills

Chlorine-releasing granules
- put on disposable gloves and apron
- cover fluid completely with chlorine granules
- leave for 2 min
- remove granules and discard into yellow waste bag
- wash the area with detergent and water

Hypochlorite solution
- put on disposable gloves and apron
- cover spill with disposable paper towels
- pour hypochlorite (10 000 ppm av.Cl) over the towels
- leave for 2 min
- remove towels and discard into a yellow waste bag
- wash area with detergent and water

Do not use either method for large spillages of urine

Urine spillage
- put on disposable gloves and apron
- soak up spill with disposable paper towels
- discard into a yellow waste bag
- wash area with detergent and water

solutions and are more portable (Plate 7.2). In the home, good quality thick bleaches, such as Domestos, contain a high concentration of available chlorine and if diluted 1 in 10 can be use to treat spills. However, chlorine compounds are corrosive to many materials and will bleach the colour from fabrics. They should not be used on carpets or furnishings and residual disinfectant should be removed from surfaces with detergent and water. If chlorine disinfectants cannot be used, spills should be removed using detergent and hot water.

Unfortunately, acidic solutions such as urine may react with the hypochorite and cause the release of chlorine vapour. Hypochlorite solutions should therefore not be used on large urine spills (DOH, 1990).

It may be impractical to treat large spills of blood or body fluid such as may occur in labour wards or operating theatres with hypochlorite. The spill should be soaked up with disposable paper towels or wipes and discarded into a yellow waste bag. The area should then be cleaned with detergent and water.

Education and Training

The adoption of a routine standard of infection control is essential for the safety of both patients and staff. Employers have an obligation to protect

Fig 7.9
*An example of a universal
precautions policy line.*

Handwashing

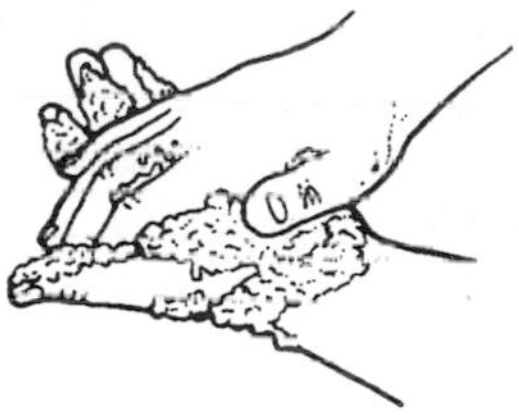

- before and after all patient contact
- after skin contamination with body fluid

Protective clothing

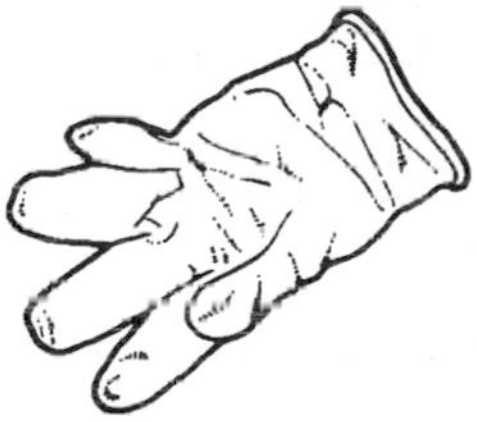

- wear gloves for direct contact with body fluid
- wear plastic apron to protect clothing
- wear eye protection and mask when splashing of body fluid is expected
- change between procedures

Keep cuts covered

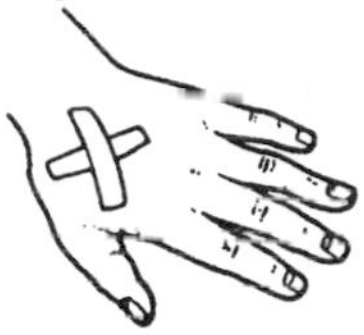

- use a waterproof dressing

Use sharps safely

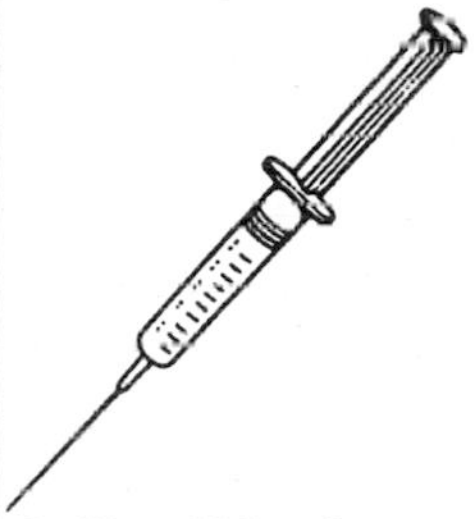

- you are responsible for disposable of sharps you use
- place directly into sharps bin
- never resheathe
- never fill bin more than $\frac{3}{4}$ full
- close bin securely before disposal
- vaccinate against hepatitis B
- follow procedure after sharps injury

Spills of blood

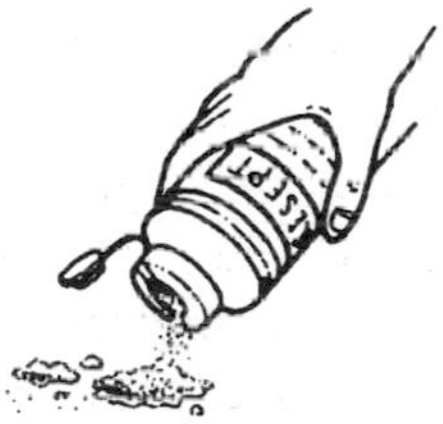

- wear gloves/apron
- cover with chlorine granules
- mop up after 2 min

Waste disposal

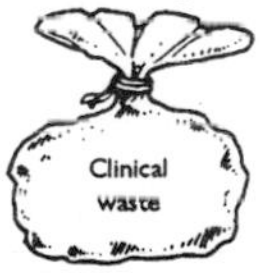

Clinical
waste

- discard excreta directly into drainage system
- use yellow bags for contaminated waste

Equipment

- decontaminate safely after each use
- refer to the disinfection policy

workers from hazards encountered during their work, including micro-biological hazards (Health and Safety at Work Act 1974; COSHH Regulations, 1988; HSE 1992a).

The Health and Safety legislation acknowledges the importance of training and the provision of suitable equipment in establishing safe working practices. The adoption of a routine standard of infection control depends on regular and appropriate education and training to ensure that all health care workers understand the procedures and know what standards are expected. Written policies or standards can help to clarify local arrangements or areas of uncertainty, for example situations where the use of protective clothing is indicated or the local arrange-ments for the disposal of sharps (Fig. 7.9). Essential equipment such as protective clothing and sharps containers must also be readily available in all clinical areas.

References

Adams D, Bagg J, Limaye M *et al.* (1992) A clinical evaluation of glove washing and re-use in dental practice. *J. Hosp. Inf.* **20**: 153–62.

Albert RK, Condie F (1981) Handwashing patterns in medical intensive care units. *New. Engl. J. Med.* **304**: 1465–6.

Ansari SA, Springthorpe VS, Sattar SA *et al.* (1991) Potential role of hands in the spread of respiratory viral infections: studies with human parainfluenza virus 3 and rhinovirus 14. *J. Clin. Micro.* **29**: 2115–19.

Ansari SA, Springthorpe US, Sattar SA *et al.* (1991a) Comparison of cloth, paper and warm air drying in eliminating viruses and bacteria from washed hands. *Am. J. Inf. Contr.* **9**: 243–9.

Ayliffe GAJ (1991) Masks in surgery? *J. Hosp. Inf.* **18**: 165–6.

Booth B (1994) Sensitivity test. Natural rubber (Latex) allergy. *Nursing Times* **90**(36): 30–2.

British Medical Association (1990) *A Code of Practice for the Safe Use and Disposal of Sharps.* BMA, London.

British Standards Institution (1990) Specification for Sharps Containers. BS 7320. British Standards Institution, London.

Burnie JP, Odd FC, Lee W *et al.* (1985) Outbreak of systemic *Candida albicans* in intensive care unit caused by cross-infection. *Brit. Med. J.* **290**: 746–8.

Casewell M, Phillips I (1977) Hands as a route of transmission for *Klebsiella* species. *Brit. Med. J.* **ii**: 1315–17.

Centers for Disease Control (1987) Recommendations for the Prevention of HIV Transmission in Health care Settings. *MMWR* (Aug 21) **36**: (2S).

Centers for Disease Control (1988) Update: Universal precautions for prevention of transmission of human immunodeficiency virus, hepatitis B virus and other blood-borne pathogens in health care settings. *MMWR* (June 24) **37**: 24.

Ciesielski C, Marianos D, Ou CY *et al.* (1992) Transmission of human immuno-deficiency virus in a dental practice. *Ann. Int. Med.* **116**: 798–805.

Coates D, Wilson M. (1989) Use of dichloroisocyanurate granules for spills of body fluids. *J. Hosp. Inf.* **13**. 241–52.

Cookson B, Peters B, Webster M *et al.* (1989) Staff carriage of epidemic methicillin-resistant *Staphylococcus aureus. J. Clin. Micro.* **27**: 1471–6.

Control of Substances Hazardous to Health Regulations (COSHH) (1988) Statutory Instrument No. 1657. HMSO, London.

Davies MS (1994) Blunt-tipped suture needles. *Inf. Contr. Hosp. Epid.*, **15**(4): 191.

Department of the Environment (1991) Environmental Protection Act 1990. *Waste Management: The Duty of Care. A Code of Practice.* HMSO, London.

Department of Health (1987) *Hospital Laundry Arrangements for Used and Infected Linen.* HC(87)30. HMSO. London.

Department of Health (1990) Spills of Urine: potential risk of misuse of chlorine-releasing disinfecting agents. *SAB* **59**(90): 41.

Department of Health (1992a) *Occupational Exposure to HIV and Use of Zidovudine: A Statement From the Expert Advisory Group on Aids.* PL/CO(92). HMSO, London.

Department of Health (1992b) *Immunisation against Infectious Disease.* HMSO, London.

Department of Health (1993) *AIDS–HIV Infected Health Care Workers: Guidance on the Management of Infected Health Care Workers* (Interim update). Expert Advisory Group on AIDS. HMSO. London.

Eisenstein HC, Smith DA (1992) Epidemiology of reported sharps injuries in tertiary care hospital. *J. Hosp. Inf.* **20**: 271–80.

Garner JS, Hierholzer WJ (1993) Controversies in isolation policies and practice. In *Prevention and Control of Nosocomial Infections*, 2nd edn (R.P Wenzel, Ed.), pp 70–81. Williams and Wilkins, Baltimore, MD.

George, Gully PR, Gill ON *et al.* (1986) An outbreak of tuberculosis in a childrens hospital. *J. Hosp. Inf.* **8**: 129–42.

Gerding DN, Johnson S, Olson M *et al.* (1988) Prospective controlled study of vinyl glove use to interrupt *Clostridium difficile* nosocomial transmission. *Abstracts 88th Annual Meeting American Society for Microbiology* **416**: L32.

Gorman LJ, Sanai L, Notman W *et al.* (1993) Cross-infection in an intensive care unit by *Klebsiella pneumoniae* form ventilator condensate. *J. Hosp. Inf.* **23**(1): 27–34.

Gould D (1993) Assessing nurses' hand decontamination performance. *Nursing Times* **89**(25): 47–50.

Greaves WL, Kraiser AB, Alford RH *et al.* (1980) The problem of herpatic whitlow among hospital personnel. *Inf. Control* **1**: 181–5.

Haley RW, Culver DH, White JW *et al.* (1985) The efficacy of surveillance and control programs in preventing nosocomial infections in US hospitals. *Am. J. Epid.* **121**: 182–205.

Hall CB (1981) Nosocomial viral respiratory infections: perennial weeds on paediatric wards. *Am. J. Med.* **70**: 670–6.

Health and Safety Executive, Health Services Advisory Committee (1992) *Safe Disposal of Clinical Waste.* HMSO, London.

Health and Safety Executive (1992a) *Personal Protective Equipment at Work. Regulations* (EEC Directive) HMSO, London.

Heptonstall J, Gill ON, Porter K *et al.* (1993) Health care workers and HIV: surveillance of occupationally acquired infection in the United Kingdom. *CDR Review* **3**(11): R147–R153.

Hoffman PN, Cooke EM, McCarville MR *et al.* (1985) Micro-organisms isolated from skin under wedding rings worn by hospital staff. *Brit. Med. J.* **290**: 206–7.

Jackson MJ, Lynch P (1985) Isolation practices: a historical perspective. *Am. J. Inf. Control.* **13**: 21–31.

Jagger J, Hunt EH, Brand-Elnaggar J *et al.* (1988) Rates of needlestick injury caused by various devices in a University hospital. *NEJM* **318**: 284–8.

Jeffries DJ (1991) Zidovudine after occupational exposure to HIV. *Brit. Med. J.* **302**: 1349–51.

Kaplan LM, McGuckin M (1986) Increasing handwashing compliance with more accessible sinks. *Inf. Cont.* **7**: 408–9.

Knittle MA, Eitzman DV, Baer H (1975) Role of hand contamination of personnel in the epidemiology of gram-negative nosocomial infections. *J. Paeds.* **86**(3): 433–7.

Larson E, Leyden JJ, McGinley KJ *et al.* (1986) Physiologic and microbiologic changes in skin related to frequent handwashing. *Inf. Contr.* **7**: 59–63.

Leclair JM, Freeman J, Sullivan BF *et al.* (1987) Prevention of nosocomial respiratory syncitial virus infections through compliance with glove and gown isolation precautions. *New. Eng. J. Med.* **6**: 317–34.

Lowbury EJL, Lilley HA (1973) Use of 4% chlorhexidine detergent solution (Hibiscrub) and other methods of skin disinfection in wards. *J. Hyg. (Camb.)* **76**: 75.

Lilley HA, Lowbury EJL, Wilkins MD (1979) Limits to progressive reduction of resident skin bacteria by disinfection. *J. Clin. Path.* **32**: 382–5.

Lynch P, Cummings MJ, Roberts PL, Herriott MJ, Yates B, Stamm WE (1990) Implementing and evaluating a system of generic infection control precautions: Body Substance Isolation. *Am. J. Inf. Control* **18**: 1–13.

Lynch P, Jackson MM, Cummings MJ *et al.* (1987) Rethinking the role of isolation practices in the prevention of nosocomial infections. *Ann. Int. Med.* **107**: 243–6.

McCleod GG (1989) Needlestick injuries at operations for trauma. Are surgical gloves an effective barrier? *J. Bone Joint Surg. Br.* **71**(3): 489–91.

Mackintosh CA, Hoffman PN (1984) An extended model for the transfer of micro-organisms and the effect of alcohol disinfection. *J. Hyg.* **92**: 345–55.

Marples RR, Towers AG (1979) A laboratory model for the investigation of contact transfer of micro-organisms. *J. Hyg.* **82**: 237–48.

Matta H, Thompson AM, Rainey JB (1988) Does wearing two pairs of gloves protect operating staff from skin contamination? *Brit. Med. J.* **297**: 597–8.

Morse LJ, Schonbek LE (1968) Hand lotions and potential nosocomial hazard. *New Engl. J. Med.* **278**: 376–8.

NHS Management Executive (1993) *Decontamination of Equipment Prior to Inspection, Service or Repair.* HSG(93)26. HMSO, London.

Ojajärvi J, Mäkelä P, Rautasalo I (1977) Failure of hand disinfection with frequent handwashing: a need for prolonged field studies. *J Hyg. (Camb.)* **79**: 107–12.

Olsen RJ, Lynch P, Coyle MB *et al.* (1993) Examination gloves as barriers to hand contamination in clinical practice. *J. Am. Med. Ass.* **270**(3): 350–3.

Palmer JD, Rickett JWS (1992) The mechanisms and risks of surgical glove perforation *J. Hosp. Inf.* **22**: 279–86.

Parry CM, Harries AD, Beeching NJ *et al.* (1991) Phlebotomy in inoculation risk patients: a questionnaire survey of knowledge and practices of hospital doctors in Liverpool. *J. Hosp. Inf.* **18**: 313–18.

Patterson JE, Vecchio J, Pantelick EL (1991) Association of contaminated gloves with transmission of *Acinetobacter calcoaceticus* var. *anitratus* in an intensive care unit. *Am. J. Med.* **91**: 479–83.

Heptonstall J, Porter K, Gill N (1993) *Occupational Transmission of HIV.* Summary of published reports. PHLS AIDS Centre, CDSC, London.

Reid JA, Breckon D, Hunter PR (1990) Infection of staff during an outbreak of viral gastro-enteritis in an elderly persons' home. *J. Hosp. Inf.* **16**: 81–6.

Reybrouck G (1983) Role of the hands in the spread of nosocomial infections. 1. *J. Hosp. Inf.* **4**: 103–110.

Saghafi L, Raselli P, Francillon C *et al* (1992) Exposure to blood during various procedures: results of two surveys before and after implementation of universal precautions. *Am, J. Inf. Contr.* **20**(2): 53–7.

Samadi AR, Huq MI, Ahmed QS (1983) Detection of rotavirus in handwashings of attendants of children with diarrhoea. *Brit. Med. J.* **286**: 188.

Sanderson PJ, Weissler S (1992) Recovery of coliforms from the hands of nurses and patients: activities leading to contamination. *J. Hosp. Inf.* **21**: 85–93.

Scanlon JW, Leikkanen M (1973) The use of fluorescein powder for evaluating contamination in a newborn nursery. *J. Paed.* **82**: 966–71.

Speller DCE, Shanson DC, Ayliffe GAJ *et al.* (1990) Acquired immune deficiency syndrome. Recommendations of a Working Party of the Hospital Infection Society. *J. Hosp. Inf.* **15**: 17–34.

Sprunt K, Redman W, Leidy G (1973) Antibacterial effectiveness of routine handwashing. *Pediatrics* **52**: 264–71.

Taylor L (1978) An evaluation of handwashing techniques. *Nursing Times* **74**: 108–10.

Tomlinson D. To clean or not to clean? *Nursing Times* **83**: 71–5.

UK Health Departments (1990) *Guidance for Clinical Health Care Workers: Protection Against Infection with HIV and Hepatitis viruses.* Recommendations of the Expert Advisory Group on AIDS. HMSO, London.

UK Health Departments (1991) *AIDS – HIV Infected Health Care Workers. Occupational Guidance for Health Care Workers, their Physicians and Employers.* Recommendations of the Expert Advisory Group on AIDS. HMSO, London.

UK Health Departments (1993) *Protecting Health Care Workers and Patients from Hepatitis B.* Recommendations of the advisory group on hepatitis. HMSO, London.

Wade JJ, Desai N, Casewell MW (1991) Hygienic hand disinfection for the removal of epidemic vancomycin-resistant *Enterococcus faecium* and gentamicin-resistant *Enterobacter cloacae.* *J. Hosp. Inf.* **18**(3): 211–18.

Webster O, Cowan M, Allen J (1986) Dirty linen. *Nursing Times* **Oct 29**: 36–7.

West DJ (1984) The risk of hepatitis B infection among health professionals in the United States: a review. *Am. J. Med. Sci.* **287**: 26–33.

Williams E, Buckles A (1988) A lack of motivation. *Nursing Times* **84**: 60–4.

Wilson J, Breedon P (1990) Universal precautions. *Nursing Times* **86**: 67–70.

Further Reading

Ayton M (1983) Continental quilts – their use in hospitals. *Nursing Times* **July 27**: 64–5.

Barrie D (1994) How hospital linen and laundry services are provided. *J. Hosp. Inf.* **27**(3): 219–36.

Jackson MM, Lynch P (1986) Education of the adult learner: a practical approach for the infection control practitioner. *Am. J. Inf. Contr.* **14**: 257–71.

Hoffman PN, Wilson JA (1995) Hands, hygiene and hospitals. *PHLS Micro Digest* **11**(4): 211-6.

Larson E (1988) A causal link between handwashing and risk of infection? Examination of the evidence. *Inf. Contr. Hosp. Epid.* **9**(1): 28–36.

Thomas L (1994) Glove story. *Nursing Times* **90**(36): 33–5.

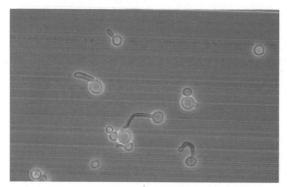

Plate 1.1 *Candida albicans*. When incubated in serum the cells produce characteristic outgrowths called germ tubes.

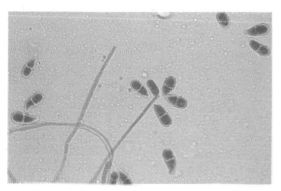

Plate 1.2 A filamentous fungi. Tubular hyphae with groups of spores.

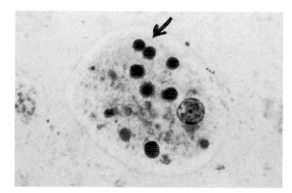

Plate 1.3 *Entamoeba histolytica*. These protozoa cause amoebic dysentry. The black dots are red blood cells which have been engulfed. The nucleus can be seen in the lower right of the cell.

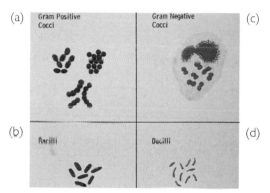

Plate 2.1 There are four main groups of bacteria: (a) Gram-positive cocci, (b) Gram-positive bacilli (rods), (c) Gram-negative cocci, and (d) Gram-negative bacilli (rods).

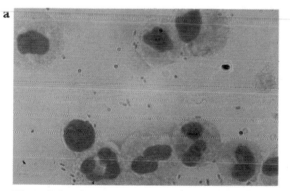

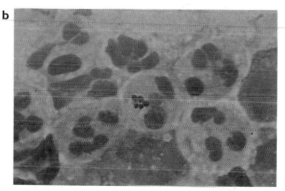

Plate 2.2 Cerebrospinal fluid from two cases of meningitis. (**a**) Large mononuclear cells and neutrophils can be seen with a number of small Gram-negative rods. Provisional diagnosis: *Haemophilus influenzae* meningitis. (**b**) Cerebrospinal fluid containing large numbers of pus cells. Some neutrophils contain small Gram-negative diplococci. Provisional diagnosis: *Neisseria meningitidis* meningitis.

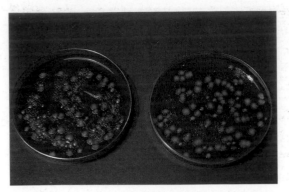

Plate 2.3 Large colonies of *Bacillus cereus*.

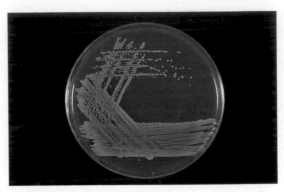

Plate 2.4 *Staphylococcius aureus*.

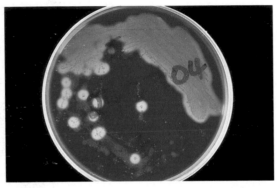

Plate 2.5 *Streptococcus* Group A. Haemolysins produced by *Streptococcus* lyse the red blood cells in blood agar, producing a clear area around the colonies.

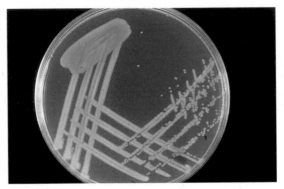

Plate 2.6 *Pseudomonas aeruginosa*. The colonies of *Ps. aeruginosa* appear green when grown on nutrient agar.

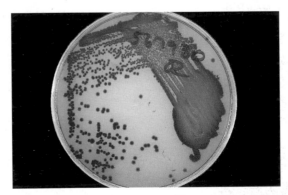

Plate 2.7 *Serratia marcescens*. The colonies of *S. marcescens* have a characteristic red coloration.

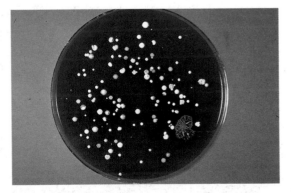

Plate 2.8 Mixed growth of organisms. Specimens often contain more than one type of bacteria, illustrated by the different forms of colony on this plate.

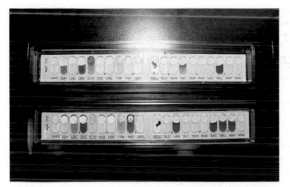

Plate 2.9 API galleries. The colour change in each chamber of the gallery helps to identify the species of bacteria present.

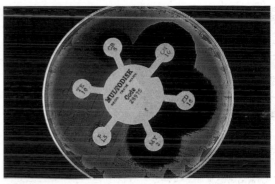

Plate 2.10 Antibiotic sensitivity testing. Antibiotics in each disc diffuse into the agar. Bacteria cannot grow around the discs unless they are resistant to the antibiotic in the disc.

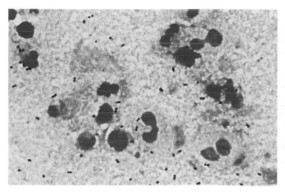

Plate 2.11 Sputum from a case of suspected pneumonia. Gram-positive cocci, mostly in pairs, can be seen amongst the numerous, large, pus cells. Provisional diagnosis: pneumococcal pneumonia.

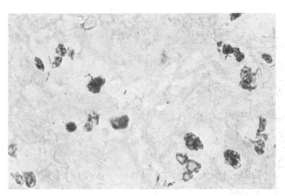

Plate 2.12 Tubercle bacilli appear as clumps of fine rods.

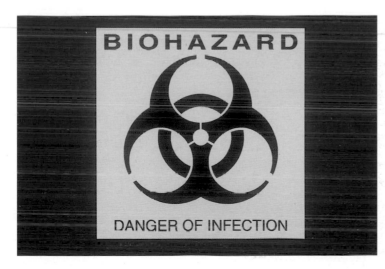

Plate 2.13 Biohazard label.

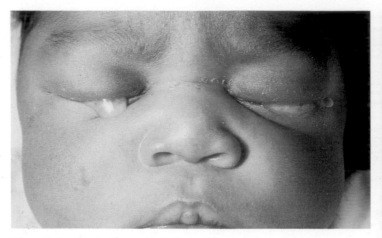

Plate 3.1 Staphylococcal infection of the eyes.

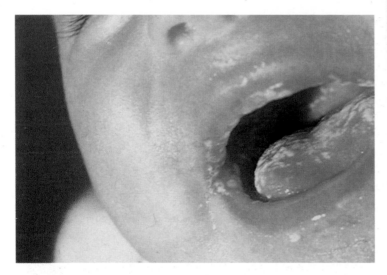

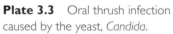

Plate 3.2 Erysipelas. An acute cellulitis caused by *Streptococcus*.

Plate 3.3 Oral thrush infection caused by the yeast, *Candida*.

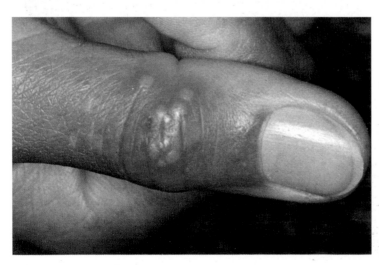

Plate 3.4 Herpatic whitlow caused by the Herpes simplex virus.

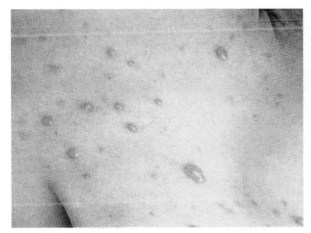

Plate 3.5 Chickenpox infection.

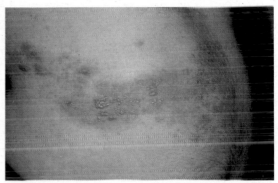

Plate 3.6 Herpes zoster (shingles).

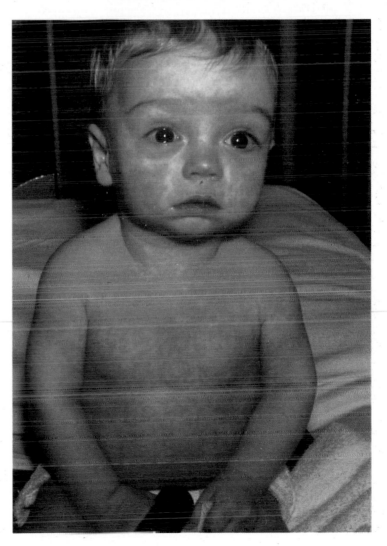

Plate 3.7 Measles infection.

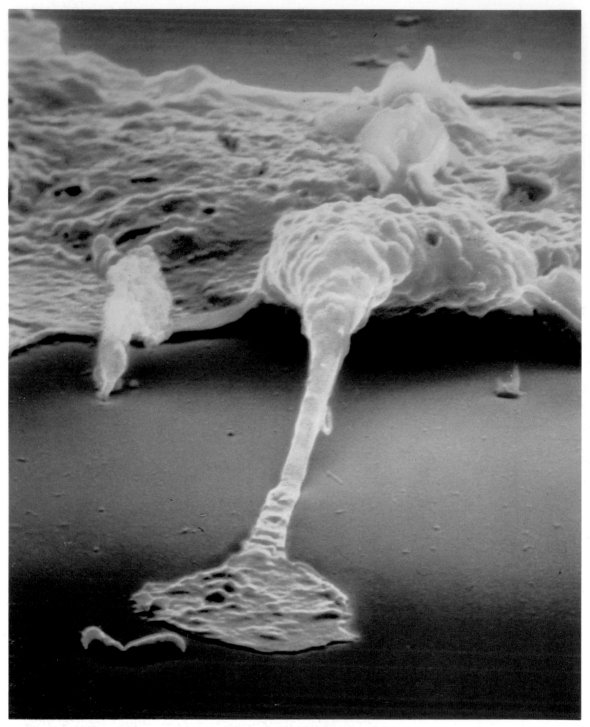

Plate 4.1   A macrophage extends a pseudopod to ingest a bacterium.

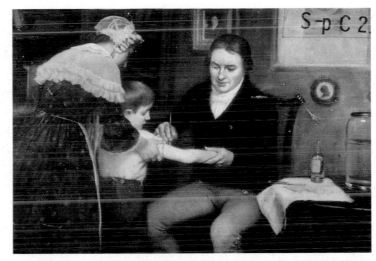

Plate 4.2 The first vaccination (Edward Jenner).

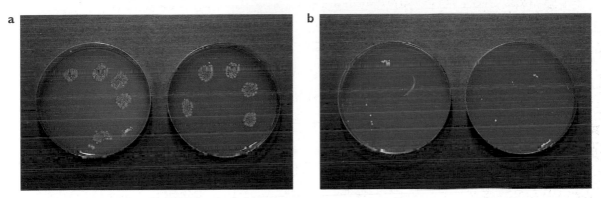

Plate 7.1 The effect of handwashing. (**a**) Fingertips pressed on to blood agar before washing. (**b**) Fingertips pressed on to blood agar after washing with soap and water.

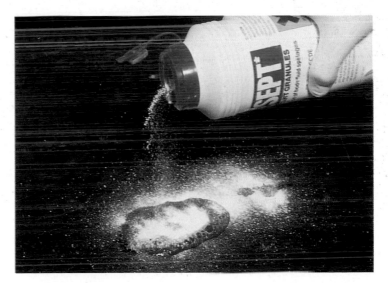

Plate 7.2 Chlorine-based granules can be used to soak up spills of blood.

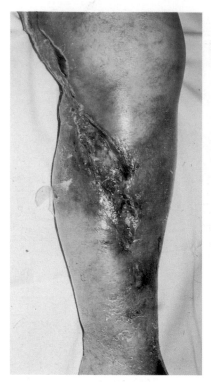

Plate 8.1 Infection in a surgical wound.

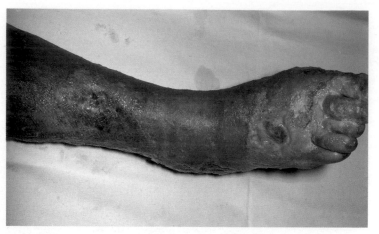

Plate 8.2 A chronic wound. Slough and superficial pus is present on the surface of the wound but without signs of infection.

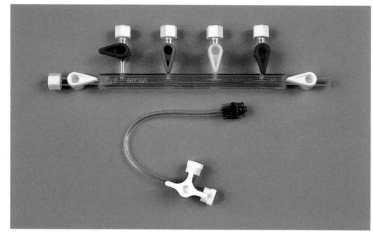

Plate 9.1 A set of access points and a three-way tap used with intravascular devices.

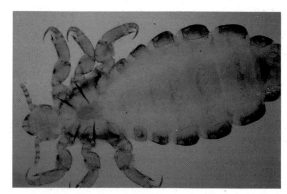

Plate 15.1 The female head louse (*Pediculus humanus capitis*).

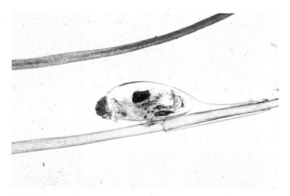

Plate 15.2 A louse egg (nit) attached to a hair.

Preventing Wound Infection

Introduction

A wound has been defined as a loss of continuity of skin or tissue (Ayton, 1985) and may result from accidental trauma, an underlying disease process (e.g. venous ulceration), or a surgical procedure. When considering the prevention of infection in wounds it is important to distinguish between wounds healing by **secondary intention** in which there is loss of tissue and the remaining tissues are exposed for many days or weeks, and the surgical wound when exposure of the underlying tissue only occurs for a few minutes or hours and healing occurs by **primary intention** (Fig. 8.1). In healing by secondary intention the gap must be gradually filled from the base by new tissue. This process is accelerated by contraction – contractile cells in the wound gradually move the edges of the wound into the centre and decrease its size.

Epithelial cells are constantly shed and replaced from the surface of the skin. When skin is damaged these cells migrate across the living tissue, towards areas where cells are lost or depleted. This process is called **epithelization** and is particularly important for healing by secondary intention.

The processes that take place in a wound as it heals are summarized in Table 8.1.

The Surgical Wound

Surgical wound infections account for around 20% of infections acquired by patients in hospital (Meers *et al.*, 1981; Haley *et al.*, 1985). There are a number of potential **sources of bacteria** that cause these infections, but the most common is the patient's own microbial flora (Table 8.2). The

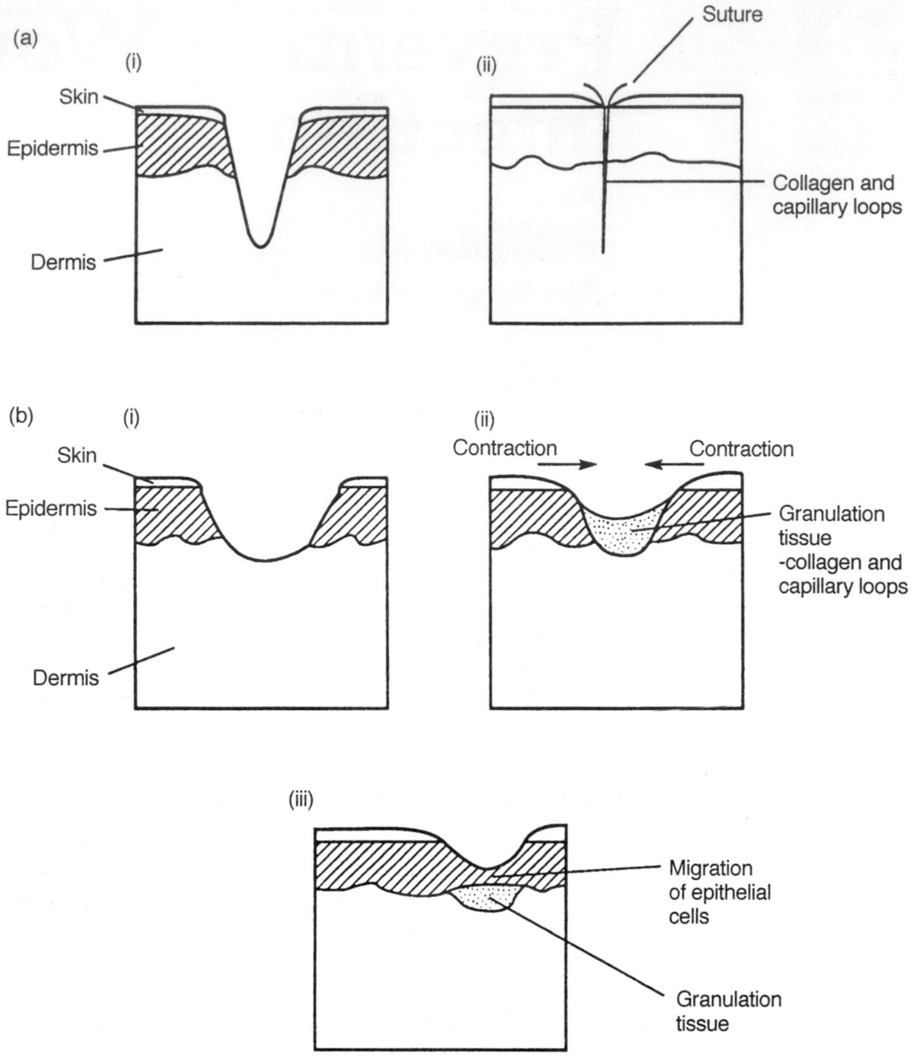

Fig. 8.1
The process of wound healing.
(a) Healing by primary
intention. (b) Healing by
secondary intention.

Table 8.1 *Stages in wound healing*	Stage 1 (0–3 days) *Inflammation phase*	Injured blood vessels thrombose, clot forms. Damaged tissue releases histamine causing vasodilation. Increased blood supply brings macrophages and polymorphonucleocytes. Epithelization begins
	Stage 2 (2–5 days) *Destructive phase*	Polymorphs and macrophages remove dead tissue and stimulate multiplication of fibroblasts
	Stage 3 (3–24 days) *Proliferation phase*	Fibroblasts begin to produce fibres of collagen (a protein which is the main constituent of structural tissue e.g. skin, bone, ligaments). New capillary loops grow into the collagen to form granulation tissue
	Stage 4 (24 days– 1 year) *Maturation phase*	More collagen fibres are made and reorganized to increase strength of the scar

Table 8.2
Surgical wound infections –
potential sources of
bacteria

Patient:
  Skin
  Colonized hollow organs
  Other infection, abscesses

Theatre:
  Staff
  Instruments
  Airborne particles

Ward:
  Staff
  Dressings
  Airborne particles

Table 8.3
Factors that increase the
risk of surgical wound
infection

In the wound	In the patient
Number of bacteria present	Debility
Dead tissue present	Malnourishment
Haematoma formation	Obesity
Tissue damage during procedure	Underlying illness eg diabetes
Foreign material present	Immune deficiency

risk of infection in a surgical wound depends on a delicate balance between the host immune defences and the number of bacteria present in the wound at the end of the operation. This balance is influenced by the condition of the wound and the susceptibility of the patient to infection (Table 8.3).

Factors Influencing the Risk of Wound Infection

Bacterial Contamination of the Wound

Wounds are able to heal despite the presence of quite large numbers of bacteria. Kriezek and Robson (1975) found that wound infection occurred only if more than 100 000 bacteria per gram of tissue were present during wound closure.

Since the bacteria that cause surgical wound infections are frequently derived from the patient's own **normal flora** the number of bacteria in the wound at the end of the procedure depends on the site of the body involved. Some parts of the body, for example the intestines, are **colonized** by large numbers of bacteria which readily enter the wound when surgery is performed on the bowel. Prior to surgery on the colon various methods are used to reduce the number of bacteria in the bowel (e.g. elemental diets, purgatives, antibiotics). Surgery that involves abscesses or necrosed tissue, when significant numbers of bacteria may already be present, is also more likely to result in wound infection. Other types of surgery, for example orthopaedic surgery, are less likely to encounter colonizing bacteria and the risk of surgical wound infection developing is correspondingly smaller (Table 8.4).

Prophylactic antibiotics are used for surgery where the risk of post-operative wound infection is high; that is, clean surgery involving the implantation of foreign material, clean-contaminated and contaminated surgery. The antibiotic should be effective against the bacteria most likely to cause infection in the wound, should be administered at the time of wound contamination or just before, and should not be prolonged for more than a few hours after surgery.

Surgical Technique

A considerable proportion of surgical wound infection has been attributed to the technique of the surgeon (Bucknall, 1985; Cruse, 1986). Tissues must be handled gently to avoid damaging the blood supply and subsequent impairment of wound healing. Bleeding points must be sealed to prevent the seepage of blood into the wound. The presence of haematomas and dead tissue in the wound encourages the multiplication of bacteria which may then be able to establish infection. Differences in infection rate for the same type of operation performed by different surgeons can frequently be accounted for by their technique (Garner, 1986).

Table 8.4
Classification of wound contamination

Category	Description	Type of surgery	Approximate infection rate (%)
Clean	Gastrointestinal and respiratory tract not entered. No inflamed tissue, no break in technique	Orthopaedic, neurosurgery	< 2
Clean-contaminated	Gastrointestinal or respiratory tract entered but no spillage of contents	Appendicec-tomy	8
Contaminated	Acute inflamed tissue, spillage from hollow organ, traumatic wounds, major break in technique	Abdominal surgery	15
Dirty	Pus encountered, perforated hollow organ. Delayed treatment of traumatic wounds	Drainage of abscess	40

Foreign Bodies

The presence in tissue of even a small foreign body has a dramatic effect on the immune defences. This was first demonstrated by Elek and Conen (1957) who inoculated the forearms of medical students with *Staphylococcus aureus*. They found that only 100 bacteria were necessary to cause infection in the presence of a silk suture compared to the 6.5 million bacteria required without a suture. Small areas of **inflammation** around skin sutures on surgical wounds are frequently observed although they rarely develop into infection.

Some bacteria are able to adhere to implanted material such as joint replacements and prosthetic heart valves where they multiply to cause infection, with devastating consequences for the patient (Sanderson, 1991).

Duration of Surgery

The longer that tissues are exposed the greater the chance that bacteria carried by airborne particles will settle onto the tissues or be carried into the wound on hands or instruments (Whyte *et al.*, 1982). Each additional hour of surgery increases the risk of postoperative wound infection (Cruse and Foord, 1973; CDC, 1991).

Susceptibility of the Patient to Infection

The risk of a patient acquiring a wound infection is influenced by their susceptibility to infection and the ability of the wound to heal.

Underlying disease may depress the response of the immune system, for example diabetes interferes with **phagocytosis** by **white blood cells** and increases the susceptibility of diabetic patients to infection. **Immunosuppressive** therapy or steroid treatment also depress the immune response and enable bacteria to multiply in the wound.

There is a significant correlation between increasing age and the risk of developing wound infection (Cruse, 1986). Poor nutrition may delay wound healing and increase the opportunity for bacteria to establish infection. Weight loss and obesity are both associated with an increased risk of infection (Cruse and Foord, 1973; Bucknall, 1985).

Patients who already have an infection, for example pneumonia or urinary tract infection, at the time of surgery are more prone to develop a wound infection and infections should be treated before surgery is performed (Valentine *et al.*, 1986).

An awareness of the underlying factors that predispose patients to infection can help the nurse to recognize patients at greatest risk, enhance their resistance to infection as much as possible before surgery and observe them closely postoperatively for early signs of infection.

Reducing the Risk of Surgical Wound Infection

Preoperative Hospitalization

From the time of admission to hospital, the normal harmless flora of the patient's skin is gradually replaced by hospital **pathogens** which may then be introduced into the surgical wound (Noone *et al.*, 1983). Cruse and Foord (1980) demonstrated that the longer a patient stayed in hospital before surgery, the greater the probability that the wound would become infected. When the pre-operative stay was one day, 1.2% of wounds became infected, whilst 3.4% of wounds became infected if the patient has been in hospital for more than 2 weeks.

Hospital stay can be reduced to a minimum by performing essential preoperative investigations in assessment clinics and admitting the patient on the day before or the day of surgery.

Preoperative Bathing

Bacteria present on the patient's skin can be introduced into the wound during surgery. *Staphylococcus aureus*, a **skin commensal**, is responsible for one-third of surgical wound infections. Reducing bacterial colonization of the skin prior to incision has therefore been advocated as a means of minimizing the risk of infection. Treatment of the skin with antiseptic can be carried out as a bath or shower before the patient reaches the operating theatre, although many studies have not demonstrated a significant reduction in wound infection rate (Ayliffe *et al.*, 1983; Lynch *et al.*, 1992).

In addition, most surgeons cleanse the skin with an alcoholic solution of iodine or chlorhexidine prior to making an incision to reduce the number of skin bacteria present when the incision is made.

Shaving the Skin

A number of studies have shown that shaving the skin prior to surgery increases the risk of wound infection (Alexander *et al.*, 1983; Cruse 1986). Bacteria multiply in micro-abrasions caused by the razor on the surface of the skin, particularly if the skin is shaved some hours prior to surgery. Removal of hair with an electric shaver is associated with a lower infection rate but shavers present their own cross-infection problems if used between patients (Millward, 1992). Hair clippers may provide a suitable alternative and cause less damage (Pettersson, 1986). The use of depilatory creams instead of razors reduces the risk of wound infection but they can cause an allergic reaction and may not remove hair of male patients (Seropian and Reynolds, 1971).

Hair is no more heavily colonized with microbial flora than the skin and the criteria for hair removal should be based on the need to view or access the operative site rather than to remove bacteria. The best solution is to remove the minimum amount of hair as near to the time of surgery as possible.

Antibiotic Prophylaxis

Prophylactic antibiotic treatment is recommended for surgery associated with a high risk of infection or when a prosthesis is inserted and an infection at the site, although unusual, would be disastrous. The aim is to inhibit bacterial growth in the wound and other areas prone to post-operative infection. For example, an appendicectomy for an inflamed appendix may be complicated by an infected wound and peritonitis, and antibiotic prophylaxis is intended to prevent both. The choice of anti-biotic is based on the species of bacteria most likely to contaminate the wound. The administration of the antibiotics should be timed to achieve the right levels in blood and tissue before bacterial contamination occurs and to maintain them during surgery.

Procedures in the Operating Department

Ventilation and Air Filtration

Air contains micro-organisms on airborne particles such as skin squames, dust, lint or respiratory droplets. In theatre, the main source of airborne bacteria are staff.

The number of airborne microbial particles in an operating room is proportional to the number of humans present and their level of activity. Each person has been estimated to emit approximately 10 000 organisms per minute at rest, increasing to 50 000 per minute during activity as friction of clothing against the skin releases more squames (Howarth, 1985). These particles may settle on to instruments, gloved hands or into the wound itself and subsequently result in wound infection (Whyte *et al.*, 1982; Hambreus, 1988). Barrie *et al.* (1992) reported an unusual outbreak of surgical wound infection caused by linen contaminated with *Bacillus cereus*. Lint from the contaminated linen was thought to have entered the wound directly or after settling on instruments, but infection occurred during two neurosurgical operations which lasted for many hours and provided ample opportunity for bacteria to enter the wound and establish infection.

Special ventilation systems are used to filter out airborne micro-organisms and prevent micro-organisms entering the theatre in the air supply from corridors or other parts of the hospital. Air is forced into the theatre through filters in the ceiling which remove particles and bacteria, the volume of air in the room will be changed approximately 20 times an hour (less frequently in scrub-up and anaesthetic rooms). Theatres are plenum ventilated; that is, a higher pressure is maintained in the room to prevent unfiltered air from outside flowing in through the doors (Fig. 8.2). Ultraclean air systems are recommended to reduce the incidence of infection in orthopaedic surgery involving the insertion of implants. These systems use a controlled flow of filtered air over the operating table and over 600 air changes per hour (Lidwell *et al.*, 1982).

The number of airborne particles can be reduced by keeping the number and activity of people present during surgery to a minimum and ensuring that the ventilation system is not disrupted by opening operating room doors during the procedure. Dust should not be allowed to collect on surfaces where it may be disturbed and become airborne.

Handwashing

The transfer of micro-organisms from the surgeon's hands to the wound may be reduced by handwashing. Whilst soap removes the transient flora of the skin, microbicidal detergents (surgical scrubs) are used to reduce the resident microbial flora of the skin (see Chapter 7). To achieve maximum reduction, the hands and arms should be washed thoroughly ensuring that all parts are covered with the detergent. Chlorhexidine and povidone–iodine have a persistent effect on skin micro-organisms there-

Fig. 8.2
Ventilation of an operating theatre. Air moves from the cleanest areas to the least clean areas. Arrows indicate direction of air flow.

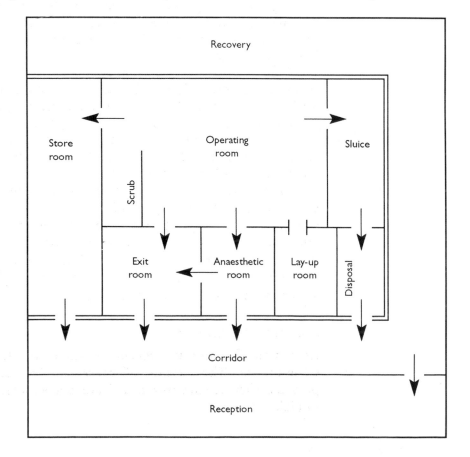

fore repeated washes through the day gradually reduce the number of bacteria on the skin (Ojajärvi, 1976). Alcohol handrub solutions containing a microbicide such as chlorhexidine are equally effective and could be used in place of surgical scrubs (Lilley *et al.*, 1979).

Operating Room Clothing

Micro-organisms are constantly shed from skin, therefore personnel directly involved in the operation wear sterile gowns to limit the transmission of their microbial skin flora into the open wound. Although gowns provide some protection against contamination by body fluid, they do not completely prevent bacteria shed from the skin escaping from the openings at the neck, ankles and wrists as well as through pores in the fabric (Whyte *et al.*, 1976). The passage of bacteria is enhanced if the material becomes wet (Hoborn, 1990). Gowns made of non-woven materials or close-woven polyester fabrics can reduce the dispersal of bacteria (Matthews *et al.*, 1985; Whyte *et al.*, 1990) and are often recommended for orthopaedic surgery.

Masks are conventionally worn to prevent bacteria from the upper respiratory tract entering the wound. There is little evidence to suggest a significant risk of transmission by this route (Ayliffe, 1991a). The mask rubbing against the skin may actually increase the shedding of skin squames (Schweizer, 1976; Mitchell and Hunt, 1991). Masks are of course necessary to protect the operator from splashes of blood or body fluid (Chapter 7).

Whilst head covers may prevent bacteria on hairs entering the operative sites they probably have limited impact on counts of bacteria in the air (Humphries *et al.*, 1991a). They are therefore probably of little value for non-scrubbed staff assisting most types of surgery. Overshoes also appear to have no effect on bacterial counts on the floor (Humphries *et al.*, 1991b) and since the open wound has no contact with the floor there seems to be no logical reason for their use.

Sterile gloves are worn to prevent the transmission of the operator's skin flora into the wound. Evidence from operations performed with punctured gloves suggests that there is no increase in the rate of wound infection as a result of bacteria leaking out of the glove from the skin (Cruse, 1986; Whyte *et al.*, 1991). Gloves are essential to protect the operator from exposure to blood and may provide some protection against needlestick injury (Chapter 7).

Instruments and Equipment

Items used for invasive procedures should be sterile when used (see Chapter 13). The sterility of packs can be maintained indefinitely provided they remain intact, and are not exposed to moisture, direct sunlight or heat.

Cleaning

In a modern, well-managed theatre the risk of infection from the environment is low (Ayliffe, 1991b). Smears of blood and body fluid on surfaces should be removed with detergent and water after each operation and spills treated with chlorine-releasing granules (see Chapter 7). Horizontal surfaces, which readily collect dust, should be cleaned daily and the minimum amount of equipment should be kept in the operating room to prevent the collection of dust and avoid unnecessary cleaning.

There is usually no need to allocate infected patients to the end of an operating list provided that spills of blood or body fluid are removed at the end of the operation, dust removed from surfaces and ventilator tubing changed. Suspended particles will be rapidly removed by the air filtration system and the next patient can be brought into the room as soon as it has been cleaned.

Wound Drains

A wound is more likely to become infected if a drain leading from the tissues out through the skin is inserted as it will provide a route through which bacteria can enter the wound (Cruse, 1986). A drain can facilitate wound healing by preventing the formation of haematomas. When required, a closed drainage system, for example emptying directly into a bag or bottle, is recommended since this reduces the risk of bacteria entering the wound. (Alexander *et al.*, 1976).

Postoperative Care

Although the first signs of infection in a surgical wound become apparent during postoperative care, usually 4–10 days after surgery, most of these infections will probably have been established during surgery. As soon as the wound has been sutured a loose mesh of fibrin is formed and is gradually infiltrated by fibroblasts and collagen. Within a few hours this structure has become impervious to the entry of bacteria and, provided the dressing applied in theatre remains undisturbed, pathogens are unlikely to gain access to the wound.

Surveillance of Wound Infection

Since there is a strong association between the surgeon's technique and the development of postoperative wound infection, continuous monitoring or audit of wound infection rates can provide useful information for surgeons to improve their practice.

Several studies have illustrated the value of providing individual surgeons with information about their infection rates. The information acts as a reminder of the risks of introducing infection during surgery and the importance of good surgical technique in preventing infection (Cruse and Foord, 1980; Haley, 1986). Major reductions in wound infection rates have been reported when such **surveillance** and feedback programmes are used (Cruse, 1986).

One of the problems associated with surgical wound infection surveillance is the difficulty of detecting infections that develop after the patient has been discharged from hospital. As many as 50% of wound infections may develop post-discharge and this can result in a significant under-reporting of infection rates unless the some form of post-discharge surveillance is included (Mishriki *et al.*, 1990).

Wounds Healing By Secondary Intention

Healing by secondary intention is a description of healing in wounds when there is tissue loss and the gap must be gradually filled from the base by new tissue. These type of wounds are often referred to as chronic wounds and include ulcers, pressure sores, burns and some surgical wounds in which closure by suture is delayed (e.g. blast injuries, dehisced wounds).

Prevention of Infection In Chronic Wounds

Exposed tissue provides an ideal growth medium for many micro-organisms and the wound rapidly becomes colonized with a variety of bacteria acquired from the patient's own normal flora and the environment. Wounds appear to be able to heal despite the presence of these bacteria provided that they do not invade the tissue and cause infection, although some species have been implicated in the poor healing of ulcers (Hutchinson and Lawrence, 1991). Attempting to discourage bacterial growth in a wound by removing exudate and keeping the wound surface dry is inappropriate. Epithelization, the formation of new granulation tissue and micro-circulation are all encouraged in the moist environment provided by an occlusive dressing on the wound (Winter, 1962; Lydon *et al.*, 1989).

Wound exudate contains white blood cells which play a major role in destroying bacteria and preventing subsequent infection in the tissues. Their activity is enhanced if the wound is occluded (Clarke, 1985; Buchan *et al.*, 1980).

The best method of preventing infection in chronic wounds is to ensure that the wound heals as rapidly as possible. Infection is more likely to occur in wounds with a poor blood supply, where the tissue is not well oxygenated and there are fewer white blood cells. **Necrotic tissue** can encourage bacterial multiplication and infection and delay healing. It should be removed from wounds by surgical means or with dressings that promote desloughing (Hutchinson and Lawrence, 1991).

Burns

Burns are always colonized by a variety of micro-organisms. Although most do not usually interfere with healing, some may invade the tissues and cause **septicaemia**, a frequent and serious complication of severely burned patients. *Streptococcus pyogenes* is associated with failure of skin grafts and *Pseudomonas aeruginosa* can interfere with skin grafting and cause invasive infections which are sometimes fatal (Lowbury and Cason, 1985).

Skin flora such as staphylococci are the predominant species in the first few days. They are often replaced by **Gram-negative** rods which proliferate in the necrotic tissue but once the **slough** has separated, **Gram-positive** bacteria again predominate on the granulation tissue.

Cross-infection is a major problem in burns units, particularly with *S. aureus*, *Pseudomonas* and other Gram-negative **bacilli** such as *Acinetobacter*. The main risk of transmission is on the hands of staff. Contaminated equipment has also been implicated in outbreaks of infection in burns units (Kolmos *et al.*, 1993). The large surface area of damaged skin increases the probability of micro-organisms being introduced from an airborne route, particularly those bacteria which are more resistant to desiccation such as staphylococci and *Acinetobacter*. Large numbers of bacteria may be released during dressing changes and the use of a dressing room supplied with filtered air at around 10 changes per hour can be used to reduce the risk of cross-infection (Ayliffe and Lilly, 1985).

Topical antimicrobial solutions are used to control colonization and reduce mortality associated with burns. Commonly used agents are silver nitrate, silver sulphadiazine and chlorhexidine creams. These agents are helpful in preventing colonization of burns by *Ps. aeruginosa* but will not remove it if already established in the burn (Lowbury and Cason, 1985). Topical antimicrobial solutions are not recommended for other types of wound.

The Care of Wounds

The nurse has a major role to play in preventing the transmission of bacteria in wounds between patients and in minimizing the risk of wound infection developing. However, the care of the wound should not be solely directed at the dressing procedure. Encouraging rapid wound healing reduces the possibility of wound infection. Adequate nutrition is essential for wound healing to take place. Collagen, the principal building material for the repair of wounds, is a protein, vitamin C is essential for collagen synthesis and other trace elements, such as zinc and copper, are also important for the healing process. Nutrition is particularly important to aid wound healing in patients with a poor nutritional state caused by malignancy, malabsorption syndromes or temporary starvation (Westerby, 1985).

Promoting a good blood supply to the wound will also aid healing. The relief of pressure from pressure sores is essential if an adequate blood supply is to reach the wound.

The Surgical Wound

The wound dressing should not be disturbed for the first 48 h as bacteria may enter the wound from adjacent skin until the wound surface has sealed. If the dressing is dislodged or cannot contain the wound exudate it should be changed using an aseptic technique (see Table 8.5).

After 48 h the dressing can be removed and wounds that are not leaking exudate and are not drained can be left exposed or protected

Table 8.5
Aseptic technique. Adapted from Riverside Health Authority nursing procedures and reprinted with permission

Aim:
To minimize the risk of introducing pathogenic organisms into a wound or other susceptible site and to prevent the transfer of potential pathogens from the wound to other patients or staff.

Indications:
Wounds healing by primary intention (before surface skin has sealed)
Intravenous cannulation
Urinary catheterization
Suturing
Vaginal examination during labour
Medical invasive procedures

Principles:
1. Ensure that all equipment required is readily available and there is a clear field in which to carry out the procedure
2. Explain the procedure to the patient, obtain verbal consent and position the patient so that the procedure can be performed easily
3. Wash hands or disinfect clean hands with an alcohol handrub
4. Open the sterile pack carefully to prevent contamination of the contents
5. Wear sterile gloves for the procedure to prevent introducing pathogenic bacteria to the site, direct contact with body fluids and cross-infection
6. Use aseptic principles to:
   Ensure that only sterile items come into contact with the susceptible site
   Sterile items do not come into contact with non-sterile objects
7. After completion discard waste contaminated with body fluid into a yellow waste bag and sharps into a sharps container. Discard protective clothing and wash hands

with a transparent film dressing and the patient allowed to shower or bathe (Chrintz *et al.*, 1989). Leaving the wound exposed enables the early signs of wound infection to be detected and saves dressing materials and nursing time.

If the wound is still leaking after 48 h, a dressing will be required to absorb excess exudate on the skin (which is not contributing to the healing process occurring under the skin). The frequency of dressing change should be dictated by the amount of exudate. The site should be cleaned, if necessary with sterile, normal saline.

Wound drains should be attached to a sterile drainage bottle which should be changed when necessary, without touching the connections and washing hands thoroughly before the procedure.

The Chronic Wound

Modern dressing materials, such as alginates, hydrocolloids and hydrogels, are designed to absorb excess exudate whilst at the same time providing a warm and moist environment in which healing can take place most effectively (Table 8.6). Research has shown that these dressings can be used safely on wounds without increasing the risk of infection or encouraging the growth of **anaerobic** bacteria (Gilchrist and Reed, 1989).

Removing the dressing reduces the temperature of the wound and may disrupt the delicate new tissue, dressing changes should therefore be kept to a minimum (Lawrence, 1982). Since bacteria are not removed from the surface of the wound by cleaning but simply redistributed (Tomlinson, 1987), dressings should not be changed simply to 'clean' the wound. Dressings on large wounds healing by secondary intention can be removed more easily and with less damage to the underlying tissue, by irrigation with a syringe of normal saline or by soaking in a bath or shower.

The use of solutions (e.g. hypochlorite, hydrogen peroxide) to debride

Table 8.6
Properties of an ideal wound dressing for wounds healing by secondary intention

- *Maintains a high humidity.* Epithelial cells require moist conditions to migrate
- *Provides thermal insulation.* Tissue repair occurs best at a constant temperature of 37°C
- *Is impermeable to bacteria.* Helps to prevent cross-infection
- *Allows gaseous exchange.* Promotes healing
- *Removes excess exudate.* There is a balance between removal of exudate to prevent tissue maceration whilst maintaining a moist environment. Exudate contains white blood cells which protect the wound from invasion by bacteria
- *Is non-adherent.* To prevent the removal of newly formed tissue and capillaries when dressings are changed
- *Is non-toxic and non-allergenic.* May interfere with healing
- *Comfortable and acceptable to the patient*

Table 8.7
Clean tech
from Ri
Auth

wounds should be avoided as there is little e
ability to remove dead tissue and some evide
delay wound healing (Gruber *et al.*, 1975; Lea
1986).

The 'Aseptic Technique'

The aseptic technique is often performed as a nursing ritual and is based
more on tradition than on rational reason or research evidence. It is often
performed without reference to the underlying principles of infection
control or to the requirements of the situation to which it is being applied
(Walsh and Ford, 1989).

The aims of aseptic technique are to prevent the introduction of
pathogens to the wound, prevent the transfer of bacteria from one
patient to another and prevent staff from acquiring infection from the
patient.

The important principles are that the open wound should not come
into contact with any item that is not sterile and that any items that have
been in contact with the wound may be contaminated and should be
discarded safely or decontaminated. Since hands are not sterile, forceps
have traditionally been used for the procedure, probably because disposable gloves are a relatively recent introduction to medical care. However,
forceps are cumbersome to use and do not prevent the transfer of bacteria
from the wound to the hands. The procedure can be performed more
easily holding sterile swabs in the hands. First, potential pathogens should
be removed from the hands with an alcohol handrub and if the wound is
extensive or the hands may come into direct contact with wound
exudate, gloves should be worn (Tomlinson, 1987).

In many situations a modified aseptic or 'clean' technique is more
appropriate (Table 8.7), for example during the removal of sutures
from a sealed surgical wound or the application of dressings to wounds
healing by secondary intention. In the latter situation the wound probably already contains large numbers of different bacterial species and will
frequently be exposed to new bacteria from the environment. The
greatest concern is to ensure that potential pathogens are not transferred
to another patient. If hydrocolloid, alginate or hydrogel dressings have
been used, the removal of the dressing is probably best achieved by
irrigation with saline or bathing, and the use of a rigorous aseptic
technique is unnecessary (Ayliffe *et al.*, 1990).

Many aseptic techniques include a ritual about cleaning the trolley.
There is no evidence that bacteria on the trolley are transferred into the
wound, or vice versa, and routine cleaning of trolleys with alcohol
between patients probably serves no useful purpose (Thompson and
Bullock, 1992).

...nique. Adapted ...erside Health ...rity nursing ...cedures and reprinted with permission

Aim:
To avoid the introduction of potential pathogens to a susceptible site, to prevent the transfer of pathogens to other patients or staff

Indications:
Dressing of wounds healing by secondary intention
Removal of sutures
Dressing intravenous lines
Removal of drains
Endotracheal suction
Dressing tracheostomy site

Principles:
1. Ensure that all equipment required is ready and that a clean area on which to place it is available
2. Explain the procedure to the patient, obtain their verbal consent and position the patient so that the procedure can be performed easily
3. Wash hands and disinfect with alcohol handrub
4. If direct contact with blood or body fluid is anticipated, wear clean gloves and a plastic apron
5. Use sterile swabs to clean the site and apply a sterile dressing
6. Avoid touching any clean area whilst performing the procedure
7. On completion of the procedure, dispose all clinical waste into a yellow plastic bag. Discard gloves and apron and wash hands.

Preventing Cross-infection

Preventing the transmission of micro-organisms from one patient to another is a particular problem with heavily colonized or **infected** wounds. An organism colonizing the wound of one patient may be transmitted and cause infection in another patient and, as illustrated by Tomlinson (1987), bacteria are easily acquired on the hands whilst cleaning a wound even if forceps are used.

The use of disposable gloves minimizes the risk of acquiring bacteria on the hands but hands should still be washed before and after dressing wounds.

Bacteria acquired on the clothing during the procedure may be transferred into the wound of another patient therefore a clean disposable apron should be used for each dressing procedure.

If dressings are removed by soaking in bathwater or bowls, the bath or bowl should be thoroughly cleaned with detergent and then dried to ensure that pathogens are removed before use by the next patient.

In the past it has been recommended that wounds should not be redressed when cleaning or bedmaking is in progress because of the risk of airborne contamination. However, it has been shown that although such activities increase the number of bacterial particles in the air, the increase is not sufficient to present a risk of infection by particles settling onto a dressing trolley (Ayliffe *et al.*, 1990).

Dressing Clinics

Particular care must be taken to prevent cross-infection between patients attending ulcer treatment or dressing clinics where there are plenty of opportunities for transmission to occur and the rapid turnover of patients may encourage inadequate cleaning of equipment between patients. Bacteria in the wound will have contaminated the dressings and the surrounding skin, hands must always be washed after touching dressings or skin. Gloves and a plastic apron should be worn for the removal and application of dressings and must be changed after each patient. Creams and dressing materials must be used for one patient only. Equipment such as buckets for soaking off dressings and scissors must be thoroughly cleaned with detergent and water and dried after each patient.

Detection and Treatment of Wound Infection

The diagnosis of wound infection is based on the presence of clinical signs (Table 8.8). The isolation of micro-organisms in a wound swab sent for culture does not necessarily indicate that a wound is infected. Surgical wounds should be inspected regularly for signs of **infection** so that prompt treatment with antimicrobial therapy can be initiated (Plate 8.1).

Detection of infection in wounds healing by secondary intention may be difficult because slough is easily mistaken for pus and in some situations pus collects on the surface of the wound but without evidence of tissue invasion (Plate 8.2). Wound swabs are not a reliable indicator of infection as bacteria may be present even in high numbers in the wound without causing infection. The most important indicator of infection is inflammation spreading from the margins of the wound, local oedema, the patient reporting a marked increase in pain in the wound or a pyrexia where no other focus of infection can be identified (Hutchinson and Lawrence, 1991).

Wound infection should always be treated with systemic antibiotics. The topical application of antiseptic solutions is unlikely to reach organisms that are invading the tissue and their antibacterial activity is probably lost rapidly in the presence of blood and tissue. Solutions such as hypochlorites are toxic to granulation tissue and delay healing (Brennan *et al.*, 1986) and chlorhexidine and povidone–iodine have been shown to destroy fibroblasts in tissue culture (Gruber *et al.*, 1975; Neidner and

Table 8.8
Signs of wound infection

- Pain
- Inflammation at wound margins
- Oedema
- Pyrexia
- Purulent exudate

Schopf, 1986; Leaper, 1986). Many antiseptic solutions have not been well researched and their effects on wound healing and on bacteria in the wound are unknown.

References

Alexander JW, Korelitz J, Alexander NS (1976) Prevention of wound infections : a case for closed suction drainage to remove wound fluids deficient in opsonic proteins. *Am. J. Surg.* **132**: 59.

Alexander JW, Fischer JE, Boyajian M *et al.* (1983) The influence of hair-removal methods on wound infections. *Arch. Surg.* **118**: 347-52.

Ayliffe GAJ (1991a) Masks in surgery? *J. Hosp. Inf.* **18**: 165-6.

Ayliffe GAJ (1991b) Role of the environment of the operating suite in surgical wound infection. *Rev. Inf. Dis.* **13**(10): 5800–4.

Ayliffe GAJ, Lilly HA (1985) Cross-infection and its prevention. *J. Hosp. Inf.* **6**(Suppl. B): 47–57.

Ayliffe GAJ, Noy ME, Davies JG *et al.* (1983) A comparison of pre-operative bathing with chlorhexidine-detergent and a non-medicated soap in the prevention of wound infection. *J. Hosp. Inf.* **4**: 237–44.

Ayliffe GAJ, Collins BJ, Taylor LJ (1990) *Hospital Acquired Infection – Principles and Prevention*, 2nd edn. Butterworth, London.

Ayton M (1985) Wounds that won't heal. *Nursing Times* **81**(46)Suppl.: 16–19.

Barrie D, Wilson JA, Hoffman PN, *et al.* (1992) *Bacillus cereus* meningitis in two neurosurgical patients: an investigation into the source of the organism. *J. Inf.* **25**: 291–7.

Brennan SS, Foster ME, Leaper DJ (1986) Antiseptic toxicity in wounds healing by secondary intention. *J. Hosp. Inf.* **8**: 263–7.

Buchan IA, Andrews JK, Lang SM *et al.* (1980) Clinical and laboratory investigation of the composition and properties of human skin wound exudate under semi-permeable dressings. *Burns* **7**: 326–34.

Bucknall TE (1985) Factors affecting the development of surgical wound infections: a surgeons view. *J. Hosp. Inf.* **6**:1–8.

Centers for Disease Control (1991) Nosocomial infection rates for interhospital comparison: Limitations and possible solutions. *Inf. Contr. Hosp. Epid.* **12**: 609–21.

Chrintz H, Vibits H, Cordtz TO *et al.* (1989) Need for surgical wound dressing. *Br. J. Surg.* **76**: 204–5.

Clarke RAF (1985) Cutaneous tissue repair: basic biological considerations I. *J. Am. Acad. Dermatol.* **13**: 701–25.

Cruse PJE, Foord R (1973) A five-year prospective study of 23 649 surgical wounds. *Arch. Surg.* **107**: 206.

Cruse PJE, Foord R (1980) The epidemiology of wound infection – a 10 year prospective study of 62 939 wounds. *Surg. Clin. N. Am.* **60**(1): 27–40.

Cruse PJE (1986) Surgical infection: incisional wounds. In *Hospital Infections*, 2nd edn (JV Bennett, PS Brachman, Eds), pp. 423–36. Little Brown, Boston.

Elek SD, Conen PE (1957) The virulence of *Staphylococcus pyogenes* for men: a study of the problems of wound infection. *Br. J. Exp. Pathol.* **38**: 573–86.

Garner JS (1986) CDC Guidelines for prevention of surgical wound infections. *Infect. Contr.* **7**(3): 193–200.

Gilchrist B, Reed C (1989) The bacteriology of leg ulcers under hydrocolloid dressings. *Br. J. Dermatol.* **121**: 337–44.

Gruber RB, Vistnes L, Pardoe R (1975) The effect of commonly used antiseptics on wound healing. *Plast. Recon. Surg.* **55**: 472–6.

Haley RW (1986) *Managing Hospital Infection Control for Cost-Effectiveness.* American Hospital Publishing, USA.

Haley RW, Culver DH, White JW *et al.* (1985) The efficacy of infection surveillance and control programs in preventing nosocomial infections in US hospitals. *Am. J. Epidemiol.* **121**: 182–205.

Hambreus A (1988) Aerobiology in operating rooms. *J. Hosp. Inf.* **11**(Suppl. A): 68–76.

Hoborn J (1990) Wet strike-through and transfer of bacteria through operating barrier fabrics. *Hyg. Med.* **15**: 15–20.

Howarth FH (1985) Prevention of airborne infection during surgery. *The Lancet* **Feb. 16**: 386–8.

Humphries H, Russell AJ, Marshall RJ *et al.* (1991a) The effect of surgical theatre head-gear on air bacterial counts. *J. Hosp. Inf.* **19**: 175–80.

Humphries H, Marshall RJ, Ricketts VE (1991b) Theatre overshoes do not reduce operating floor bacterial counts. *J. Hosp. Inf.* **17**: 117–24.

Hutchinson JJ, Lawrence JC (1991) Wound infection under occlusive dressings. *J. Hosp. Inf.* **17**: 83–94.

Kolmos HJ, Thuesen B, Nielsen SV *et al.* (1993) Outbreak of infection in a burns unit due to *Pseudomonas aeruginosa* originating from contaminated tubing used for irrigation of patients. *J. Hosp. Inf.* **24**: 11–21.

Kriezek TJ, Robson MC (1975) Biology of surgical infection. *Surg. Clin. N. Am.* **55**: 1262–7.

Lawrence JC (1982) What materials for dressings? *Injury* **13**: 500–12.

Leaper DJ (1986) Antiseptics and their effect on healing tissue. *Nursing Times* **82**(22): 45–7.

Lidwell OM, Lowbury EJL, Whyte W *et al.* (1982) Effect of ultraclean air in operating rooms on deep sepsis in the joint after total hip or knee replacement; a randomised study. *Br. J. Med.* **285**: 10–14.

Lilley HA, Lowbury EJL, Wilkens MD (1979) Limits to progressive reduction of resident skin bacteria by disinfection. *J. Clin. Path.* **32**: 382–5.

Lowbury EJL, Cason JS (1985) Aspects of infection control and skin grafting in burned patients. In *Wound Care* (S. Westerby, Ed.), pp. 170–89. Heinemann Medical, London.

Lydon MJ, Hutchinson JJ, Rippon M *et al.* (1989) Dissolution of wound coagulum and promotion of granulation tissue under DuoDERM™. *Wounds* **1**: 95–106.

Lynch W, Davey PG, Malek M *et al.* (1992) Cost-effectiveness analysis of the use of chlorhexidine detergent in preoperative whole-body disinfection in wound infection prophylaxis. *J. Hosp. Inf.* **21**: 179–91.

Matthews J, Slater K, Newsom SWB (1985) The effect of surgical gowns made with barrier cloth on bacterial dispersal. *J. Hyg.* **95**: 123–30.

Miles AA, Miles EM, Burke J. (1957) The value and duration of defence reactions of the skin to primary lodgement of bacteria. *Br. J. Exp. Pathol.* **38**: 79.

Millward S (1992) The hazards of communal razors. *Nursing Times* **88**(6): 58–62.

Mitchell NJ, Hunt S (1991) Surgical face masks in modern operating rooms – a costly and unnecessary ritual? *J. Hosp. Inf.* **18**: 239–42.

Meers PD, Ayliffe GAJ, Emmerson AM *et al.* (1981) National survey of infections in hospital, 1980. *J. Hosp. Inf.* **2**(Suppl.): 23–8.

Mishriki SF, Law DJW, Jeffrey PJ (1990) Factors affecting the incidence of post-operative wound infection. *J. Hosp. Inf.* **11**: 253–62.

Neidner R, Schopf E (1986) Inhibition of wound healing by antiseptics. *Br. J. Derm.* **115**(S31): 41–4.

Noone MR, Pitt TL, Bedder M *et al.* (1983) *Pseudomonas aeruginosa* colonisation in an intensive therapy unit: role of cross infection and host factors. *Brit. Med. J.* **286**: 341–4.

Ojarjärvi J (1976) An evaluation of antiseptics used for hand disinfection in wards. *J. Hyg. (Camb.)* **76**: 75–82.

Pettersson E (1986) A cut above the rest? *Nursing Times* **31**(5): 68–70.

Sanderson PJ (1991) Infection in orthopaedic implants. *J. Hosp. Inf.* **18**(Suppl. A): 367–75.

Schweizer RT (1976) Mask wiggling as a potential source of wound contamination. *Lancet* **2**: 1129–30.

Seropian R, Reynolds BM (1971) Wound infections after preoperative depilatory versus razor preparation. *Am. J. Surg.* **121**: 251–6.

Tomlinson D. (1987) To clean or not to clean? *Nursing Times* **83**(9): 71–5.

Thompson G, Bullock D (1992) To clean or not to clean? *Nursing Times* **88**(34): 66–8.

Valentine RJ, Weigelt JA, Dryer D *et al.* (1986) Effect of remote infection on clean wound infection rates. *Am. J. Inf. Contr.* **14**: 64–7.

Walsh M, Ford P (1989) *Nursing Rituals, Research and Rational Actions*. Butterworth-Heinemann, Oxford.

Westerby S (1985) *Wound Care*. Heinemann Medical, London.

Whyte W, Hamblen DL, Kelly IG *et al.* (1990) An investigation of occlusive polyester surgical clothing. *J. Hosp. Inf.* **15**: 363–74.

Whyte W, Hambreus A, Laurell G *et al.* (1991) The relative importance of routes and sources of wound contamination during general surgery. 1. Non-airborne. *J. Hosp. Inf.* **18**: 93–107.

Whyte W, Hodgson R, Tinkler J (1982) The importance of airborne bacterial contamination of wounds. *J. Hosp. Inf.* **2**: 349–54.

Whyte W, Vesley D, Hodgson R. (1976) Bacterial dispersion in relation to operating room clothing. *J. Hyg.* **76**: 367–78.

Winter GD (1962) Formation of the scab and the rate of epithelialisation of superficial wounds in the skin of the young domestic pig. *Nature* **193**: 293–4.

Further Reading

Dowding CM (1986) Nutrition in wound healing. *Nursing* **4**: 174–6.

Humphries H (1993) Infection control and the design of a new operating theatre suite. *J. Hosp. Inf.* **23**: 61–70.

Johnson A (1989) Preparing for elective surgery. *Nurs. Stand.* **3**(23): 22–5.

Morison MJ (1987) Wound assessment. *Prof. Nurse* **2**(10): 315–7.

Morison M (1990) Pressure sores: a risk assessment and prevention plan. *Prof. Nurse* **5**: 12 (Wallchart).

Morison M (1992) *A Colour Guide to the Nursing Management of Wounds*. Wolfe, London.

Nichols RL (1991) Surgical wound infection. *Am. J. Med.* **91**(Suppl. 3B): 54S–63S.

Stewart A, Foster M, Leaper D (1985) Cleaning v. healing. *Community Outlook* **August**: 22–6.

Thomas S (1994) *Handbook of Wound Dressings.* Macmillan Magazines, London.

Williams CM (1986) Wound healing: a nutritional perspective. *Nursing* **7**: 249–51.

9 Preventing Infection Associated with Intravascular Therapy

Introduction

Intravascular (IV) devices are now widely used in medical care for the administration of fluids, blood products, nutritional support and haemo-dynamic monitoring. Infections associated with IV devices are reported relatively infrequently but are often life-threatening, particularly in the critically ill, **immunocompromised** or neonate, and can largely be prevented by good infection control practice (Maki, 1986).

Sources of Infection

Micro-organisms may enter the IV device along the outside of the cannula or along the inside of the hub. They may be introduced at the time of cannulation or in contaminated infusion fluids (Fig. 9.1).

Most IV-device-related infections are caused by the micro-organisms that commonly **colonize** the skin, especially *Staphylococcus epidermidis*, which accounts for about 70% of infections (Elliot, 1988) and has been found to increase the risk of mortality in an infected patient by about 15% (Daschner and Frank, 1989). It has a particular ability to adhere to plastic cannula and is resistant to many antibiotics (Fig. 3.1). These organisms are usually derived from the patient's skin or from staff who handle the device (Table 9.1).

Fig. 9.1
Sources of infection in IV devices. A schematic cross-section of the skin and underlying tissue at the site of cannulation. Reprinted with permission from Elliot (1988).

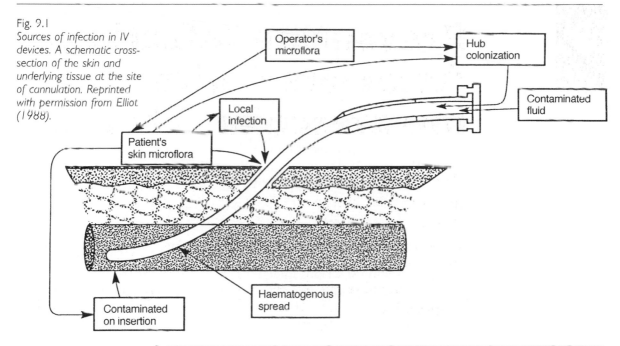

Table 9.1
Micro-organisms most commonly responsible for IV-device-related infection

Micro-organism	Source
Staphylococcus epidermidis	Common skin commensal
Staphylococcus aureus	Skin commensal
Enterococcus sp.	Gut flora
Klebsiella	
Pseudomonas	Gram-negative organisms, colonize the skin of hospitalized
Escherichia coli	patients and carried transiently on the hands of staff
Serratia	
Candida	May colonize skin when normal flora altered by antibiotic therapy or immunosuppression

Types of Infection Associated with IV Devices

Infection associated with intravenous therapy can be difficult to diagnose and cannulae are frequently not recognized as the cause of the symptoms of infection in the patient (Maki, 1991). A range of infectious complications can be identified:

Local Site Infection

Infection of the skin may develop where the cannula enters, indicated by **inflammation** or the presence of pus. There is considerable evidence to suggest a link between the growth of bacteria at the insertion site and subsequent infection of the cannula (Cercenardo *et al.*, 1990; Mermel *et al.*, 1991). Surveillance cultures of insertion sites may be of some value in early identification and treatment of IV device related infections in some patients at particular risk of infection such as the **immunosuppressed** (Syndman *et al.*, 1982).

Inflammation of the Vein (Phlebitis)

This is usually caused by chemicals in the infusate or mechanical irritation of the cannula. However, infection may subsequently develop in the damaged tissue to cause suppurative phlebitis.

Bacteraemia and Septicaemia

These are the most serious infections associated with IV therapy and are frequently life-threatening. **Bacteraemia** is the presence of micro-organisms in the blood and where this is accompanied by symptoms of infection (e.g. fever, rigors, hypotension) is described as **septicaemia**.

Diagnosis of Infection Related to IV Devices

One of the difficulties of quantifying the risks of IV therapy is the range of definitions of what constitutes a catheter-related infection. Some studies use the incidence of septicaemia as a measure, others the occurrence of phlebitis or the colonization of the cannula (Tager *et al.*, 1983; Ricard *et al.*, 1985; Maki and Ringer, 1987; Weightman *et al.*, 1988). Often the main indication of a line-associated infection is a pyrexia which has no other apparent cause and is unresponsive to antibiotic therapy (Elliot, 1993).

The standard method for diagnosing cannula-related infection is by culture of the tip of the cannula. The method used is semi-quantitative; that is it involves an estimation of the number of bacteria present and takes account of inadvertent contamination when the cannula is removed (Maki *et al.*, 1977). Growth is considered significant when more than 15 bacteria are found and this information may confirm the cannula as the source of clinical symptoms of infection.

Blood cultures can also be used to indicate IV device infection. Blood should be taken from a peripheral vein and through the cannula. If the same organism is isolated from both sources, particularly if more organisms are obtained from the cannula specimen, then this is suggestive of a device-related infection (Wing *et al.*, 1979).

Major Factors that Influence the Risk of Infection
Duration of Cannulation

The length of time that a cannula is in place probably has most effect on the risk of infection. The longer a device is in place the more likely an infection will develop (Elliot, 1988). To take account of this many studies report infections related to the number of days of cannulation. For example, if 100 cannulae are under study and each in place for 10 days, the total number of days of cannulation is 1000. If two become infected then the rate of infection is two per 1000 cannula days. Tager *et al.* (1983) found that the risk of phlebitis related to peripheral cannulae increased after 96 h and recommended that the peripheral cannula site should be changed at this time interval. Weekly resiting or replacement of central cannulae has been advocated as a means of reducing the risk of infection. Eyer *et al.* (1990) however reported no difference in catheter-related infection between patients, whose cannulae were neither resited or changed weekly and patients whose cannulae were either resited or changed over a guidewire every 7 days.

Type of Cannula

Peripheral cannulae are associated with a much lower rate of infection than central venous or arterial cannulae (Nystrom *et al.*, 1983). The risk of infection is increased by the use of multi-lumen catheters. In one study the rate was 8% for single lumen compared to 32% for multi-lumen cannulae (Weightman *et al.*, 1988). Haemodynamic monitoring and the administration of parenteral nutrition (PN) fluids also increase the risk of infection (Mughal, 1989; Mermel *et al.*, 1991). Table 9.2 illustrates the approximate risks of infection associated with different types of IV device.

Site of Insertion

More infections are associated with cannulation of the femoral vein than the subclavian vein. Infection rates as high as 34% have been associated with femoral cannulation (Collingnon *et al.*, 1988). The tunnelling of the central cannula so that the place at which it exits on to the skin is a

Table 9.2
Approximate incidence of IV-device-related septicaemia. Adapted from Maki (1991).

Type of device	Incidence* (%)	Range* (%)
Peripheral	<0.2	0–1
Central venous		
multi-lumen	3	1–7
Swan–Ganz	1	0–5
Hickman	0.2	0.1–0.5
Subcutaneous	0.04	0–0.1

* Based on a combination of recently published data.

considerable distance from the vein seems to be a particularly effective method of reducing the incidence of infectious complications (Garden and Sim, 1983). Recent evidence also suggests that central venous cannulae inserted into a peripheral vein are associated with fewer infections (Graham *et al.*, 1991).

Cannula Material

In common with all foreign material in contact with tissue, IV devices become covered with a film of proteins such as albumin, fibrinogen and **immunoglobulin**, mixed with micro-organisms and known collectively as a '**biofilm**'. This biofilm helps the bacteria adhere to the cannula and resist the effect of antibiotics circulating in the blood. The smooth surface of teflon and polyurethane cannulae are the most resistant to bacterial adherence, whilst polyvinylchloride (PVC), polyethylene and silicone are more susceptible to colonization by bacteria (Sheth *et al.*, 1985).

Cannulae with surfaces that discourage bacterial adhesion or containing antibacterial substances which will inhibit them are being developed and may help to reduce the risk of device-related infection (Elliot and Faroqui, 1992).

Preventing Infection in Intravascular Devices

Nurses are largely responsible for the care of IV-devices and many infections could be prevented by improvements in practice. Education and training is an essential part of this process and several studies have demonstrated a substantial reduction in the numbers of infections where IV devices have been maintained by specially trained personnel (Keohane *et al.*, 1983; Puntis *et al.*, 1990).

Insertion of the Cannula

The cannulation procedure may introduce bacteria from the skin into the vein. These bacteria may be derived either from the patient or from the hands of the person inserting it. The cannula site has been described as 'not unlike an open wound containing a foreign body' (Maki *et al.*, 1973) and insertion should therefore be considered a minor surgical procedure carried out with a high standard of asepsis. This is particularly important for central cannula insertion which is a more invasive procedure and the use of sterile gloves, gowns and drapes has been shown to reduce the risk of infection significantly (Mermel *et al.*, 1991).

The cannula should be firmly anchored to prevent movement, which may both carry micro-organisms from the skin into the wound and

Insertion of a Cannula

- Use teflon or polyurethane cannulae where possible
- Wash hands before insertion. Use sterile gloves, gowns and drapes to insert central venous and arterial cannula
- Use chlorhexidine to clean skin, allow to dry before insertion
- Avoid shaving the site of insertion
- Secure cannula but do not cover insertion site with non-sterile tape

increase the risk of mechanical phlebitis (Maki *et al.*, 1973). Tape has been implicated as a source of infection and tape that is in direct contact with the insertion site should be sterile (Sheldon and Johnson, 1979).

Skin Preparation

Recent studies by Maki *et al.* (1991a) suggest that cleaning the site with 2% chlorhexidine prior to the insertion of central or arterial cannula is associated with a lower rate of infection than 10% povidone–iodine or 70% alcohol. To ensure maximum disinfection of the skin, the disinfectant should be applied for about 30 s and allowed to dry before starting the procedure.

Effective skin preparation will remove bacteria from hair as well as the skin. Shaving the skin causes microscopic damage which can increase microbial colonization. Shaving around the insertion site should therefore be avoided. See practice guidelines for the insertion of a cannula.

Care of the Insertion Site

The conventional method of protecting the insertion site is with a dressing but there is conflicting evidence about which type of dressing is most effective. Gauze dressings do not protect the site from moisture and do not allow the insertion site to be visualized easily. Transparent film dressings enable the insertion site to be viewed easily to detect early signs of phlebitis or infection. A build-up in bacteria on the skin under transparent film dressings has been reported although most studies have not demonstrated an increased risk of device-related infection. Ricard *et al.* (1985) found no difference in skin colonization or cannula-related infection between films left on for 7 days and gauze changed every 2–3 days. Maki and Ringer (1987) found no increase in the incidence of infection when films were left on for the lifetime of the cannula.

However, Conly *et al.*, 1989 have reported an increase in site infections and bacteraemias associated with transparent films. A five-fold increase in bacteraemias has been demonstrated when film dressings have been used

Guidelines for Practice

Care of the Insertion Site

- Use sterile gauze or transparent film to cover the insertion site. Do not use transparent films on arterial cannulae
- Change dressing when no longer intact, when moisture collects at the site and at least every 7 days
- Clean central venous or arterial insertion sites with aqueous chlorhexidine each time the dressing is changed. Peripheral cannulae are unlikely to benefit from cleaning with antiseptic
- Inspect the site every 2–3 days for signs of infection (e.g. inflammation, pain, pus)

on arterial catheters, possibly because blood collecting at the insertion site provides a rich medium for bacterial growth (Maki and Will, 1984). One of the explanations for this conflicting information is the variation in moisture vapour permeability of dressings made by different manufacturers. New transparent films with a high vapour permeability may reduce skin colonization (Maki *et al.*, 1991b).

Skin disinfectants used to clean the skin when the dressing is changed may reduce the rate of infection associated with central venous and arterial cannulae. A 2% aqueous solution of chlorhexidine, which has a residual antibacterial effect on the skin for several hours after application, has been shown to be most effective (Maki *et al.*, 1991a). Antiseptic-impregnated dressings do not appear to reduce the rate of infection (Maki and Ringer, 1987). See practice guidelines for the care of the insertion site.

Management of Administration Sets

Some bacteria, notably *Klebsiella* and *Enterobacter*, grow rapidly in IV solutions, especially 5% Dextrose (CDC, 1971). A number of outbreaks of infection in the 1970s were caused by IV fluids contaminated during manufacture but improvements in quality control methods have now made this an unlikely source of infection.

However, infusion fluids may become contaminated during use when drugs are added, or when infusion fluids or administration sets are changed. Units of blood or platelets may contain bacteria which can contaminate the infusion set (Walsh *et al.*, 1993).

Table 9.3
Contamination of infusion fluids. From Maki et al. (1987).

Type/location of IV device	% Infusions contaminated
Peripheral	0.6
Central venous	1.5
Central–TPN	3.6
Devices on ITU	2.5
Devices on general wards	0.9

The extent to which fluids are accessed affects the risk of infection (Table 9.3). Administration sets in intensive care units, where lines are accessed frequently for haemodynamic monitoring and drug administration, are more likely to become contaminated (Maki *et al.*, 1987; Mermel *et al.*, 1991). Bacteria introduced from contaminated infusate or during manipulation of the line will multiply over time and, to prevent this, regular changing of the administration sets has been recommended (DHSS, 1972). Some studies have shown that lines can be changed every 4 days without increasing the risk of infection (Sitges-serra *et al.*, 1985, Maki *et al.*, 1987), although frequently accessed lines should be changed more often. The number of infections associated with IV therapy is usually low and in most circumstances the use of gloves to manipulate administration sets or administer drugs is probably unnecessary. Where parenteral nutrition is being administered, it may be preferable to use sterile gloves to attach new bags of fluid because the risk of infection is much greater (see below).

IV Filters

A filter placed between the cannula and the fluid administration set can be used to prevent bacteria in the fluid gaining access to the vein and is probably cost effective with administration sets that are frequently accessed (Spencer, 1990). Filters cannot be used on Swan–Ganz catheters or where blood, blood products, lipid emulsion and amphotericin are being infused (Quercia *et al.*, 1986).

Bacteria have frequently been recovered from cannula hubs and stopcocks such as those illustrated in Plate 9.1 (Grabe and Jakobsen, 1983; Cheeseborough and Finch, 1985). Although the significance of these bacteria in subsequent infection of the line is open to debate the number of access points should be kept to a minimum (Mermel *et al.*, 1991). There is no evidence that wrapping hub joints with gauze soaked in

Guidelines for Practice

Care of the Administration Set

- Wash hands before accessing IV devices. Do not touch IV line connections or allow them to come into contact with non-sterile surfaces. Sterile gloves are not usually necessary provided sterile connections are not touched by hand
- Keep the number of access points on an intravenous line to a minimum. If a tap or stopcock is not in use then remove it
- Administer IV drugs through the latex membrane on peripheral lines to avoid the use of ports
- Change administration sets at least every 4 days, every 24–48 h if frequently accessed, and always after the infusion of blood products
- Consider use of IV filters where lines are frequently accessed

antiseptic prevents infections and alcohol-based solutions may damage the cannula material (Hazard Notice, 1993). Practice guidelines for the care of administration sets are described on page 209.

Parenteral Nutrition

The administration of elemental nutrients into a vein is used to feed patients who are unable to meet their nutritional requirements by oral or nasogastric feeding. Conventionally, parenteral nutrition is administered via a central venous catheter where the high blood flow reduces the thrombophlebitic effects of glucose. Bacteria can multiply easily in PN fluid and infection is a frequent complication of PN therapy, with an infection rate of around 14% (Mughal, 1989). Particular care must therefore be taken to avoid contamination of IV devices used to administer PN.

Peripheral cannulae have been used successfully for short-term feeding using a lower concentration of glucose and are associated with a lower risk of infection (Hansell, 1989). Glyceryl trinitrate patches applied close to the insertion site can prolong the life of peripheral PN cannulae by increasing vasodilation (Khawaja *et al.*, 1988). See practice guidelines for the management of parenteral nutrition.

Guidelines for Practice

Management of Parenteral Nutrition

The risks of infection associated with the infusion of parenteral nutrition are much greater than other fluids and extreme care must be taken to avoid contamination

- The catheter should be inserted under aseptic conditions in theatre or treatment room by an experienced doctor
- Designate the cannula for PN only (avoid using multi-lumen catheters), do not add drugs or withdraw blood from the line
- Do not connect ports, stopcocks or taps and should preferably be a single-lumen line
- Change the infusion fluid and administration set every 24 h using sterile gloves and a non-touch technique
- Inspect the insertion site daily for signs of infection and clean with chlorhexidine when dressing is changed
- Record temperature and pulse 4 hourly to detect early signs of sepsis
- Take blood cultures through the line and from a peripheral vein if the patient becomes pyrexial

---

Hickman and Subcutaneous Lines

Intravenous catheters made of an inert material, silicone elastomer, were pioneered by Broviac and developed by Hickman. These catheters are inserted into a central vein and tunnelled under the skin to exit on the chest wall (Fig. 9.2). Tissue grows into a dacron cuff positioned in the skin tunnel and this stabilizes the catheter so that a securing suture is not necessary and prevents bacteria migrating from the skin into the vein.

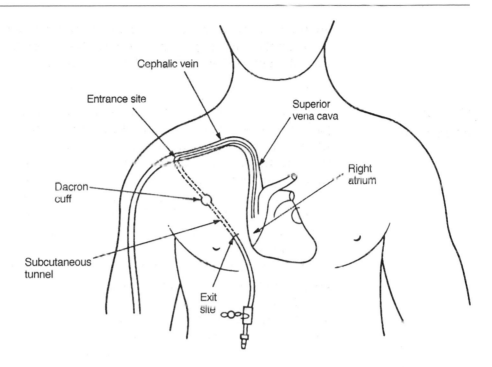

Fig. 9.2
A tunnelled right atrial catheter.

Cephalic vein

Entrance site

Superior vena cava

Right atrium

Dacron cuff

Subcutaneous tunnel

Exit site

Cuffs added to conventional central catheters reduce the incidence of infection (Flowers *et al.*, 1989).

Hickman catheters are used extensively in the management of patients requiring prolonged venous access, particularly for chemotherapy. They are associated with low rates of infection if the length of time they are in the vein is accounted for. Decker and Edwards (1988) reported a rate of 1.7 cases of septicaemia per 1000 catheter days. Infections in Hickman catheters used in patients with AIDS may occur more frequently (Raviglione *et al.*, 1989).

Initially insertion site care should be the same as for other central catheters but approximately 10 days after insertion the dacron cuff has been secured by tissue ingrowth, the exit site suture can be removed and the site left exposed without a dressing (Johnstone, 1982). In common with other central catheters, provided that a good non-touch technique is used, gloves are not necessary to manipulate the administration set or administer intravenous drugs except perhaps where parenteral nutrition is being infused and the risk of introducing infection through line manipulation much greater.

Totally implanted or subcutaneous central venous catheters (e.g. Port-a-Cath) with a self sealing septum are being used increasingly, particularly for patients cared for in their own home. These devices have been reported to reduce the risk of infection, although occasionally infection of the subcutaneous pocket occurs (Decker and Edwards, 1988).

The
Management
of Intravascular
Devices in the
Home

It is often difficult to translate the care of IV devices in hospital to the environment of the home, where the patient may be responsible for most of the care and the facilities and equipment available are less sophisticated. The risks of introducing infection may be lower because cross-infection from other patients is unlikely to occur. The plan of care should be as simple as possible but considerable distress can be caused by forcing patients to adopt unfamiliar procedures and is unnecessary provided the general principles of infection control are adhered to.

References

Centers for Disease Control (1971) Nosocomial bacteremias associated with intravenous fluid therapy. *MMWR* **20** (Suppl. 9): 1–2.

Cercenardo E, Ena J, Rodriguez-Creixems M *et al.* (1990) A conservative procedure for the diagnosis of catheter-related infections. *Arch. Int. Med.* **150**: 1417–20.

Cheeseborough JS, Finch RG.(1985) Studies on the microbiological safety of the valved side-port of the 'venflon' cannula. *J. Hosp. Inf.* **6**: 201–8.

Collingnon P, Soni N, Pearson T *et al.* (1988) Sepsis associated with central vein catheters in critically ill patients. *Int. Care Med.* **14**: 277–31.

Conly JM, Grieves K, Peters B (1989) A prospective randomised study comparing transparent and dry gauze dressings for central venous catheters. *J. Inf. Dis.* **159**: 310–19.

Daschner FD, Frank U (1989) Intravenous catheter and device-related infection. *Curr. Opin. Inf. Dis.* **2**: 663–7.

Decker MD, Edwards KM (1988) Central venous catheter infections. *Paed. Clin. N. Am.* **14**: 503–9.

DHSS (1972) *Guidelines on the Administration of Parenteral Infusion Fluids*. DS 216/72. HMSO, London.

Elliot TSJ (1988) Intravascular device infections. *J. Med. Micro.* **27**: 161–7.

Elliot TSJ (1993) Line-associated bacteraemias. *Comm. Dis. Rep.* **3**(7): R91–5.

Elliot TSJ, Faroqui MH (1992) Infection and intravascular devices. *Br. J. Hosp. Med.* **48**(8): 496–503.

Eyer S, Brummitt C, Crossley K *et al.* (1990) Catheter-related sepsis: prospective randomised study of three methods of long-term catheter maintenance. *Crit. Care Med.* **18**(10): 1073–9.

Flowers RH, Schwezer KJ, Kopel RJ *et al.* (1989) Efficacy of an attachable subcutaneous cuff for the prevention of intravascular catheter-related infection. *JAMA* **261**: 878–3.

Garden OJ, Sim AJW (1983) A comparison of tunnelled and non-tunnelled subclavian catheters: a prospective study of complications during parenteral feeding. *Clin. Nutr.* **2**: 51–4.

Grabe N, Jakobsen CJB (1983) Bacterial contamination of Venflon intravenous cannulae with valved injection sideport. *J. Hosp. Inf.* **4**: 291–5.

Graham DR, Keldermans MM, Klemm LW *et al.* (1991) Infectious complications among patients receiving home intravenous therapy with peripheral, central or peripherally placed central venous catheters. *Am. J. Med.* **91**(Suppl. B): 95S–101S.

Hansell DT (1989) Intravenous nutrition: the central or peripheral route? *Intravenous Therapy and Clinical Monitoring* **July**: 184–90.

Hazard Notice (1993) *Degradation of Silicone Tubing by Alcohol-based Antiseptics.* HN(93) 7. Medical Devices Directorate, 22 March.

Johnstone JD (1982) Infrequent infections associated with Hickman catheters. *Cancer Nursing* **April**: 125–9.

Keohane PP, Jones BJM, Attrill H *et al.* (1983) Effect of catheter tunnelling and a nutrition nurse on catheter sepsis during parenteral nutrition. A controlled trial. *Lancet* **ii**: 1388–90.

Khawaja HT, Campbell MJ, Weaver PC (1988) Effect of transdermal glyceryl trinitrate on the survival of peripheral intravenous infusions: a double-blind prospective clinical study. *Br. J. Surg.* **75**: 1212–15.

Maki DG (1986) Infections due to infusion therapy. In *Hospital Infection Control* (JV Bennett, PS Brachman, Eds), pp. 561–80. Little Brown, Boston.

Maki DG (1991). Infection caused by intravascular devices: pathogenesis, strategies for prevention. In *Improving Catheter Site Care*. Proceedings of a symposium, Series 179, March 1991. Royal Society of Medicine Services, London.

Maki DG, Band JD (1981) A comparative study of polyantibiotic and iodophor ointments in prevention of catheter-related infection. *Am. J. Med.* **70**: 739–44.

Maki DG, Ringer M. (1987) Evaluation of dressing regimens for prevention of infection with peripheral intravenous catheters, gauze, a transparent polyurethane dressing and an iodophor-transparent dressing. *JAMA* **258**: 2396–403.

Maki DG, Will L (1984) Colonisation and infection associated with transparent dressings for central venous, arterial and hickman catheters: a comparative trial. In *24th Interscience Conference on Antimicrobial Agents and Chemotherapy*. Abstract 991. American Society for Microbiology, Washington.

Maki DG, Goldman DA, Rhame FS (1973) Infection control in intravenous therapy. *Ann. Int. Med.* **79**: 867–87.

Maki DG, Hassemer C, Sarafini HW (1977) A semi-quantitative culture method for identifying intravenous catheter-related infection. *New. Engl. J. Med.* **296**: 1305–9.

Maki DG, Botticelli JT, Le Roy ML *et al.* (1987) Prospective study of replacing administration sets for intravenous therapy at 48 hour versus 72 hour intervals. 72 hours is safe and cost-effective. *JAMA* **258**: 1777–81.

Maki DG, Ringer M, Alvarado CJ. (1991a) Prospective randomised trial of povidone–iodine, alcohol and chlorhexidine for prevention of infection associated with central venous and arterial catheters. *Lancet* **338**: 339–43.

Maki DG, Stolz S, Wheeler S. (1991b) A prospective, randomised, three-way clinical comparison of a novel, highly impermeable, polyurethane dressing with 206 Swan–Ganz pulmonary artery catheters: Opsite IV3000 vs Tegaderm v gauze and tape. I. Cutaneous colonisation under the dressing, catheter-related infection. In *Improving Catheter Site Care*. Proceedings of a symposium, Series 179, pp. 61–6. Royal Society of Medicine Services, London.

Mermel L, Stolz S, Maki DG (1991). Epidemiology and pathogenesis of infection with Swan–Ganz catheters. A prospective study using molecular epidemiology. *Am. J. Med.* **91** (3b): 197.

Mughal MM. (1989) Complications of intravenous feeding catheters. *Br. J. Surg.* **76**: 15–21.

Nystrom B, Larson SO, Dankert J *et al.* (1983) Bacteraemia in surgical patients with intravenous devices: a European multicentre incidence study. The European Working Party on the Control of Hospital Infections. *J. Hosp. Inf.* **4**: 338–49.

Puntis JWL, Holden CE, Smallman S (1990) Staff training: key factor in reducing intravascular catheter sepsis. *Arch. Dis. Child.* **65**: 335–7.

Raviglione MC, Battan R, Pablos-Mendez A *et al.* (1989) Infections associated with Hickman catheters in patients with acquired immune deficiency syndrome. *Am. J. Med.* **86**: 780–6.

Ricard P, Martin R, Marcoux JA (1985) Protection of indwelling vascular catheters; incidence of bacterial contamination and catheter-related sepsis. *Crit. Care Med.* **13**: 541–3.

Sheldon DL, Johnson WC (1979) Cutaneous mucormycosis: two documented cases of suspected nosocomial infection. *JAMA* **241**: 1032–3.

Sheth NK, Franson TR, Sohnle PG (1985) Influence of bacterial adherence to intravascular catheters on *in vitro* activity antibiotic susceptibility. *Lancet* **2**: 1266–8.

Sitges-serra A, Linares J, Perez JL *et al.* (1985) A randomised trial on the effect of tubing changes on hub contamination and catheter sepsis during parenteral nutrition. *J. Paren. Enter. Nut.* **9**: 322–5.

Spencer RC (1990) Use of in-line filters for intravenous infusions in intensive care units. *J. Hosp. Inf.* **16**: 281.

Syndman DR, Pober BR, Murray SA *et al.* (1982) Predictive value of surveillance skin cultures in total-parenteral nutrition-related infection. *Lancet* **ii**: 1385–8.

Tager IB, Ginsberg MB, Ellis SE (1983) An epidemiologic study of the risks associated with peripheral intravenous catheters. *Am. J. Epid.* **118** (6): 839–51.

Quercia RA, Hills SW, Klimek JJ *et al.* (1986) Bacteriologic contamination of intravenous infusion delivery systems in an intensive care unit. *Am. J. Med.* **80**: 364–8.

Walsh R, Gurevich R, Cunha SA (1993) *Listeria*: a potential cause of febrile transfusion reactions. *J. Hosp. Inf.* **24**: 81–2.

Weightman NC, Simpson EM, Speller DCE *et al.* (1988) Bacteraemia related to indwelling central venous catheters: prevention, diagnosis, and treatment. *Eur. J. Clin. Microbiol. Inf. Dis.* **7(2):** 125–9.

Wille JC, Blusse A, Van Oud Ablas *et al.* (1993) A comparison of two transparent film-type dressings in central venous therapy. *J. Hosp. Inf.* **23**: 113–22.

Wing EJ, Norden CW, Shadduck RK *et al.* (1979) Use of quantitative bacteriological techniques to diagnose catheter-related sepsis. *Ann. Intern. Med.* **139**: 482.

10 Preventing Infection Associated with Urethral Catheters

Introduction

Urinary tract infections (UTI) are the most common infection acquired in hospital, accounting for between 30 and 40% of all such infections (Meers *et al.*, 1981; Krieger *et al.*, 1983). The major predisposing factor is the presence of an indwelling urethral catheter. Three-quarters of hospital-acquired UTI are related to indwelling urethral catheters and approximately one in every 10 patients admitted to hospital receives a catheter (Crow *et al.*, 1988). UTI is also a major problem in nursing homes and rehabilitation centres where the elderly, debilitated and others catheterized for prolonged periods are at greater risk of acquiring recurrent UTIs and of the long-term complications associated with the infection (Warren *et al.*, 1982).

Definition of Urinary Tract Infection

In a non-catheterized individual the diagnosis of a UTI is usually based on clinical symptoms: frequency of micturition, pain on micturition (dysuria), fever and sometimes loin or suprapubic pain. These symptoms reflect **inflammation** of the bladder or kidneys. In the catheterized patient, frequency and dysuria will not be apparent and other symptoms may be absent, particularly in the elderly or confused patient.

The diagnosis of UTI may be confirmed in the microbiology laboratory by the isolation of more than 10^5 organisms per ml from a specimen of urine. The presence of **white blood cells** in the urine can provide evidence of an inflammatory process in the bladder, which may be caused by **infection** but could be related to the presence of the catheter or urological surgery.

Bacteria may also **colonize** the urinary tract without invading the tissues; this is referred to as **bacteriuria**. Bacteriuria can occur in both catheterized and non-catheterized people but is particularly associated with catheterization. Bacteria may initially be present in the urine in low numbers but if the patient is not receiving antibiotics, will increase to more than a million per ml of urine within a few days (Stark and Maki 1984). If more than one type of bacteria is found in the urine of a non-catheterized patient this is often attributed to contamination of the specimen by bacteria from the skin or perineum. In the catheterized patient, two or more types of bacteria are frequently identified. The longer the catheter is *in situ* the greater the variety of bacteria isolated from the urine (Warren *et al.*, 1982). Treatment of asymptomatic bacteriuria is usually unsuccessful but the colonization will frequently disappear after the catheter is removed.

The Routes of Infection

Bacteria enter the bladder of the catheterized patient in one of three ways; firstly, they may be introduced with the catheter at the time of insertion; secondly, they may travel along the outside of the catheter; and thirdly, they may travel along the inside lumen of the catheter (Fig. 10.1). There are important differences between men and women in the significance of each route of infection.

The perineum is frequently colonized by micro-organisms from the intestinal tract, especially **Gram-negative** bacteria. The presence of these bacteria is particularly significant in women because they are able to travel along the relatively short urethra to establish infection in the bladder more easily than in men. The elderly are particularly vulnerable to infection by this route and up to 50% of non-catheterized elderly residents in nursing homes have bacteria in their urine (Nicolle, 1987).

When a urethral catheter is in place the bacteria which colonize the perineum travel along the outside of the catheter into the bladder. Kass and Schneiderman (1959) demonstrated that *Serratia marcescens* inoculated onto the urethral meatus of catheterized patients could be isolated in the urine a few days later. This route accounts for around 70% of episodes of bacteriuria in women (Daifuku and Stamm, 1984). Gram-negative **bacilli** predominate in the perineal flora of the long-term catheterized patient and are frequently recovered from their urine (Kunin and Steel, 1985).

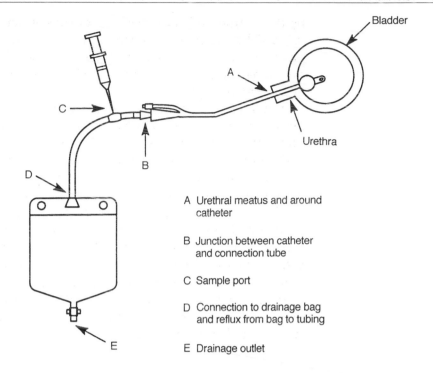

Fig. 10.1
*Potential points of entry of
micro-organisms into the
bladder of a catheterized
patient.*

Bladder

A

Urethra

C

B

D

E

A Urethral meatus and around
   catheter

B Junction between catheter
   and connection tube

C Sample port

D Connection to drainage bag
   and reflux from bag to tubing

E Drainage outlet

In men, infection from perineal flora is less important because the urethra is longer and further away from the rectum. Generally, bacteria gain access to the bladder via the lumen of the catheter, frequently as a result of cross-infection from enteric bacteria carried on the hands of staff which enter the urine system when it is disconnected or handled (Daifuku and Stamm, 1984).

Nickel *et al.* (1985) suggest that in the patient catheterized for less than 7 days, most bacteria enter the drainage system from the drainage tap or following disconnection of the system. As the duration of catheterization increases, bacteria are more likely to enter the bladder alongside the catheter.

The Duration of Catheterization

Garibaldi *et al.* (1974) demonstrated the strong relationship between the length of time the catheter was in place and the risk of UTI. He found that the risk of acquiring infection increased by 5% for each additional day of catheterization and after 10 days 50% of patients have bacteria in the urine. It is therefore not surprising that virtually all chronically catheterized patients have bacteria in their urine (Warren *et al.*, 1982).

One of the most crucial measures to prevent catheter-associated UTI is the removal of the catheter as quickly as possible. This is particularly important where prolonged catheterization is not necessary (e.g. the post-surgical patient). Patients who require a permanent or long-term catheter will ultimately acquire bacteria in the urine and in this group of patients it is important to recognize and treat *symptomatic* infection, to prevent the introduction of new bacteria and to prevent cross-infection of bacteria in the urine to other patients.

The Effect of Urinary Tract Infections

The bladder usually relies on mechanical defence mechanisms, including flushing the urinary tract with urine and regular emptying of the bladder, to prevent bacteria multiplying in the bladder. When a catheter is inserted, the retention balloon prevents complete emptying of the bladder and by damaging the epithelial lining enables bacteria to adhere to the surface (Stamm, 1991). Bacteria may subsequently invade the bladder wall and enter the blood stream (**bacteraemia**). If the catheter or drainage tubing is kinked, the build-up of urine in the bladder may result in infected urine entering the ureters or kidneys and causing pyelonephritis.

Generally, catheterized patients with bacteriuria remain asymptomatic with no evidence of bacteria invading the bladder tissues, ureters or kidneys. However, in up to 30% of catheterized patients with bacteriuria, the bacteria invade the tissues and the patient develops symptoms of UTI (Garibaldi *et al.*, 1982). Patients with long-term catheters have approximately one episode of unexplained fever every 100 days (Peterson and Roth, 1989).

A study by Platt *et al.* (1982) demonstrated that catheterized patients who acquired a UTI in hospital were three times more likely to die than those who did not, even if other factors such as age, duration of catheterization and the severity of their illness were taken into account. This increased mortality is probably related to consequences of UTI:

Bacteraemia

The most serious outcome of bacteria colonizing the urinary tract is bacteraemia – the presence of bacteria in the bloodstream but without apparent symptoms. Symptomatic invasion of the bloodstream (**septicaemia**) occurs much less frequently.

Bacteraemia probably goes unrecognized in many catheterized patients. It has been found to occur in up to 10% of patients during catheterization, when trauma to the mucosa during the procedures enables bacteria to enter the bloodstream. The urinary tract is a common source of bacteraemia, especially those caused by Gram-negative bacilli. In about one-third of cases, the patient dies as a result (Bryan and Reynolds, 1984).

Secondary Infections

Bacteria from the urinary tract may also cause secondary infections at other sites of the body for example wounds and central venous cannulae (Garibaldi, 1993).

Damage to the Urinary Tract

Evidence from autopsies suggests that acute inflammation of the kidneys occurs in over one-third of patients who have been catheterized for prolonged periods. These patients are also at risk of developing urinary stones, epididymitis and prostate infection (Warren *et al.*, 1988).

Measures to Prevent Infection in the Catheterized Patient

Since the urethral catheter has become a routine feature of medical care it is easy to forget the importance of prevention of infection in its management. The impact of good catheter management has been demonstrated by the reduction in catheter-associated UTI over the last few decades. In the 1960s urethral catheters drained into open buckets or bottles and over 90% of catheterized patients developed bacteriuria. In the 1970s, the system of closed drainage system into a plastic bag was introduced and the rate dropped to 25%. In the 1980s and 1990s even lower rates of around 10% have been reported, reflecting improved infection control and decreasing duration of catheterization (Stamm, 1991).

Practices to prevent infection, based on research evidence, should be applied to the insertion of the catheter, the management of the urine drainage system and the care of the urethral meatus. Recommended practices are summarized in the Guidelines for Practice and are discussed in more detail below.

Insertion of the Catheter

The development of bacteriuria after a single insertion and removal of a catheter ranges from 0.5% to 30% in the severely debilitated (Garibaldi, 1993). Since the risk of infection increases with each additional day of catheterization, the catheter should be removed as soon as possible.

To minimize the risk of infection the catheter should be inserted directly into the urethra without touching other parts of the perineum which may be heavily colonized with bacteria. This probably explains

Guidelines for Practice

Insertion of a Urethral Catheter

- Wash hands and use sterile gloves
- Prepare the patient and position comfortably
- Instil anaesthetic lubricating gel into the urethra
- Clean perineum and external meatus with soap and water
- Use sterile equipment
- Insert catheter directly into urethra
- Select catheter appropriately
- Inflate balloon with correct amount of sterile water
- Remove the catheter as soon as possible

why catheters inserted in the operating theatre, where the procedure is more easily performed, are associated with fewer infections (Castle and Osterhout, 1974). It is impossible to remove completely the perineal flora prior to the procedure but the number of bacteria can be reduced by washing with soap and water before insertion. A thorough explanation to the patient and the use of anaesthetic gel will improve patient compliance and reduce the risk of contamination of the catheter and trauma to the urethra (Boore, 1978).

Securing the catheter to the patient's thigh has been recommended to prevent it moving in the urethra (Jenner 1983). There is no evidence that this reduces the infection rate but it is probably more comfortable for the patient.

Intermittent Catheterization

In patients who need long-term catheterization, periodic emptying of the bladder by a single catheterization has been shown to be effective and reduces the risk of infection associated with long-term catheterization (Perkush and Giroux, 1993). The patient can be taught to self-catheterize safely using a clean, re-usable catheter washed between each use (Lapides *et al.*, 1975). Self-catheterization is an accepted form of management for some spinal injury patients enabling them to lead a more normal life in the community. If hospitalized, patients using self-catheterization should be facilitated to manage their catheterization using the technique with which they are familiar. The value of intermittent catheterization in other groups of patients has yet to be determined (Garibaldi, 1993).

Suprapubic catheterization

The risk of bacteria entering the bladder along the outside of the catheter can be avoided by insertion of a catheter directly into the bladder through the abdominal wall. The catheters are inserted under local or general anaesthetic, can be self-retaining or stitched to the abdominal wall. There is some evidence to suggest that suprapubic catheters are less frequently associated with bacteriuria (Sethia *et al.*, 1987).

Penile sheaths

Drainage of urine into a penile sheath attached to a drainage bag should reduce the risk of bacteria entering the bladder alongside the catheter, but they have been associated with high rates of bacteriuria and local skin infection (Johnson, 1983).

Type of Catheter

Urine catheters are available in a wide range of sizes and materials, appropriate selection is essential to minimize the trauma to the delicate mucosa of the bladder and urethra.

Catheter Size

The diameter of a catheter is measured in Charriere, 8–10 Ch for paediatric catheters and 12–30 Ch for adult catheters. The lumen of even the smallest catheter is sufficient to cope with the volume of urine produced and the larger catheters are only indicated where the lumen may become blocked by an unusual amount of debris (e.g. following bladder or prostate gland surgery). To minimize trauma to the urethra only 12 and 14 Ch catheters should be used for routine catheterization in adults, unless the urine contains a considerable amount of debris. Whistle-tip catheters have large drainage holes to accommodate clots and debris.

Catheters are now also available in a shorter length for female patients. Male length catheters used in female patients result in a considerable amount of excess tubing which is more likely to kink and cannot be easily concealed under skirts when used with leg bags.

The most common sizes of retention balloon are 10 ml and 30 ml. Large balloons irritate the bladder mucosa, causing pain and discomfort to the patient (Roe and Brocklehurst, 1987). They also increase the

Fig. 10.2
The urine catheter retention balloon. (a) A 30 ml balloon. (b) A 10 ml balloon.

(a)   (b)

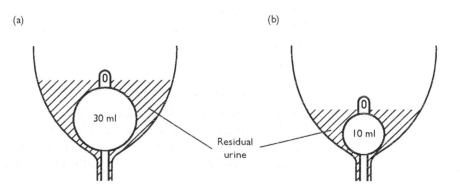

30 ml

Residual
urine

10 ml

Fig. 10.3
An underinflated retention balloon. The distorted balloon is more likely to damage the bladder mucosa.

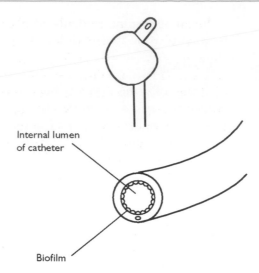

Fig. 10.4
Biofilm formation inside a urethral catheter.

Internal lumen
of catheter

Biofilm

volume of urine remaining in the bladder, providing nutrients in which bacteria can multiply (Fig. 10.2). The 30 ml balloon is therefore usually only indicated following prostate surgery where its size and weight may reduce bleeding from the prostatic bed. All other catheters should be retained in the bladder with a 10 ml balloon. It is also essential to inflate the balloon with the correct amount of sterile water. Balloons that are under- or over-inflated become misshapen and increase the risk of irritating the bladder mucosa (Fig. 10.3).

Catheter material

Bacteria attach to the internal surface of the catheter, secrete a matrix of sugars and proteins (glycocalyx) which together with salts, proteins and cell debris from the urine form a **biofilm**. The biofilm, commonly referred to as encrustation can build up to such an extent that it obstructs the lumen of the catheter and prevents the flow of urine (Fig. 10.4). Patients who are expected to have a catheter in place for more than 3 weeks require a catheter that will cause the minimum of irritation and be resistant to encrustation (Table 10.1).

Table 10.1
Selection of a catheter for routine urine drainage

Catheter material	Indication	Comments
Plastic	Very short-term use only, avoid if possible	Rigid material, irritates mucosa
Latex coated with silicone or teflon	For up to 3 weeks of catheterization e.g. post surgery	Reasonably non-irritant but prone to encrustation
Latex coated with hydrogel and all silicone	For more than 3 weeks of catheterization	Minimal mucosal irritation. Resistant to encrustation

Note : examine the packaging carefully for a description of the catheter material. Some trade names such as 'silastic' refer to latex-coated not all-silicone catheters.

Urine catheters are made of plastic, latex coated with inert materials such as silicone or teflon, or all-silicone. The bladder mucosa tolerates these materials to a variable extent and the material can also influence the rate at which biofilms develop. Plastic catheters are associated with bladder spasm, urethral pain and leakage and their use should be avoided (Blannin and Hobden 1980). Silicone is a very inert material, causes minimal irritation and is fairly resistant to encrustation (Kunin *et al.*, 1987). Latex is a highly irritant material but when coated with a more inert material, such as silicone, can be tolerated for longer. Hydrogel coating absorbs liquid to become soft and slippery and therefore causes minimum damage to the urethral mucosa and has a similar resistance to encrustation as all-silicone catheters (Cox *et al.*, 1988). Silver is antibacterial and non-toxic and, recently, silver-coated catheters have been developed with the aim of reducing bacteriuria. Currently, there is limited evidence to support their use (Johnson *et al.*, 1990)

Frequency of Catheter Replacement

A transient bacteraemia can occur during re-catheterization and long-term catheters should therefore not be changed unless necessary (Bryan and Reynolds, 1984). Provided the most appropriate size and type of catheter has been selected, the main indication for catheter change is when the lumen becomes blocked by debris or encrustation. The rate at which the catheter encrusts depends on the catheter material and the urine. An alkaline urine which contains high concentrations of proteins and calcium salts causes biofilms to develop more rapidly (Kunin *et al.*, 1987). The presence of certain types of bacteria in the urine, especially *Proteus* and *Pseudomonas*, also encourages the formation of biofilms. Some solutions are recommended for regular instillations into the bladder to prevent biofilm formation but the efficacy of these solutions has yet to be demonstrated (Roe, 1989).

A catheter blocked by encrustation may cause urine to leak around the side of the catheter. Irritation of the bladder mucosa initiating bladder spasm may also force urine out of the bladder around the catheter. Large catheters are particularly associated with irritation and leakage (Blannin and Hobden, 1980).

Reducing Colonization of the Perineum

A considerable amount of advice about the management of urine catheters has related to preventing bacteria colonizing the perineum gaining access to the bladder from the urethral opening. Regular cleansing with an antiseptic solution has been recommended (Seal *et al.*, 1982) and a survey in the UK indicated that meatal cleansing is still widely practised (Crow *et al.*, 1986). However, a controlled trial found that catheterized patients who received no meatal cleansing had the lowest infection rate and that cleansing with soap was associated with fewer infections than with povidone–iodine (Burke *et al.*, 1981). The conclusion to be drawn from this study is that bacteria are more likely to be introduced to the urethra during the cleaning procedure and a specific meatal cleansing procedure should be avoided. Meatal care using soap and water and clean wipes should therefore be based on the usual hygiene requirements of individual patients.

There is little evidence that bathing increases the incidence of UTI in catheterized patients. Degroot (1979) in a study on 10 catheterized patients, used a dye in the bathwater to indicate that the water did not pass into the bladder during bathing.

Although antimicrobial creams applied to the urethral opening have been shown to reduce the incidence of bacteriuria the additional costs of cream and nursing time do not make this procedure cost effective (Classen *et al.*, 1991).

Guidelines for Practice

Perineal Cleansing

- Should be part of daily hygiene, particularly in women
- Perineum should be cleaned more frequently in faecally incontinent patients
- Retract prepuce and clean underneath it
- Use soap/water and clean wipes
- Wash hands before and after procedure
- Antimicrobial creams are not cost-effective
- Patient may take baths

Management of the Drainage System

Bacteria enter the drainage system in the drainage bag or at the junction between the catheter and the drainage bag. These bacteria reach the bladder along the tubing after a few days (Garibaldi *et al.*, 1974).

The significance of a closed system of urinary drainage to the prevention of UTI was not really appreciated until the 1960s. Prior to this time, catheter urine had commonly flowed into an open container and infection rates as high as 95% within 24 h of catheterization were common. The plastic, drainable urine drainage bags with which we are now familiar were introduced in the early 1970s and have had a significant impact on reducing the rate of UTI (Thornton and Andriole, 1970).

Breaks in the closed system have been reported to occur frequently (Burke *et al.*, 1986). Crow *et al.* (1988) found that the catheter/drainage bag junction was disconnected in 42% of patients and in 52% of patients the bag was not properly positioned to ensure downward flow of urine.

The importance of not opening the drainage system was demonstrated in a study by Platt *et al.* in 1983 who used catheters which had been pre-sealed to a drainage bag. The seals could be removed and the bag disconnected but none the less a 17% reduction in disconnection was recorded. The control group of patients whose catheters were not sealed had three times more UTIs than the group with sealed catheters. These studies suggest that there is considerable room for improvement in the management of urinary drainage systems which may prevent the development of bacteriuria in the short-term catheterized patient.

Bacteria easily gain access to the drainage bag from the tap and multiply very rapidly in urine at room temperature (Bradley *et al.*, 1986). Bacteria remaining in the bag after it is emptied inoculate fresh urine entering the bag. The bacterial biofilm that adheres and spreads over the surface of the catheter and drainage bag enables bacteria in the bag to travel through non-return valves in the bag and along the lumen of the catheter into the bladder (Nichel *et al.*, 1985). Flutter valves, drip chambers or airlocks are of no value in preventing bacteriuria.

Incorrect positioning of the drainage bag can assist the transfer of bacteria to the bladder. Roberts *et al.* (1965) found that bacteria could be transported distances of 0.9–1.2 m in rising air bubbles, often generated when the tubing is kinked and columns of urine formed.

Bacteria grow less readily in dilute urine which has scarce nutrients (Asscher *et al.*, 1966). Encouraging the catheterized patient to drink plenty of fluid has the practical value of maintaining a constant downward flow of urine and reducing bacterial multiplication in the drainage bag. Some fluids (e.g. cranberry juice) are considered to reduce bacteria in the urine by changing its acidity (Rogers, 1991). The insertion of antiseptic solutions is not recommended as resistant bacteria emerge rapidly (Stickler, 1990).

Maintenance of the Drainage System

- Use bag with an integral measuring chamber if monitoring of urine output required
- Do not change bag routinely
- Do not disconnect the catheter from the drainage bag unless absolutely necessary
- Empty bag as infrequently as possible
- Wash hands before and after procedure
- Use gloves to empty bag into clean container
- Take urine specimens from sample port, not drainage bag
- Ensure urine always flows downwards
- Avoid kinks in tubing
- Hang bag evenly on stand
- Do not change leg bags at night but connect to an overnight drainage bag
- Avoid use of bladder instillations

Guidelines for Practice

Catheter valves have also been proposed as a method of preventing bacteria gaining access to the bladder via the drainage bag. They enable the bladder to fill and to be emptied intermittently without the use of a drainage system. They may benefit the catheterized patient by reducing the incidence of infection, restoring bladder tone and improving their quality of life (Roe, 1990a).

Cross-infection between catheterized patients has been frequently reported but the extent of the problem is probably underestimated (Schaberg *et al.*, 1980). Bacteria contaminating the drainage bag and the junction between catheter and bag are easily transferred to the hands when the bag is emptied or the drainage system is handled. The design of the tap influences the extent to which urine contaminates the hands during the emptying of the bag (Glenister, 1987). Inadequately cleaned collection containers may also transmit infection between catheterized patients. Antibiotic-resistant strains of bacteria, which often have an ability to survive and transmit easily in the hospital environment, are commonly associated with outbreaks of infection amongst catheterized patients.

Bladder Instillations

The administration of a bladder instillation involves disconnection of the closed drainage system which, as illustrated earlier, has been clearly demonstrated to increase the incidence of UTI.

There is some evidence that antiseptics instilled in the bladder may prevent infection in patients who have had urological surgery, but they are ineffective in treating established infections (Slade and Gillespie, 1985). The extensive use of these solutions has also been associated with the emergence of resistant bacteria (Stickler, 1990).

Instillation of antiseptic solutions such as chlorhexidine and noxythiolin should therefore not be used as part of routine management of the catheterized patient. A catheter blocked with debris should be flushed with saline taking great care not to contaminate the connections.

Other bladder instillations containing weak acids are intended to remove or control crystal formation (e.g. Suby-G). These are indicated only for patients who have particular problems with rapidly encrusting catheters where they may remove or prevent encrustation may reduce the need for frequent recatheterization (Roe, 1990c).

Leg drainage bags

Until recently, patients with a leg bag to collect urine changed it for a larger overnight drainage bag to collect the volume of urine produced at

Fig. 10.5
Overnight drainage system for a leg drainage bag.

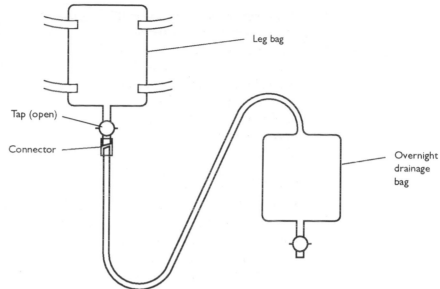

Leg bag

Tap (open)

Connector

Overnight drainage bag

night. This frequent disconnection of the drainage system increased the risk of introducing bacteria. Leg bag systems which enable an overnight drainage bag to be connected directly to the leg bag without incurring a break in the closed system are now available (Fig. 10.5)

Patient Education

Teaching patients to care for their own urinary catheters can minimize the risk of cross-infection. The long-term catheterized patient in the community can benefit from education on how to manage his/her catheter and minimize the risk of introducing bacteria. Instruction should include advice on careful hand hygiene, perineal cleansing, positioning of the drainage bag and recognizing symptoms of infection (Roe, 1990b).

Treatment of Catheter-associated UTI

Treatment of asymptomatic bacteriuria is not usually recommended; it will only have a temporary effect and may encourage the emergence of antibiotic-resistant bacteria. Bacteriuria normally resolves spontaneously once the catheter has been removed and the best treatment is for the catheter to be removed as soon as possible. The catheterized patient who develops symptoms of UTI or symptoms of infection which are thought to be associated with the catheter requires treatment with systemic antibiotics if the catheter cannot be removed. Since bacteria in a biofilm on the catheter may be protected from the antibiotic, the catheter should changed once treatment has commenced (Garibaldi, 1993).

References

Asscher AW, Sussman M, Waters WE *et al.* (1966) Urine as a medium for bacterial growth. *Lancet* **1**: 1039–41.

Blannin JP, Hobden J (1980) The catheter of choice. *Nursing Times*. **76**: 2092–3.

Boore JRP (1978) *Prescription for Recovery*. Nursing Research Series. Royal College of Nursing, London.

Bradley C, Babb J, Davies J *et al.* (1986) Taking precautions. *Nursing Times* **5th March**: 70–3.

Burke JP, Garibaldi RA, Britt MR *et al.* (1981) Prevention of catheter-associated urinary tract infections – efficacy of daily meatal care regimes. *Am. J. Med.* **70**: 655–8.

Burke JP, Larsen RA, Stevens LE (1986) Nosocomial bacteriuria: estimating the potential for prevention by closed sterile urinary drainage. *Inf. Contr.* **7**: 96–9.

Bryan CS, Reynolds KL (1984) Hospital-acquired bacteremic urinary tract infection. Epidemiology and outcome. *J. Urol.* **132**: 494–8.

Castle M, Osterhout S (1974) Urinary tract catheterisation and associated infection. *Nurs. Research* **23**: 170–4.

Classen DC, Larsen RA, Burke JP *et al.* (1991) Daily meatal care for prevention of catheter-associated bacteriuria: results using frequent applications of poly-antibiotic cream. *Inf. Contr. Hosp. Epid.* **12**: 157–62.

Cox A, Hukins D, Sutton T (1988) Comparison of *in vitro* encrustation on silicone and hydrogel-coated latex catheters. *Brit. J. Urol.* **61**: 156–61.

Crow RA, Chapman RG, Roe BH, Wilson JA (1986) *A Study of Patients with an Indwelling Urethral Catheter and Related Nursing Practice*. Nursing Practice Research Unit. University of Surrey.

Crow RA, Mulhall A, Chapman RG (1988) Indwelling catheterisation and related nursing practice. *J. Adv. Nurs.* **13**: 489–95.

Daifuku R, Stamm W (1984) Association of rectal and urethral colonisation with urinary tract infection in patients with indwelling urethral catheters. *JAMA* **252**: 2028–30.

Degroot JE (1979) Entrance of water into the bladder during Sitz bath in elderly catheterised and non-catheterised females. *Invest. Urol.* **117**: 207–8.

Garibaldi RA (1993) Hospital-acquired urinary infections. In *Prevention and Control of Nosocomial infections*, 2nd edn (RP Wenzel, Ed.), pp. 600–13. Williams and Wilkins, Baltimore MD.

Garibaldi RA, Burke JP, Dickman ML *et al.* (1974) Factors predisposing to bacteriuria during indwelling urethral catheterisation. *New Engl. J. Med.* **291**: 215–19.

Garibaldi RA, Mooney BR, Epstein BJ *et al.* (1982) An evaluation of daily bacteriologic monitoring to identify preventable episodes of catheter-associated urinary tract infection. *Inf. Control* **3**: 466–70.

Getliffe K (1990) Catheter blockage in the community. *Nurs. Stand.* **5**(9): 33–6.

Glenister H (1987) The passage of infection. *Nursing Times* **83**(22): 68–73.

Jenner EA (1983) Prevention of catheter associated urinary tract infection. *Nursing* **2**(13)Suppl: 1–3.

Johnson ET (1983) The condom catheter: urinary tract infection and other complications. *South. J. Med.* **76**: 579–82.

Johnson JR, Roberts PL, Olsen RJ *et al.* (1990) Prevention of catheter-associated urinary tract infections with a silver oxoid-coated urinary catheter: clinical and microbiological correlates. *J.Inf. Dis.* **162**: 1145–50.

Kass EH, Schneiderman LJ (1959) Entry of bacteria into the urinary tract of patients with inlying catheters. *New Engl. J. Med.* **256**: 556–7.

Krieger JN, Kaiser DL, Wenzel RP (1983) Nosocomial urinary tract infections:

secular trends, treatment and economics in a university hospital. *J. Urol.* **130**: 102–6.

Kunin CM (1987) *Detection, Prevention and Management of Urinary Tract Infections*. Lea and Febiger, Philadelphia.

Kunin CM, Steele C (1985) Culture of the surfaces of urinary catheters to sample urethral flora and study the effect of antimicrobial therapy. *J. Clin. Micro.* **21**: 902–8.

Kunin CM, Chin QF, Chambers S (1987) Formation of encrustations on indwelling urinary catheters in the elderly: a comparison of different types of catheter materials in blockers and non-blockers. *J. Urol.* **138**: 899–902.

Lapides J, Diokono AC, Gould FR *et al.* (1975) Further observations on self-catheterisation. *Transactions of the American Association of Genito-Urinary Surgeons* **67**: 15–17.

Meers PD, Ayliffe GAJ, Emmerson AM *et al.* (1981) National survey of infections in hospital, 1980. *J. Hosp. Inf.* **2**(Suppl.): 23–8.

Nickel JC, Grant SK, Costerton JW (1985) Catheter-associated bacteriuria an experimental study. *Urology* **36**: 369–75.

Nicolle LE (1987) Urinary tract infections in long-term care facilities. *Inf. Contr. Hosp. Epid.* **14**: 220–5.

Perkush I, Giroux J (1993) Clean intermittent catheterisation in spinal cord injury patients. A follow-up study. *J. Urol.* **149**(5): 1068–71.

Peterson JR, Roth EJ. (1989) Fever, bacteriuria and pyuria in spinal cord injured patients with indwelling urethral catheters. *Arch. Phys. Med. Rehab.* **70**: 839–41.

Platt R, Polk BF, Murdock B *et al.* (1982) Mortality associated with nosocomial urinary tract infection. *New Engl. J. Med.* **307**: 939–43.

Platt R, Murdock B, Polk BF (1983) Reduction of mortality associated with nosocomial urinary tract infection. *Lancet* **1**: 1893–7.

Roberts JMB, Linton KB, Pollard BR *et al.* (1965) Long term catheter drainage in the male. *Brit. J. Urol.* **37**: 63–72.

Roe BH (1989) Use of bladder washouts: a study of nurses recommendations *J. Adv. Nurs.* **14**: 494–500.

Roe B (1990a) Do we need to clamp catheters? *Nursing Times* **86**(43): 66–7.

Roe BH (1990b) Study of the effects of education on the management of urine drainage systems by patients and carers. *J. Adv. Nurs.* **15**: 223–31.

Roe B (1990c) Bladder instillations. *Nursing Standard* **4**(51): 25–7.

Roe BH, Brocklehurst JC (1987) Study of patients with indwelling catheters. *J. Adv. Nurs.* **12**: 713–18.

Rogers J (1991) Pass the cranberry juice. *Nursing Times* **87**(Nov. 27): 36–7.

Schaberg DR, Haley RW, Highsmith AK *et al.* (1980) Nosocomial bacteriuria: a prospective study of case clustering and antimicrobial resistance. *Ann. Intern. Med.* **93**: 420–4.

Seal DU, Wood S, Barret S *et al.* (1982) Evaluation of aseptic techniques and chlorhexidine on the rate of catheter-associated urinary-tract infection. *Lancet* **i**: 89–92.

Sethia KK, Selkon JB, Berry AR *et al.* (1987) Prospective randomised controlled trial of urethral versus suprapubic catheterisation. *Br. J. Surg.* **74**: 624–5.

Slade N, Gillespie WA (1985) *The Urinary Tract and the Catheter: Infection and Other Problems*. John Wiley, Chichester.

Stamm WE (1991) Catheter-associated urinary tract infections: epidemiology, pathogenesis and prevention. *Am. J. Med.* **91**(Suppl. 3B): 65S–71S.

Stark RP, Maki D (1984) Bacteriuria in the catheterised patient. What quantitative level of bacteriuria is relevant? *New Engl. J. Med.* **311**: 560–4.

Stickler DJ (1990) Antiseptics in bladder catheterization. *J. Hosp. Inf.* **16**: 89–108.

Thornton GF, Andriole VT (1970) Bacteriuria during indwelling catheter drainage II: effect of a closed sterile drainage system. *J. Am. Med. Ass.* **214**: 339–42.

Warren JW, Muncie HL, Hall-Craggs M (1988) Acute pyelonephritis associated with bacteriuria during long-term catheterisation: a prospective clinico-pathological study. *J. Inf. Dis.* **158**: 1341–6.

Warren JW, Tenney JH, Hoopes JM, Muncie HL (1982) A prospective microbiological study of bacteriuria in patients with chronic indwelling urethral catheters. *J. Inf. Dis.* **146**: 719–23.

Further Reading

Berman P, Hogan DB, Fox RA (1987) The atypical presentation of infection in old age. *Age & Aging* **16**: 201–7.

Winder A (1990) Intermittent self-catheterisation. *Nursing Times* **86**(43): 63–4.

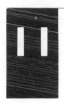

Preventing Infection of the Respiratory Tract

Introduction

The respiratory tract is divided into the upper part, from the nostrils to the larynx and the lower part, from the larynx to the alveoli (Fig. 11.1).

Infections of the upper respiratory tract (URT) are usually minor; most are caused by viruses and are acquired in the community (e.g. influenza, respiratory syncytial virus). Occasionally they may progress to more serious lower respiratory tract infection, particularly in the very young or the elderly (Breuer and Jeffries, 1990). Cross-infection between hospitalized patients and staff may occur.

Infections of the lower respiratory tract (LRT) are more serious and can be life-threatening. They include bronchitis and tracheitis, but the most important infection is pneumonia when the alveoli are filled with pus, air is excluded and the lung described as 'consolidated'. Pneumonia accounts for approximately 20% of infections acquired in hospital and is a serious problem – as many as 30% of the patients may die as a consequence (Leu *et al.*, 1989). Hospital-acquired pneumonia may be caused by inhalation of micro-organisms (e.g. *Legionella*, *Aspergillus* and respiratory viruses) from the environment or from infected individuals. However, the principal cause is the aspiration of bacteria from the oropharynx or their inhalation in aerosols from contaminated respiratory equipment (Tablan *et al.*, 1994).

Fig. 11.1
The respiratory tract.

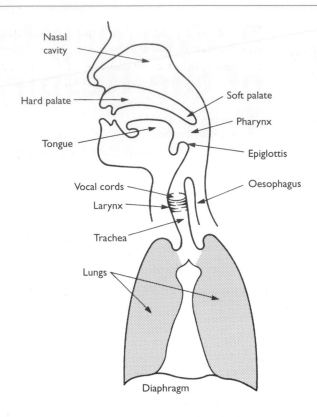

Micro-organisms can enter the respiratory tract on particles of dust or droplets of moisture carried in the air. Hairs in the nose filter some of the particles as they are breathed in. Most of the respiratory tract is lined by ciliated cells covered with sticky mucus. The mucus traps small particles preventing micro-organisms reaching the lungs. The **cilia**, which are hair-like structures, beat rhythmically in a co-ordinated fashion, propelling mucus upwards towards the larynx from the LRT and downwards from the nasal passages towards the larynx. When the mucus reaches the pharynx it is swallowed or coughed out of the respiratory system. If very small particles reach the alveoli they are engulfed by **phagocytic** cells of the immune system.

The cough reflex is stimulated by larger particles on the larynx or trachea and is an important mechanism for the expulsion of micro-organisms.

Natural Defences Against Infection of the Respiratory Tract

Factors Predisposing to Hospital-acquired Pneumonia

The risk of a patient developing pneumonia depends on the number of bacteria that enter the respiratory tract, the susceptibility of the patient to infection and the **virulence** of the organism. The risk of developing pneumonia is not the same for all patients. Some of the underlying conditions which make patients particularly vulnerable are illustrated in Table 11.1.

A number of factors influence the acquisition of hospital-acquired pneumonia and are summarized in Fig. 11.2 and discussed in detail below.

Aspiration

The most common cause of bacterial pneumonia is the aspiration of **pathogens colonizing** the surface of the oropharyngeal mucosa (Pugliese and Lichtenberg, 1987). Forty-five per cent of healthy people aspirate secretions from their oropharynx whilst they are asleep; however,

Table 11.1
Host factors that increase the risk of respiratory tract infection

- Elderly (over 70 years)
- Obesity
- History of smoking
- Immunosuppression
- Impaired consciousness
- Low birth weight infant (<1500 g)
- Abdominal or thoracic surgery
- Viral respiratory infection
- Serious underlying illness
- Underlying respiratory disease

Fig. 11.2
Factors that influence the acquisition of hospital-acquired pneumonia.

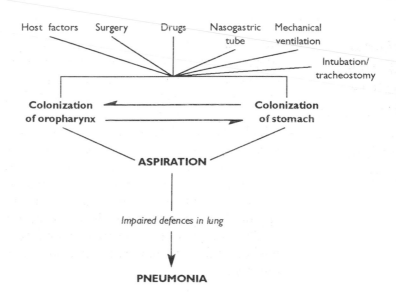

the natural defences are usually able to remove bacteria introduced to the respiratory system in this way (Huxley *et al.*, 1978).

In hospital patients the risk of aspiration is increased by invasive procedures which by-pass the natural defences, for example endotracheal and tracheostomy tubes. Aspiration is also more likely in patients with reduced levels of consciousness, for example in cerebrovascular accidents, drug overdose or general anaesthesia.

Colonization of the Oropharynx

The oropharynx in healthy people is frequently colonized by *Streptococcus pneumoniae* and *Haemophilus influenzae* and these two organisms are responsible for most pneumonia acquired in the community.

In hospitalized patients with serious underlying illness and who have been exposed to **antibiotics**, the **normal flora** of the oropharynx tends to be replaced with **aerobic Gram-negative bacilli** such as *Pseudomonas*, *Klebsiella* and *Enterobacter*. Where the organism causing the hospital-acquired pneumonia has been identified, Gram-negative bacilli account for approximately 60% of the infections (Table 11.2). After surgery or during severe illness, a protein, fibronectin, which prevents bacteria adhering to cells in the oropharynx, appears to be depleted. In its absence, Gram-negative bacteria are able to establish. The degree of colonization is particularly high in critically ill patients and is strongly associated with the development of pneumonia (Johanson *et al.*, 1972).

Colonization of the Stomach

Drugs such as antacids or cimetidine, which neutralize or block the production of gastric acid, are frequently used to prevent stress ulcers in ventilated patients and their use is associated with an increased

Table 11.2
Pathogens associated with hospital-acquired pneumonia. From Horan et al. (1988).

Pathogen	% Pneumonias
Gram-negative bacilli	60
Ps. aeruginosa	17
Enterobacter spp.	10
K. pneumoniae	7
E. coli	6
H. influenzae	6
Other	14
Gram-positive cocci	18
S. aureus	15
Strep. pneumoniae	3
Fungi	4

incidence of pneumonia (Craven *et al.*, 1991). In healthy people the stomach is normally sterile because the hydrochloric acid destroys micro-organisms entering with ingested food. If the acidity is reduced to a pH of around 4, the stomach rapidly becomes colonized by large numbers of Gram-negative bacilli (Craven *et al.*, 1986). Bacterial colonization of the stomach is also more likely to occur in elderly or malnourished patients and those with gastrointestinal disease. Once in the stomach bacteria may ascend the oesophagus to colonize the oropharynx and subsequently cause pneumonia (Du Moulin *et al.*, 1982).

Mechanical Ventilation and Respiratory Equipment

The highest incidence of hospital-acquired pneumonia occurs amongst patients who have received respiratory therapy. Continuous ventilatory support has been reported to increase the incidence of pneumonia by more than 7% (Cross and Roup, 1981). The entry of bacteria into the respiratory tract may be facilitated by contaminated aerosols, increased

Fig. 11.3
An endotracheal tube.

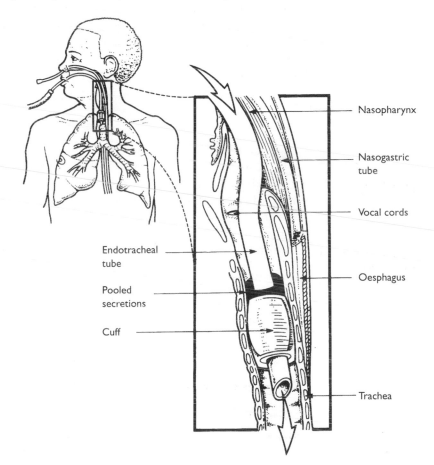

Nasopharynx

Nasogastric tube

Vocal cords

Endotracheal tube

Pooled secretions

Cuff

Oesophagus

Trachea

oropharyngeal colonization and impairment of the mechanisms that normally clear the airway (Garibaldi *et al.*, 1981).

The endotracheal and tracheostomy tubes by-pass the nose filter and impair swallowing of secretions. They also cause irritation and injury to the mucosa, enhancing the ability of Gram-negative bacilli to colonize the oropharynx. Heavily contaminated secretions may leak around the tube cuff, particularly when it is deflated, or enter the bronchi during suctioning procedures (Fig. 11.3). Like other types of invasive tubing, endotracheal tubes are susceptible to the formation of **biofilms**, a covering of bacteria and proteins which adheres firmly to the surface of the tube (Sottile *et al.*, 1986).

Bacteria may colonize ventilation equipment and deliver contaminated air directly into the lungs. This is a particular problem when gases are mixed with aerosolized water from nebulizers or humidifiers because

Fig. 11.4
Nebulization and humidification.

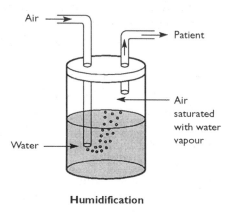

Humidification

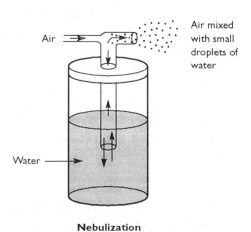

Nebulization

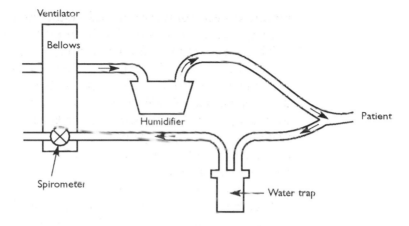

Fig. 11.5
Ventilator tubing with a heated-water humidifier.

bacteria, particularly Gram-negative bacilli, are able to survive and multiply in the moist environment (Figs 11.4, 11.5).

Epidemics of hospital acquired pneumonia related to contaminated nebulizers have been reported since the introduction of respiratory therapy equipment in the 1950s (Reinarz *et al.*, 1965). Nebulizers present a particular problem as they create an aerosol of small droplets, 1–2 μm in diameter, that can be inhaled into the lower respiratory tract. Contamination of small-volume medication nebulizers has been reported and has been associated with increased oropharyngeal colonization and ventilator-associated pneumonia (Craven *et al.*, 1984a; Botman and de Kreiger 1987).

Humidifiers increase the amount of water vapour in the inhaled gas but, unlike nebulizers, should not produce an aerosol of water droplets. Therefore, although the humidification reservoir may become contaminated with bacteria the organisms are not as likely to be inhaled in to the respiratory tract. None the less, humidified circuits are prone to the condensation of water in the tubing. Bacteria from the patient may colonize and multiply in this moisture and if the tubing is inadvertently raised the condensate will drain into the patient's trachea and increase the risk of pneumonia (Craven *et al.* 1984b). Stucke and Thompson (1980) found 45% of ventilator tubing was contaminated before the same organism appeared in the tracheal aspirates implicating cross-infection as the source of contamination of the tubing.

Recently, the development of heat–moisture exchange filters, which recycle the moisture in exhaled air, has eliminated the need for a humidifier in the ventilation of many patients (Make *et al.*, 1987).

Surgery

Three-quarters of hospital-acquired pneumonias have been found to occur in patients who had undergone surgery (Haley *et al.*, 1985). This increased risk is related to several factors: the defences of the respiratory tract are impaired by endotracheal intubation and anaesthetic gases, and aspiration is more likely to occur during anaesthesia. One-third of healthy patients develop oropharyngeal colonization with Gram-negative bacilli within 48 h of major surgery (Johanson *et al.*, 1980). Coughing is often difficult and painful following abdominal surgery and respiration may be depressed by the use of narcotics for pain relief.

Nasogastric Tubes

The presence of a nasogastric tube increases reflux of fluid from the stomach, providing a route for bacteria to migrate from the stomach to colonize the oropharynx and subsequently cause pneumonia (Craven *et al.*, 1991). The risk of pneumonia is further increased if the patient is receiving enteral feeding as bacteria are more likely to enter and colonize the stomach (Pingleton *et al.*, 1986). Maintaining the patient in an upright position may reduce reflux and hence the incidence of pneumonia.

The Prevention of Hospital-acquired Pneumonia
Postoperative Pneumonia

The patients most at risk of developing pneumonia postoperatively should be identified (see Table 11.1) and a programme of breathing exercises to encourage lung expansion and coughing, implemented before surgery. Lung expansion will also be helped by early ambulation. Some patients may need postural drainage and percussion postoperatively to assist expectoration of sputum. Pain that interferes with deep breathing or coughing should be controlled using analgesics together with appropriate wound support.

If oxygen therapy is required it should always be humidified to prevent drying of respiratory secretions and subsequent impairment of the normal clearance mechanisms.

The Management of Respiratory Therapy Equipment

Contaminated respiratory equipment has been frequently incriminated in outbreaks of respiratory tract infection and an organized approach to its decontamination is essential (Cefai *et al.*, 1990; Gorman *et al.*, 1993). For most equipment, high level **disinfection** is required to remove or substantially reduce microbial contamination. This can be achieved by **autoclave**, automated washing machine or, when these are unavailable, by chemical **disinfectants** (see Chapter 13). Tap water can be used to rinse off chemical disinfectants provided that the equipment is then allowed to dry completely, preventing the growth of any remaining bacteria.

Ventilators

Filters can often be used to protect both the inspiratory and expiratory circuits so that routine **sterilization** or disinfection of ventilators is not considered necessary (Gallagher *et al.*, 1987).

The level of contamination does not differ significantly after 24 or 48 h of mechanical ventilation. Disinfection or disposal of circuits every 48 h is therefore recommended (Craven *et al.*, 1982). If a heat–moisture exchange filter is fitted at the patient end instead of humidification, only the filter need be changed every 48 h. The tubing of anaesthetic machines can also be protected with heat–moisture exchange filters or heat-disinfected, preferably in an automated washing machine. Corrugated tubing is particularly difficult to dry and it should be washed and dried in a anaesthetic washing machine or hung vertically until dry.

Spirometers and resuscitation bags have been associated with the transmission of infection and should be changed with the ventilator circuits (Irwin, *et al.*, 1980). Resuscitation bags can be protected from contamination by the use of a filter.

Prevention of Hospital-acquired Pneumonia

Handwashing and Gloves
- Wear clean gloves for all contact with the respiratory tract secretions (including oral hygiene)
- Wash hands after every contact with an intubated patient even if gloves are worn

Maintenance of Respiratory Therapy Equipment
- Replace ventilator breathing circuits every 48 h
- Protect expiratory circuit with filter
- Fill nebulizers and humidifiers with sterile fluid
- Replace all opened fluid containers daily
- Decontaminate cascade humidifiers and nebulizers every 48 h (unless disposable)
- Clean and dry medication nebulizers between each treatment and discard between patients
- Change oxygen masks and tubing between patients

Suctioning
- Use clean gloves and wash hands before and after procedure
- Use sterile suction catheter and sterile fluid to flush catheter
- Insert catheter directly into airway and discard after each use
- Change suction collection canisters between patients (or daily in short-term care units)
- Change suction tubing between patients

Postoperative Care
- Implement breathing exercises prior to surgery
- Early ambulation post-surgery
- Control pain with analgesia
- Support wound to aid coughing

Guidelines for Practice

The condensate that tends to accumulate in ventilator tubing when cascade humidification is used is often contaminated and these bacteria are easily transmitted by staff handling the circuits. The condensate should be drained regularly from the tubing, although not into the nebulizer reservoir, and hands washed each time the tubing is handled (Gorman *et al.*, 1993).

Nebulizers and Humidifiers

Nebulizers and humidifiers should always be filled with sterile water to prevent colonization by *Legionella* or other bacteria. They may become contaminated by backflow of condensate from the delivery tubing and should be decontaminated every 48 h (Craven *et al.*, 1982). In cascade humidifiers bacteria will usually be prevented from multiplying as the temperature of the water is maintained at over 50°C (Christopher *et al.*, 1983). Medication nebulizers have been reported to become easily contaminated and should be cleaned with detergent and thoroughly dried after each treatment (Simmonds and Wong, 1983). This is also important for patients receiving respiratory therapy in their own home (Pitchford *et al.*, 1987).

Nebulizers and humidifiers should always be stored clean and dry when not in use and tubing and masks changed between patients.

Disposable humidification systems (e.g. Aquapak) have not been shown to reduce the incidence of pneumonia but are a useful alternative when access to autoclaving facilities is not possible (Daschner *et al.*, 1988).

Respiratory Suction

Bacteria colonizing the oropharynx will be easily acquired on the hands and catheter during suctioning. To minimize the risk of cross-infection a sterile suction catheter should be used, inserted directly into the trachea or pharynx and discarded after each use. Hands should be washed thoroughly before and after the procedure but clean gloves should also be worn to protect hands from contamination. There is no evidence that bacteria in suction canisters can reach the suction catheter, although a filter should be used on the canister to prevent release of bacteria into the environment. Studies comparing multi-use closed suction systems with the conventional single-use suction catheter system suggest that there is little difference in risk of pneumonia between the two (Deppe *et al.* 1990).

Cross-infection　　Bacteria that colonize the oropharynx of one patient may be easily transferred on the hands of staff to other patients (Lowbury *et al.*,

1970). This is a particular problem in intensive care or neonatal units where contact with respiratory excretions is extensive and where colonization of the oropharynx with Gram-negative bacteria is very common. In one study, the hands of staff were found to be contaminated with Gram-negative bacilli after changing ventilator tubing and were rarely washed before new tubing was attached (Cadwallader *et al.*, 1990). The routine use of gloves in intensive care units for contact with respiratory secretions has been associated with a decrease in the incidence of hospital-acquired pneumonia (Green *et al*, 1987).

Often outbreaks of infection are caused by bacteria resistant to a number of antibiotics. Controlling their spread usually requires isolation of colonized patients and rigorous use of protective clothing and hand-washing to interrupt spread (Sakata *et al.*, 1989).

Equipment must be decontaminated after each use. The level of decontamination required depends on the type of equipment; for example, low-risk items such as reusable oxygen masks should be washed with detergent and water and dried after each use. Other items that may be contaminated by blood or body fluid (e.g. laryngoscopes, airways) should be decontaminated by autoclaving or washing at a temperature of at least 70°C. See Chapter 13 for further information.

Monitoring the Incidence of Hospital-acquired Pneumonia

Awareness of the problem of hospital-acquired pneumonia and the need to consider its prevention when planning postoperative care and the management of respiratory therapy can significantly reduce the incidence of infection. Regular feedback of information to clinical staff on the incidence of hospital-acquired pneumonia in their ward has been shown to reduce the infection rate considerably (Haley *et al.*, 1985).

Airborne Transmission of Hospital-acquired Pneumonia

Most reported cases of hospital-acquired pneumonia are caused by bacteria and are not transmitted by an airborne route. Airborne transmission is of significance in the spread of respiratory viruses, tuberculosis and on rare occasions, *Legionella*. Severely **immunocompromised** patients may be susceptible to a range of unusual respiratory pathogens, notably *Aspergillus* and atypical *Mycobacterium*, which may be associated with outbreaks of **hospital-acquired infection** in certain circumstances (see Chapter 3). Tuberculosis is transmitted by the inhalation of airborne droplets expelled from the lungs of an infected person, but prolonged, close contact is usually necessary for transmission to occur (see Chapter 3).

Respiratory Viruses

Viral respiratory infections are commonly not diagnosed because the laboratory techniques that such diagnosis requires are frequently not requested by clinical staff. However, viruses have been found to be responsible for 20% of lower respiratory tract infections acquired in hospital (Valenti *et al.*, 1981). They often reflect the prevalence of the virus in the community, and in contrast to bacterial infections, most are acquired **exogenously** from other patients, staff or visitors. Viral respiratory infections are not particularly associated with debilitated patients although they may cause serious disease in them.

A large proportion of hospital-acquired viral pneumonias are caused by respiratory syncytial virus (RSV), influenza and parainfluenza viruses (Hall, 1981). In healthy adults these viruses cause a mild respiratory illness but may cause pneumonia in the very young or old or those with severe underlying disease. Community epidemics of RSV regularly occur in winter and children admitted with the infection are a source of infection to other patients in the ward (Madge *et al.*, 1992). Outbreaks of **nosocomial** influenza also usually occur when influenza is **epidemic** in the community.

The principal route of transmission of these viruses is contaminated hands and subsequent transferral to the eyes, nose or mouth. Virus may be acquired on the hands either directly from respiratory secretions or indirectly via contaminated surfaces or equipment (Ansari *et al.*, 1991). Virus may be shed from the infected person for up to 7 days after the onset of symptoms (Breese-Hall *et al.*, 1980). Influenza is thought to be transmitted by airborne droplets as well as on hands (Breuer and Jeffries, 1990).

To prevent transmission, patients admitted with suspected viral respiratory infection should be nursed in a single room with isolation precautions (see Chapter 14). Masks are not necessary as they are unlikely to protect the wearer. The greatest risk is from direct contact with secretions from the mouth and nose, and hands should therefore always be washed before leaving the patient's room.

Staff with respiratory infections also present a risk to patients and they should not care for patients who could develop serious illness if they acquired the infection.

Legionnaires' Disease

Legionella pneumophilia is commonly found in natural sources of water and in water supply systems. Under some conditions it multiplies in water systems and can be transmitted by an aerosol or spray of water from water cooling towers or whirlpool spas. It has been responsible for a number of outbreaks of nosocomial pneumonia, principally affecting the elderly or

immunosuppressed, although it may cause less serious disease in healthy people (Timbury et al., 1986; Bartlett et al., 1986). Infection is thought to be acquired by inhalation of Legionella in small water droplets. The risk from Legionella infection can be minimized by chlorination of the water supply, regular cleaning of the system, prevention of water stagnation in pipework and ensuring water is kept at temperatures at which the organism cannot multiply (less than 20°C or more than 60°C). Unfortunately, this means that the temperature of the hot water supply in hospitals must not fall below 50°C and care must be taken to avoid scalds to patients or staff. Showerheads do not require disinfecting if the water supply system is properly maintained (NHS Estates, 1993).

Respiratory therapy equipment has also been implicated in hospital-acquired legionellosis. Humidifiers or nebulizers contaminated with tap water can result in inhalation of aerosolized Legionella (Arnow et al., 1982). Other studies have implicated re-breathe bags attached to ventilators as a source of Legionella if rinsed with tap water (Woo et al., 1986) and ice-making machines (Medical Services Directorate, 1993). There is no evidence that Legionella can be transmitted from person to person and therefore isolation of infected patients is not necessary.

References

Ansari SA, Springthorpe S, Sattar SA et al. (1991) Potential role of hands in the spread of respiratory viral infections: studies with human para-influenza virus 3 and rhinovirus 14. J. Clin. Micro. **29**: 2115–19.

Arnow P, Chou T, Weil D et al. (1982) Nosocomial Legionnaires disease caused by aerosolised tap water from respiratory devices. J. Inf. Dis. **146**: 460–7.

Bartlett CLR, Macrae AD, Macfarlane JD (1986) Legionella Infections. Edward Arnold, London.

Botman MJ, de Krieger RA (1987) Contamination of small volume medication nebulisers and its association with oropharyngeal colonisation. J. Hosp. Inf. **10**: 204–8.

Breese-Hall C, Doughlas RG, Gelman JM (1980) Possible transmission by fomites of respiratory syncytial virus. J. Inf. Dis. **141**: 98–102.

Breuer J, Jeffries DJ (1990) Control of viral infections in hospital. J. Hosp. Inf. **16**: 191–221.

Cadwallader HL, Bradley CR, Ayliffe GAJ (1990) Bacterial contamination and frequency of changing ventilator circuitry. J. Hosp. Inf. **15**: 65–72.

Cefai C, Richards J, Gould FK et al. (1990) An outbreak of Acinetobacter respiratory tract infection resulting from incomplete disinfection of ventilatory equipment. J. Hosp. Inf. **15**. 177–82.

Christopher KL, Saravoltatz LD, Bush TL et al. (1983) The potential role of respiratory therapy equipment in cross-infection. Am. Rev. Resp. Dis. **128**: 271.

Craven DE, Connolly MG, Lichtenberg DA et al. (1982) Contamination of mechanical ventilator with tubing changes every 24 or 48 hours. New Eng. J. Med. **306**: 1505–8.

Craven DE, Lichtenberg DA, Goularte TA (1984a) Contaminated medication nebulisers in mechanical ventilatory circuits: a source of bacterial aerosols. *Am. J. Med.* **77**: 834–8.

Craven DE, Goularte TA, Make BJ (1984b) Contaminated condensate in mechanical ventilator circuits: a risk factor for nosocomial pneumonia? *Am. Rev. Resp. Dis.* **129**: 625–8.

Craven DE, Kunches LM, Kilinsky V *et al.* (1986) Risk factors for pneumonia and fatality in patients receiving continuous mechanical ventilation. *Am. Rev. Resp. Dis.* **133**: 792–6.

Craven DE, Steiger KA, Barber TW (1991) Preventing nosocomial pneumonia: state of the art and perspectives for the 1990s. *Am. J. Med.* **91**(Suppl. 3B): 44S–53S.

Cross AS, Roup B (1981) Role of respiratory assistance devices in endemic nosocomial pneumonia. *Am. J. Med.* **70**: 681–5.

Daschner FD, Kappstein I, Schuster F *et al.* (1988) Influence of disposable ('Conchapak') and reusable humidifying systems on the incidence of ventilation pneumonia. *J. Hosp. Inf.* **11**: 161–8.

Deppe SA, Kelly JW, Thoi LL *et al.* (1990) Incidence of colonization, noscomial pneumonia and mortality in critically ill patients using TrachC are closed suction system versus open suction system: prospective randomised study. *Crit. Care Med.* **18**: 1389–93.

Du Moulin GC, Paterson DG, Hedley-White J *et al.* (1982) Aspiration of gastric bacteria in antacid treated patients: a frequent cause of post-operative contamination of the airway. *Lancet* **1**: 242–5.

Gallagher J, Strangeways JEM, Allt-Graham J (1987) Contamination control in long-term ventilation. *Anaesthesia* **42**: 476–81.

Garibaldi RA, Britt MR, Coleman ML *et al.* (1981) Risk factors for post-operative pneumonias. *Am. J. Med.* **70**: 677–80.

Gorman LJ, Sanai L, Notman W *et al.* (1993) Cross-infection in an intensive care unit by *Klebsiella pneumoniae* from ventilator condensate. *J. Hosp. Inf.* **23**: 17–26.

Green SL, Overton S, Procter C (1987) The effect of glove wearing on the ICU nosocomial infection rates. *14th Annual APIC Educational Conference.* Abstract 1.

Haley RW, Culver DH, White JW *et al.* (1985) The efficacy of infection surveillance and control programs in preventing nosocomial infections in US hospitals *Am. J. Epidemiol.* **121**: 182.

Hall CB (1981) Nosocomial viral respiratory infections: perennial weeds on pediatric wards. *Am. J. Med.* **70**: 670–6.

Horan T, Culver D, Jarvis W *et al.* (1988) Pathogens causing nosocomial infections. *Antimicrob. Newsletter* **5**: 65–7.

Huxley EJ, Viroslav J, Gray WR *et al.* (1978) Pharyngeal aspiration in normal adults and patients with depressed consciousness. *Am. J. Med.* **64**: 564–8.

Irwin RS, Demars RR, Pratter MR *et al.* (1980) An outbreak of *Acinetobacter* infection associated with the use of a ventilator spirometer. *Resp. Care* **25**: 232–7.

Johanson WG, Pierce AK, Sanford JP *et al.* (1972) Nosocomial respiratory infections with Gram negative bacilli: the significance of colonisation of the respiratory tract. *Ann. Int. Med.* **77**: 701–6.

Johanson WG, Higuchi JG, Chaudhuri TR *et al.* (1980) Bacterial adherence to epithelial cells in bacillary colonisation of the respiratory tract. *Am. Rev. Resp. Dis.* **121**: 55–63.

Leu HS, Kaiser DL, Mori M *et al.* (1989) Hospital-acquired pneumonia: attributable mortality and morbidity. *Am. J. Epid.* **129**: 1258–67.

Lowbury EJL, Thorn BT, Lilly HA *et al.* (1970) Sources of infection with *Pseudomonas aeruginosa* in patients with tracheostomy. *J. Med. Micro.* **3**: 39–56.

Madge P, Payton JY, McColl JH *et al.* (1992) Prospective controlled study of four infection control procedures to prevent nosocomial infection with respiratory syncitial virus. *Lancet* **340**: 1079–83.

Make BJ, Craven DE, O'Donnell C *et al.* (1987) Clinical and bacteriologic comparison of hydroscopic and cascade humidifiers in ventilated patients. *Am. Rev. Resp. Dis.* **135**: A212.

Medical Services Directorate (1993) Ice cubes: Infection caused by *Xanthomonas maltophia.* **Hazard**(93): 42.

NHS Estates (1993) *The Control of* Legionella *in Healthcare Premises – a Code of Practice. Health Technical Memorandum* **240**. HMSO, London.

Pingleton SK, Hinthorn DR, Liu C (1986) Enteral nutrition in patients receiving mechanical ventilation: multiple sources of tracheal colonisation include the stomach. *Am. J. Med.* **80**: 827–32.

Pitchford KC, Corey M, Highsmith AK *et al.* (1987) *Pseudomonas* species contamination of cystic fibrosis patients' home inhalation equipment. *J. Paeds.* **111**: 212–16.

Pugliese G, Lichtenberg DA (1987) Nosocomial bacterial pneumonia: an overview. *Am. J. Inf. Contr.* **15**: 249–65.

Reinarz JA, Pierce AK, Mays BB *et al.* (1965) The potential role of inhalation therapy equipment in nosocomial pulmonary infections. *J. Clin. Invest.* **44**: 831–9.

Sakata H, Fujita K, Maruyama S *et al.* (1989) *Acinetobacter calcoaceticus* biovar *anitratus* septicaemia in a neonatal intensive care unit: epidemiology and control. *J. Hosp. Inf.* **14**: 15–22.

Suttile FD, Marrie TJ, Prough DS *et al.* (1986) Nosocomial pulmonary infection: possible etiologic significance of bacterial adhesion to endotracheal tubes. *Crit. Care. Med.* **14**: 265–70.

Stucke VA, Thompson REM (1980) Infection transfer by respiratory condensate during positive pressure respiration. *Nursing Times* **76**(9): 3–4.

Tablan OC, Anderson LJ, Arden NH *et al.* (1994) Guideline for the prevention of nosocomial pneumonia. *Am. J. Inf. Contr.* **22**: 247–92.

Timbury MC, Donaldson JR, McCartney AC *et al.* (1986) Outbreak of legionnaires' disease in Glasgow Royal Infirmary: microbiological aspects. *J. Hyg. (Camb.)* **97**(3): 393–403.

Valenti WM, Hall CB, Douglas RG *et al.* (1981) Nosocomial viral infections I: epidemiology and significance. *Infect. Control* **1**. 33–7.

Woo AH, Yu VL, Goetz A *et al.* (1986) Potential in-hospital modes of transmission of *Legionella pneumophilia*. Demonstration experiments for dissemination by showers, humidifiers and rinsing of ventilation bag apparatus. *Am. J. Med.* **80**. 567–73.

Further Reading Harrison L (1993) Factors influencing the frequency of ventilator circuit changes. *Brit. J. Nurs.* **2**(16): 793–801.

Hovig B (1981) Lower respiratory tract infection associated with respiratory therapy and anaesthetic equipment. *J. Hosp. Inf.* **2**: 301.

12 Preventing Gastrointestinal Infection: The Principles of Food Hygiene

- Introduction
- Principles of Food Hygiene
- Preventing the Spread of Gastrointestinal Infection
- Outbreaks of Gastrointestinal Illness
- References and Further Reading

Introduction
The source of micro-organisms which cause hospital-acquired gastrointestinal infection are contaminated food or **infectious** faeces and vomit. These micro-organisms may be easily transferred from person to person on hands or equipment. A hospital kitchen provides food for most of the patients and many staff. Poor personal and food hygiene may result in large numbers of people developing food poisoning which in debilitated and elderly patients may cause severe disease or death. Hospital patients are particularly susceptible to gastrointestinal infection because of reduced gastric acid production in the stomach associated with illness or old age. Table 12.1 illustrates the wide variety of micro-organisms associated with food poisoning and the most common sources from which they are derived.

Although outbreaks of gastrointestinal illness in hospital are usually assumed to be food-borne they can also result from cross-infection. Person-to-person transmission of enteric viruses occurs particularly easily. Even infections that are originally food-borne may be transmitted by cross-infection to other patients. Despite these problems, hospital-acquired gastrointestinal illness can be prevented. This chapter discusses the basic principles of food and personal hygiene that should be observed

Table 12.1
*Common causes of food-
borne illness*

Bacteria	Common source	Symptoms	Incubation period
Bacillus cereus[a]	Rice, cereals, dried foods, dairy products, meat, vegetables	V	1–6 h
Campylobacter spp.	Raw meat, poultry, untreated milk, water	D, fever, abdominal pain	3–5 days
Clostridium perfringens[b]	Cooked meat, gravy, fish, stews, pies, dried foods, vegetables	D, abdominal pain	8–24 h
Escherichia coli (enteropathic and toxogenic strains)	Raw food, water	D	12–72 h
Listeria spp.	Chilled food, soft cheese, raw and prepared meats, poultry, vegetables	Variable; D, V, abdominal pain, fever	1 day–3 weeks
Salmonella spp.	Meat, especially poultry, eggs, dairy products	D, fever, abdominal pain	12–36 h
Shigella spp.	Faecally contaminated water, food especially salads. Faecal–oral spread common	Variable: D, fever, abdominal pain	1–7 days
Staph. aureus[a]	Cold foods handled during preparation, dairy products	V, D, abdominal pain	1–6 h
Viruses (especially SRSV)	Shellfish, contaminated water, cold foods handled during preparation	V (sometimes projectile), D	24–48 h

[a] = symptoms caused by ingested toxin.
[b] = symptoms caused by toxin produced in the gut during sporulation.
D, diarrhoea; V, vomiting; SSRV, small round structured virus

to prevent food-borne gastrointestinal infection. Also discussed are the infection control precautions required to prevent cross-infection and control outbreaks of gastrointestinal infection.

Principles of Food Hygiene

There has been a marked increase in the number of cases of food-borne illness caused by bacteria during the 1980s, in particular by *Salmonella* spp., *Campylobacter* spp., *Clostridium perfringens* and *Bacillus cereus* (Cooke, 1990; Eley, 1992). Table 12.2 describes the 10 most common causes of food poisoning, all reflecting poor food hygiene. This section discusses these principles and emphasizes those measures that are most relevant to the role of the nurse in the delivery of food to the patient.

Table 12.2
The ten most common causes of food poisoning. From Roberts (1982)

1. Food prepared too far in advance
2. Food stored at room temperature
3. Cooling food too slowly before refrigeration
4. Not reheating food to 70°C
5. Cooked food contaminated with bacteria
6. Undercooking meat and meat products
7. Incomplete thawing of frozen meat and poultry
8. Cross-contamination from raw to cooked foods
9. Storing hot food below 63°C
10. Infected food handlers

The food-handling responsibilities of nurses vary enormously with different health care systems and with the type of food delivery. In a large general hospital the nurse may only distribute meals on trays, whilst in small hospitals, nursing homes or rehabilitation centres the nurse may participate in all stages of food preparation. More detailed information about food handling can be obtained by referring to the DHSS publication *Health Services Catering* (DHSS, 1986a).

It is also worth noting that a large proportion of food poisoning probably occurs as a result of food preparation in the home, where principles of food safety are frequently ignored. Nurses are often required to advise patients on the prevention of gastrointestinal illness, particularly people who are **immunosuppressed**, pregnant or who have suffered an episode of food poisoning. An understanding of the following principles of food hygiene and infection control is therefore essential for appropriate advice to be offered.

Food Preparation

Raw food is frequently contaminated with potential **pathogens**. *Campylobacter*, *Clostridium perfringens* and *Salmonella* are commonly found in the intestines of animals. Around a half of raw chicken carcasses have been found to be contaminated with *Salmonella*, although contamination of red meat is much lower at around 1% (Mackey, 1989). *Bacillus cereus* and *Cl. perfringens* are also widely found in the environment and may therefore contaminate a variety of produce including rice and vegetables.

Most intestinal pathogens must be ingested in very large numbers, at least several hundred in each gram of food to establish infection in the gut. Bacteria in raw food should be destroyed by thorough cooking and the few bacteria remaining should be insufficent to cause infection.

Bacteria transferred on to food that has already been cooked, for example cold meats, may multiply and cause infection. *Campylobacter* is particularly likely to be transmitted in this way. Although they are easily destroyed by cooking, infection can follow the ingestion of only a few hundred organisms as they multiply rapidly in the gut (Eley, 1992).

One of the essential principles of safe food handling is to ensure that cooked food is never contaminated by uncooked food. Bacteria may be transferred from raw to cooked food on hands and equipment such as knives and chopping boards. Such equipment must always be washed with hot water and detergent after each use and have smooth surfaces to enable easy cleaning. Cloths used to clean surfaces or equipment will become contaminated rapidly and should be discarded or washed frequently. Raw and cooked food should be stored separately because raw food may touch or drip on to other food.

Food that is eaten raw is not decontaminated by heat and must be washed under running water to remove potential pathogens. Salads prepared in hospitals have been found to be contaminated with various **Gram-negative bacilli**, which, although unlikely to cause infection in healthy people, may be harmful to the **immunocompromised** patient (Houang *et al.*, 1991). People who handle food may be carrying food-borne pathogens and may transfer them to prepared foods such as fruit, salads or sandwiches. Small round structured viruses (SRSV) or Norwalk viruses are a common cause of gastroenteritis and outbreaks of infection are frequently associated with the handling of this type of food by a chef recently recovered from gastroenteritis (Adak *et al.*, 1991).

The important guidelines for practice when preparing food are summarized below.

Preparation of Food

- Always wash hands before and after handling food, after using the toilet
- Use separate utensils for raw and cooked food, clean thoroughly with detergent and water after each use
- Clean preparation surfaces thoroughly with detergent and water after each use
- Blenders, mixers and slicing machines must be dismantled and thoroughly cleaned with detergent and water after each use
- Wash all salads, fruit and vegetables in running water
- Do not store raw and cooked food together
- Keep food in the refrigerator covered to prevent inadvertent contamination

Guidelines for Practice

Cooking Food

Destruction of bacteria in food by cooking depends on the exposure of bacteria to heat for a sufficient period of time. However, there is a balance between destroying bacteria and spoiling the taste and nutrient value of food by over-cooking. Most bacteria are destroyed at temperatures of around 60°C and prolonged heating may be needed to ensure that these temperatures are achieved throughout the food. It may take a long time for heat to penetrate the centre of the food, particularly if the food is dense (e.g. mashed potato, raw meat) or is still frozen in the middle. Standard cooking times are based on the heating of food from room temperature and food that is incompletely defrosted may be undercooked. This is particularly dangerous with some types of food, such as poultry, which are prone to contamination.

The same principles should be applied to reheating food before consumption. Different foods take different times to reheat and it can therefore be difficult to estimate the reheating time. For example, the gravy in a stew will heat more rapidly than the meat and a bubbling gravy does not mean that the meat has been reheated to the correct temperature. A thermometer should be used to check that the centre of the food is at 70°C before it is safe to serve. The important guidelines for practice when cooking or reheating food are summarized in the guidelines for practice.

Microwave Ovens

Microwave ovens heat food from the inside outwards and vegetative bacteria are unlikely to survive provided that all parts of the food reach 70°C. Unfortunately, heating in microwave ovens tends to be uneven so that some parts of the food may become extremely hot whilst other parts remain cool (Knutson *et al.*, 1987). Food should therefore be allowed to stand for 5 min after heating to ensure that the heat is evenly distributed by conduction (Lund *et al.*, 1989). Precooked chilled foods should be reheated in the manner specified by the manufacturer. The time necessary to heat other foods is extremely difficult to estimate and a thermometer should be used to ensure that the food has been heated throughout.

Guidelines for Practice

Cooking

- Defrost meat thoroughly before cooking
- Adhere to standard or recommended cooking times
- Use a thermometer to check the temperature in the centre of the food
- Reheat food thoroughly and use a thermometer to check the temperature

Food Storage

Bacteria can multiply in most foods provided there is moisture present and the temperature is between 20 and 40°C, (e.g. at room temperature). At refrigeration temperatures of between 5 and 10°C, multiplication occurs extremely slowly so that food can be stored for a few days without spoiling. Bacteria cannot multiply at all below 0°C and food can be stored for prolonged periods. *Listeria monocytogenes* presents particular problems as it can multiply in the refrigerator. It is transmitted by food and, although rare, may cause serious infection in the immuno-compromised, elderly and unborn child or neonate. It can survive drying, freezing and even cooking. *Listeria* is frequently isolated from freshly cut salads, paté and soft cheeses (Lund *et al.*, 1989). Outbreaks of infection associated with coleslaw, milk and cook–chill chicken have also been reported (Jones, 1990).

B. cereus and *Staphylococcus aureus* cause food poisoning by producing a heat-stable toxin. If food is stored at ambient temperatures these organisms may multiply and produce significant amounts of toxin that will not be destroyed during subsequent reheating (Eley, 1992).

To prevent bacterial multiplication, food should not be stored at room temperature for more than 1.5 h. It should always be stored at temperatures below 4°C or above 63°C where cell multiplication cannot take place.

If cooked food is to be refrigerated, it must be cooled quickly and not held at room temperature for long periods (DHSS, 1986). Food poisoning with *Salmonella* and *Cl. perfringens* is frequently associated with meat which has cooled slowly and not eaten until many hours later (see Table 12.1).

Meals should not be saved for more than an hour if a patient is not on the ward at meal times. Bacteria may multiply in the food and the food may not be reheated sufficiently to destroy them (DHSS, 1986a) (Figure 12.1).

The method of delivering meals to wards must ensure that the food is kept either hot or cold. Heated trolleys should maintain a temperature of

Fig. 12.1
Bacteria multiply in food at room temperature.

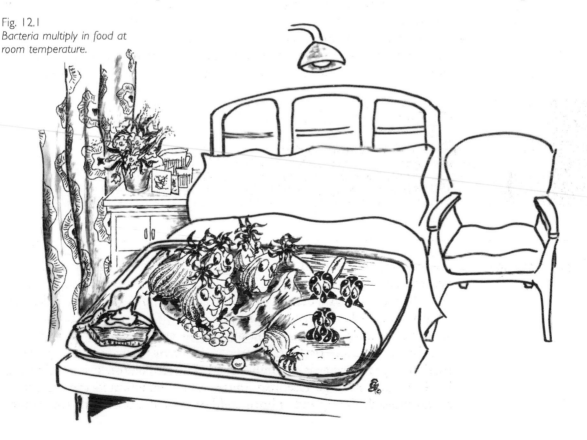

at least 63°C and should incorporate a refrigerated compartment for cold desserts and salads. The meals should be served as rapidly as possible to reduce the risk of bacterial multiplication (DHSS, 1986a).

Food stored in the refrigerator should be dated and discarded after its sell-by or use-by date. The temperature of the refrigerator must be maintained between 1 and 4°C (Food Hygiene Regulations, 1990). Immunocompromised patients and pregnant women should not eat foods likely to be contaminated with *Listeria*. Particular care should be taken with the storage and reheating of ready-to-eat chilled foods. Eggs should be stored in the refrigerator to prevent *Salmonella enteritidis*, which has been isolated from a small proportion of eggs, from multiplying to a potentially infectious dose (De Louvois, 1993).

Dry foods should be protected from moisture and whilst dry will not be able to support the growth of bacteria.

The principles of safe food storage are summarized in the guidelines for practice.

Guidelines for Practice

Storage of Food

- Do not keep prepared food at room temperature for more than 1.5 h
- Plug heated food trolleys in as soon as they arrive on the ward and serve the food immediately
- Do not keep meals in a warm oven
- Do not save and reheat meals for patients absent at mealtimes
- Do not use chilled meals or food beyond its sell-by date
- Ensure the refrigerator is fitted with a thermometer and is maintained between 1 and 4°C
- Date items stored in the fridge and discard after 3 days

Ward Kitchens

These are subject to the Food Hygiene Regulations (see 'Food Safety Act' p. 256) and may be inspected during visits by the Environmental Health Officer. The ward manager is responsible for ensuring that the regulations are complied with. The fittings should be designed to be cleaned easily, with smooth surfaces to prevent the collection of dirt or grease. A handwash basin with soap and hand towels must be available. The refrigerator must be checked daily to ensure that food is covered, labelled and discarded when appropriate. Drugs, blood or specimens should never be kept in the food refrigerator. The refrigerator should be sited away from a heat source and out of direct sunlight. A thermometer inside the refrigerator should be used to check the temperature regularly. Goldthorpe *et al.* (1991) found that very few ward fridges maintained a temperature of between 5 and 7°C and recommended the use of commercial larder refrigerators in place of the domestic fridge.

To minimize the risk of cross-contamination separate colour-coded

Ward Kitchens

- Check that the ward kitchen is clean
- Ensure the refrigerator is sited out of direct heat or sunlight
- Monitor the refrigerator regularly, discard unlabelled or outdated items and check the temperature
- Ensure soap and handtowels are available
- Use disposable cloths and paper towels when washing and drying dishes

mops, buckets and cloths should be used to clean kitchen areas and should not be confused with equipment used to clean other areas. Patients and their relatives should be discouraged from bringing food into the hospital because there is no control on how it is prepared (see guidelines for practice).

Crockery and Cutlery

Bacteria are easily removed from crockery and cutlery by washing in hot water and detergent. This is best done in a central wash-up area where dishes can be washed in an automatic machine at very high temperature. If items have to be washed at ward level, use clean hot water and detergent, rinse, and leave to drain rather than dry with a cloth which may easily become contaminated with potential pathogens. If dishcloths are necessary they should be disposable.

Personal Hygiene

Food is easily contaminated by bacteria carried on the hands. *Staphylococcus aureus* is commonly carried on the skin and is present in high numbers in an abscess or infected skin lesion. Other pathogens, such as *Salmonella* or *Campylobacter* may be acquired on the hands after handling raw meat. People suffering from gastrointestinal infection or excreting food poisoning pathogens (e.g. *Salmonella*) may transfer the organism to their hands after using the toilet. Staff who develop gastrointestinal infection must be particularly scrupulous about hand hygiene prior to handling food and should seek advice from the occupational health department before returning to work.

Personal Hygiene

- Wash hands before handling food
- Wash hands after using the toilet, after handling raw meat and vegetables, after cleaning procedures and after handling waste food
- Use a clean plastic apron to handle food
- Keep hair tied back
- Report any gastrointestinal illness to the occupational health department

Hands must always be washed after using the toilet and before handling any food. Cold or cooked food such as salads and cold meats should be handled with gloves or utensils. (See guidelines for practice).

Cook–Chill Catering

This system of food production is increasingly used in institutions as it is efficient and flexible. Food is prepared and cooked in the conventional manner, cooled very rapidly, kept chilled (between 0 and 3°C) and reheated immediately before eating. The maximum life of the food must not exceed 5 days, which includes the day of cooking and the day of consumption. If the food reaches a temperature of 5–10°C it must be consumed within 12 h, if 10°C is exceeded it must be discarded (DOH 1989). Although this system of food production has the potential to cause food poisoning, meals are microbiologically safe provided that strict quality control checks are employed, particularly in relation to temperature control (Chudasama *et al.*, 1991). The food is kept chilled until delivered at the ward when reheating takes place within the trolley at a set temperature and time.

Enteral Feeds

Feeding via a nasogastric tube is increasingly used as an alternative to parenteral nutrition when patients are unable to feed themselves. However, there are significant microbiological hazards associated with it (Anderton, 1985). Many types of bacteria, including *Salmonella*, *Klebsiella*, *Enterobacter*, *Escherichia coli* and *Staphylococcus aureus*, have been found in high concentrations in enteral feeds. These have been responsible for gastroenteritis and, by **colonization** of the gut, for subsequent **septicaemia** and **pneumonia** (Casewell *et al.*, 1981; Thurn *et al.*, 1990).

The liquid nutrients provide a favourable medium in which bacteria can grow and are easily contaminated during assembly and manipulation of the administration sets. Once the adminstration reservoir or tubing is contaminated, the bacteria can multiply rapidly in the feed at room temperature. If feeds are administered over several hours bacteria may multiply to high numbers. Contamination of enteral feeds occurs frequently, despite strict protocols for their management. Crocker *et al.* (1986) found that the onset of contamination is delayed if the feed is supplied in pre-filled, ready-to-use administration reservoirs. Where feeds were transferred to an administration reservoir, the rate of contamination was much higher and, if the mixture had to be reconstituted before adding to the reservoir, 75% were contaminated after 12 h and 100% after 24 h in use. The standards used in the preparation and handling of enteral feeds must therefore be even higher than with conventional meals.

Currently there are no accepted recommendations concerning the management of enteral feeds but the strong association between infection and contaminated feeds suggests that a rigorous non-touch technique must be used when assembling the administration sets and handling the feed. The risk of contamination may be reduced by the use of clean, disposable gloves (Anderton and Aidoo, 1991). Commercially prepared feeds in ready-to-use administration reservoirs are preferable as they are supplied as sterile liquids.

If separate administration reservoirs are used they should be discarded after a maximum of 24 h in use. Attempts to decontaminate these containers with detergent and water or disinfectants may not be successful. Tubing experimentally inoculated with *Klebsiella* was decontaminated only after 10 min of flushing with soapy water followed by 7 h immersion in 125 ppm hypochlorite (Anderton and Nwoguh, 1991).

There is considerable potential for feeds prepared in a hospital kitchen or ward to become contaminated through contact with equipment such as blenders, mixers or liquidizers. Feeds must be prepared under controlled conditions, preferably in the dietary department, using an extremely high standard of hygiene (Thurn *et al.*, 1990). Once a container of feed has been opened it must be stored in the refrigerator and discarded after 24 h.

Enteral feeds prepared by patients at home are also susceptible to contamination and these patients should be prepared with a rigorous education programme prior to discharge (Anderton *et al.*, 1993).

The important guidelines for practice for the management of enteral feeding are summarized below.

The potential for contamination during preparation also applies to infant milk feeds. Most milk feeds can be supplied safely in commercial sterile, pre-filled bottles. When special milk diets are required, the milk

The Management of Enteral Feeds

- Use commercially prepared feeds in pre-filled administration reservoirs where possible
- Pay scrupulous attention to principles of food hygiene if feeds are mixed on the ward
- Blenders used to prepare feed must be dismantled, thoroughly washed with detergent and dried after each use
- Wash hands before handling enteral feeding systems
- Avoid direct contact between the administration set connections and any non-sterile object
- Administer feed over as short a time as possible
- Store opened feeds in the refrigerator and discard after 24 h
- Replace administration sets and reservoirs every 24 h. Do not wash out and re-use
- Flush tubing with plenty of water after administering intermittent feeds

Guidelines for Practice

should be prepared using an extremely high standard of hygiene (Burnett *et al.*, 1989).

Food Safety Act

The Food Safety Act (1990) and the Food Hygiene (General) Regulations (1970) are designed to ensure that premises where food is prepared are clean and properly maintained and that the handling and storage of food is safe. They stipulate that hot food must be kept at temperatures above 63°C and cold food below 5°C. All staff who are involved in handling food should receive training in the principles of food hygiene.

Any premises involved in the production, supply or storage of food must be registered with the Local Authority and their Environmental Health Departments are responsible for enforcing the regulations. Environmental Health Officers have a right of entry into all premises where food is stored, prepared and handled, including hospitals and ward kitchens. The officers inspect the premises, check records and may take samples of food. They can issue informal warnings, *improvement notices*, which specify remedial action to be taken within a given period, or *prohibition notices* which require the immediate closure of the premises, and they may also prosecute for breaches of the food legislation. The Food Safety Act specifies that anyone who is involved in handling food must receive both initial and refresher training in food hygiene.

Preventing the Spread of Gastro-intestinal Infection

Some micro-organisms that cause gastrointestinal infection mainly spread from person to person following contact with excreta (e.g. rotavirus, *Clostridium difficile*).

Micro-organisms transmitted by food can also be spread to others by cross-infection. In outbreaks of food-borne illness, cross-infection may cause what are described as secondary cases of infection, occurring several days after the main outbreak. Joseph and Palmer (1989) reported that 30% of outbreaks of *Salmonella* infection in hospitals affecting two or more patients or staff, resulted from cross-infection rather than food poisoning. Person-to-person transmission occurred particularly frequently in elderly care, maternity, or paediatric units where contact with faecal material is more likely. Faulty bedpan washers were implicated in four outbreaks and contaminated gastroscopes in a further two outbreaks. Person-to-person transmission of *Shigella* occurs readily because the ingestion of only a very few organisms may result in infection (Benenson, 1990). Cross-infection of *Clostridium perfringens* amongst the elderly has also been reported

(Cooke, 1990). Cross-infection by *Campylobacter* is not thought to occur (Skirrow, 1990).

Viruses, notably the small round structured viruses, are readily spread from person to person through aerosols and environmental contamination from vomiting (Adak *et al.*, 1991; Owen Caul, 1994). Outbreaks of infection in hospitals caused by cross-infection are frequently reported (Riorden and Wills, 1986). Rotavirus is a very common cause of diarrhoea in children and extensive outbreaks of infection amongst susceptible groups of patients such as children and the elderly have been reported (Lewis *et al.*, 1989). During the acute stage of the illness millions of virus particles are excreted in the stools, and virus continues to be shed for several days following recovery. Transmission of the infection on hands following contact with excreta, bedding or nappies can therefore occur extremely easily (Breuer and Jeffries, 1990).

Clostridium difficile causes a serious disease of the colon called **pseudo-membranous colitis** (PMC). This usually occurs in patients whose normal intestinal flora has been altered by antibiotic therapy, enabling *Cl. difficile* to multiply and produce toxins. Hospital outbreaks of infection associated with the transmission on the hands of staff and the accumulation of spores in the environment have been reported (Hall, 1993).

Spread of gastrointestinal infections occurs particularly easily amongst children or other groups of patients or clients who have a poor understanding of hand hygiene and where staff may have considerable contact with excreta. The routine use of blood and body fluid precautions should prevent the transmission of gastrointestinal illness in most health care settings (see Chapter 7). Wearing disposable gloves and aprons for contact with excreta or vomit and scrupulous handwashing after contact with affected patients are particularly important control measures. Staff may acquire infection from patients with gastrointestinal infection (Reid *et al.*, 1990). Since the pathogen may be excreted for several days or weeks after the infection, advice should be sought from the occupational health department before affected staff return to clinical duties.

Preventing the Spread of Gastrointestinal Infections

- Nurse patient in a single room whilst symptomatic
- Wear gloves and apron for direct contact with faeces/vomit and discard after use
- Wash hands after any contact with the patient
- Remove spills of body fluid promptly and clean the area thoroughly
- Instruct the patient to wash hands thoroughly after using the toilet
- Place bedpans directly into bedpan washer/macerator without emptying the contents first

The measures required to prevent cross-infection of gastrointestinal infections are summarized on p. 257.

Patients may remain infectious for several days after the symptoms have resolved and, in the case of *Salmonella*, the bacteria may be excreted in faeces for many months. Provided the patient has a good standard of personal hygiene the risk of cross-infection is minimal once asymptomatic (Pathar and Scott, 1982).

Outbreaks of Gastro-intestinal Illness

A sudden increase in unexplained diarrhoea or vomiting amongst patients or staff may indicate an outbreak of infection. Outbreaks are commonly caused by viruses, which can be highly infectious and spread extremely rapidly, particularly amongst the elderly (Mitchell *et al.*, 1989).

Food poisoning, in particular salmonellosis, also causes many outbreaks of gastrointestinal illness in hospitals (Abbott *et al.*, 1980). The most notorious outbreak occurred in 1984 at the Stanley Royd psychogeriatric hospital in Wakefield, where *Salmonella typhimurium* in cold beef infected 355 residents, 19 of whom died, and 106 members of staff (Fig. 12.2). The severity of this outbreak culminated in the removal in 1987 of immunity from prosecution previously enjoyed by NHS premises.

Control of outbreaks of gastrointestinal illness requires prompt notification of the Infection Control Team, who will then investigate the source and advise on the management of patients to minimize the risk of further spread (Table 12.3). Specimens of faeces should be taken from all symptomatic patients as soon as possible and examined in the laboratory for both bacteria and viral pathogens. The specimens can provide crucial evidence to indicate the source of the infection. Patients who no

Table 12.3
Action to be taken in the event of a suspected outbreak of gastrointestinal illness

A suspected outbreak of gastrointestinal illness is when 2 or more patients or staff are affected by unexplained diarrhoea or vomiting

- Inform the doctor in charge of the affected patients
- Inform the infection control nurse and/or infection control doctor
- Ensure sufficient disposable gloves and aprons are available
- Collect stool specimens from affected patients, *even if they no longer have symptoms*, and send for bacterial and viral culture
- Transfer affected patients into single rooms if possible and follow standard isolation precautions
- Ensure all affected members of staff report to the occupational health department

If a considerable number of patients are affected the Infection Control Team will form an Action Group to co-ordinate the control measures, provide instruction to staff and identify the source of the outbreak

Fig. 12.2
*Press reports of an outbreak
of food poisoning at the
Stanley Royd Hospital.*

PUBLIC INQUIRY INTO SALMONELLA OUTBREAK

SOCIAL SERVICES SECRETARY Norman Fowler has set up a full-scale public inquiry into the outbreak of food poisoning which has killed 27 patients at the Stanley Royd psychiatric hospital in Wakefield.

Announcing his decision last week, Mr Fowler said there was a need to establish 'the full facts surrounding the outbreak', although priority had been to bring it under control. Eight patients were still suffering from salmonella symptoms and three of them were seriously ill as *NT* went to press, but no new cases had been reported for 48 hours.

Investigation into the infection has shown that cold roast beef left out for 10 hours on a warm day had caused the rapid spread of the bacteria, according to Wakefield health authority, although the actual source of the infection is still not known.

District medical officer Dr Geoffrey Ireland said last week that the meat had been taken out of the refrigerator in the morning to be sliced and been left out until it was served later that afternoon. This has been denied by the hospital's kitchen staff. NUPE branch secretary George Rusling told *NT* the meat had been left out of the refrigerator no longer than four hours.

longer have symptoms may still excrete the organism and specimens should be sent to the laboratory to identify the causative organism.

The Infection Control Team may involve the Consultant for Communicable Disease Control or Director of Public Health and local Environmental Health Officers in measures to control outbreaks of gastrointestinal illness.

References   Abbott JD, Hepner ED, Clifford C. (1980). Salmonella infections in hospital. A report from Public Health Laboratory Service Salmonella Subcommittee. *J. Hosp. Inf.* **1**: 307–14.

Adak GK, Caul EO, Cowden JM (1991) Infection with small round structured viruses: England and Wales 1981–1990. *CDR* **1**(13): R141–3.

Anderton A (1985) Growth of bacteria in enteral feeding solutions. *J. Med. Micro.* **20**: 63–8.

Anderton A, Aidoo KE (1991) The effect of handling procedures on microbial contamination of enteral feeds – a comparison of the use of sterile vs non-sterile gloves. *J. Hosp. Inf.* **17**(4): 297–301.

Anderton A, Nwoguh CE (1991) Re-use of enteral feeding tubes – a potential hazard to the patient? A study of the efficacy of a representative range of cleaning and disinfection procedures. *J. Hosp. Inf.* **18**: 131–8.

Anderton A, Nwoguh CE, McCune I *et al.* (1993) A comparative study of the numbers of bacteria present in enteral feed prepared and administered in hospital and the home. *J. Hosp. Inf.* **23**: 43–9.

Benenson AS (1990) *Control of Communicable Diseases in Man*, 15th edn. American Public Health Association, Washington.

Breuer J, Jeffries DJ (1990) Control of viral infections in hospital. *J. Hosp. Inf.* **16**: 191–221.

Burnett IA, Wardley BL, Magee GS (1989) The milk kitchen, Sheffield children's hospital, before and after a review. *J. Hosp. Inf.* **13**: 179–86.

Casewell MW, Cooper JE, Webster M (1981) Enteral feeds contaminated with *Enterobacter cloacae* as a cause of septicaemia. *Br. J. Med.* **282**: 973.

Chudasama Y, Hamilton-Miller JMT, Maple PAC (1991) Bacteriological safety of cook-chill food at the Royal Free Hospital, with particular reference to Listeria. *J. Hosp. Inf.* **19**: 225–30.

Cooke EM (1990) Epidemiology of foodborne illness: UK. *Lancet* **336**: 790–3.

Crocker KS, Krey SH, Markovic M *et al.* (1986) Microbial growth in clinically used enteral delivery systems. *Am. J. Inf. Control* **14**: 250–6.

De Louvois J (1993) Salmonella contamination of eggs. *Lancet* **342**: 366–7.

Department of Health (1989) *Chilled and Frozen. Guidelines on Cook–Chill and Cook–Freeze Catering Systems*, HMSO, London.

DHSS (1986a) *Health Service Catering, Hygiene.* HMSO, London.

Eley AR (Ed.) (1992) *Microbial Food Poisoning.* Chapman & Hall, London.

Food Hygiene (General) Regulations (1970) S.I. 1970, No. 1172. ISBN 0–11–001172–4. HMSO, London.

Food Hygiene (Amendment) Regulations (1990) S.I. 1990 No. 1431. ISBN 0–11–004431–2. HMSO, London.

Food Safety Act (1990) ISBN 0–10–541690–8. HMSO, London.

Goldthorpe G, Kerry P, Drabu YJ (1991) Refrigerated food storage in hospital ward areas. *J. Hosp. Inf.* **18**: 63–6.

Hall S (1993) *Clostridium difficile* – epidemiological aspects. *PHLS Micro. Digest.* **10**(2): 87–90.

Houang E, Bodnarak P, Ahmet Z (1991) Hospital green salads and the effects of washing them. *J. Hosp. Inf.* **17**: 125–31.

Joseph CA, Palmer SR. (1989) Outbreaks of Salmonella infection in hospitals in England and Wales 1978–87. *Brit. Med. J.* **298**: 1161–4.

Jones D (1990) Foodborne listeriosis. *Lancet* **336**: 1171–4.

Knutson KM, Marth EH, Wagner MK (1987) Microwave heating of food. *Food Sci. Technol.* **20**: 101–10.

Lewis DC, Lightfoot NF, Cubitt WD *et al.* (1989) Outbreaks of astrovirus type 1 and rotavirus gastroenteritis in geriatric inpatient populations. *J. Hosp. Inf.* **14**: 9–14.

Lund BM, Knox MR, Cole MB (1989) Destruction of *Listeria monocytogenes* during microwave cooking. *Lancet* **i**: 218.

Mackey BM (1989) The incidence of food poisoning bacteria in red meat and poultry in the United Kingdom. *Food Sci. Technol. Today* **3**: 246–9.

Mitchell E, O'Mahoney M, McKeith I *et al.* (1989) An outbreak of viral gastro-enteritis in a psychiatric hospital. *J. Hosp. Inf.* **14**(1): 1–8.

Owen Caul E (1994) Small round structured viruses: airborne transmission and hospital control. *Lancet* **343**: 1240–2.

Pethar JVS, Scott RJD (1982) Salmonella carriers; are they dangerous? A study to identify finger contamination with salmonellae by convalescent carriers. *J. Inf.* **5**: 81–8.

Reid JA, Breckon D, Hunter PR (1990) Infection of staff during an outbreak of viral gastroenteritis in an elderly persons' home. *J. Hosp. Inf.* **16**: 81–6.

Riorden T, Wills A. (1986) An outbreak of gastroenteritis in a psychogeriatric hospital associated with a small round structured virus. *J. Hosp. Inf.* **8**: 296–9.

Roberts D (1982) Factors contributing to outbreaks of food poisoning in England and Wales 1970–79. *J. Hyg.* **89**: 491–8.

Roberts D (1990) Sources of infection: food. *Lancet* **336**: 859–61.

Skirrow MB (1990) Campylobacter. *Lancet* **336**: 921–3.

Thurn J, Crossley K, Gerdts A *et al.* (1990) Enteral hyperalimentation as a source of nosocomial infection *J. Hosp. Inf.* **15**: 203–18.

Further Reading

Baird-Parker AC (1990) Foodborne salmonellosis. *Lancet* **336**: 1231–5.

Collee JG (1990) Bovine-spongiform encephalopathy. *Lancet* **336**: 1300–3.

Department of Health (1990) *Management of Food Services and Food Hygiene in the National Health Service.* National Health Service Management Executive. HMSO, London.

DHSS (1986b) *The Report of the Committee of Inquiry into an Outbreak of Food Poisoning at Stanley Royd Hospital.* HMSO, London.

Hobbs BC, Roberts D (1993) *Food Poisoning and Food Hygiene,* 6th edn. Edward Arnold, London.

Lund BM (1990) Foodborne disease due to *Bacillus* and *Clostridium* species. *Lancet* **336**: 982–6.

Noah ND (1985) Food poisoning. *Brit. Med. J.* **291**: 879–83.

Schlech WF (1991) Listeriosis: epidemiology, virulence, and significance of contaminated foodstuffs. *J. Hosp. Inf.* **19**: 211–24.

Tranter HS (1990) Foodborne staphylococcal illness. *Lancet* **336**: 1044–6.

Wilkenson PJ (1988) Food hygiene in hospitals. *J. Hosp. Inf.* **11** (Suppl. A): 77–81.

13 Cleaning, Disinfection and Sterilization

- **Introduction**
- **Levels of Decontamination**
- **Methods of Decontamination**
- **References and Further Reading**
- **Appendix: A Policy for the Decontamination of Equipment**

Introduction

Cleaning, **disinfection** and **sterilization** are used to remove micro-organisms from the hospital environment and from equipment used for patient care. The risk presented by these micro-organisms depends on the number of bacteria present and the extent of contact with susceptible sites on the patient. The environment is commonly perceived as a more important source of infection than evidence suggests. Microbes cannot multiply in dry environments and most die fairly rapidly on surfaces or in the air. The few that remain will be unlikely to be present in sufficient numbers to initiate infection even if they could reach a susceptible site on the patient. The environment does provide a more important microbiological hazard where moisture is present, for example in food, solutions or equipment containing water. Here, bacteria may multiply rapidly to create a source of infection, provided that a suitable vehicle transfers them to a susceptible site on the patient.

The transmission of infection in association with equipment has been recognized as a problem since germs were first perceived as the cause of infection. Inadequate decontamination has frequently been responsible for outbreaks of infection in hospital (Cefai *et al.*, 1990; Kolmos *et al.*, 1993). The emergence of human immunodeficiency virus has focused attention on the potential of medical equipment to transmit infection. Safe decontamination of equipment between patients is an essential part of routine infection control (see Chapter 7).

The method of decontamination selected should consider the risk of the item acting as a source or vehicle of infection and the processes that it will tolerate.

Levels of Decontamination

The levels of decontamination are defined in Table 13.1. Micro-organisms are destroyed by physical methods such as heat, or by chemicals such as **disinfectants**. Chemical disinfectants exhibit a wide variation in their effect on different micro-organisms and are susceptible to inactivation by organic material and instability. Decontamination by heat is a more efficient process which is easier to regulate and is the preferred method.

When equipment is exposed to heat or chemical agents there is a delay in effect on micro-organisms whilst the agent penetrates the cells. The penetration time is extended if organic material is present. Micro-organisms are then steadily destroyed, rapidly by some methods, more slowly by others. If the process destroys all micro-organisms, including spores it is described as *sterilization*. Physical processes, such as steam sterilization, are the most effective method of sterilization, although a few chemicals, used in a specific way, can be used to sterilize. Other processes will not destroy all micro-organisms, particularly bacterial spores and are described as *disinfection*.

Cleaning involves the use of detergent to remove visible contamination from equipment but also removes a large proportion of the micro-organisms. Cleaning alone is an adequate method of decontamination of a wide range of equipment. Cleaning, by removing organic material and reducing the number of micro-organisms present, is an essential preparation for most equipment undergoing sterilization or disinfection. The terms sterilization and disinfection are often used incorrectly. For example, it is not correct to refer to the immersion of baby bottles in hypochlorite solution as sterilization. In fact, this is a disinfection procedure which destroys some, but not all, micro-organisms present.

Selecting the Level of Decontamination

The decision to clean, disinfect or sterilize depends on the risk of the equipment transmitting infection(Table 13.2).

As a general rule, methods of sterilization or disinfection employing heat, such as autoclaves and bedpan washers, are more reliable than

Table 13.1
Levels of decontamination

Sterilization	A process that removes or destroys all micro-organisms, including spores
Disinfection	A process that reduces the number of micro-organisms to a level at which they are not harmful. Spores will not usually be destroyed
Cleaning	A process that physically removes contamination (blood, faeces, etc.) and many micro-organisms using detergent

Table 13.2
Categories of decontamination

Category	Indication	Level of contamination	Methods
High-risk	Items that penetrate skin/mucous membranes or enter sterile body areas	Sterilize	Autoclave and use sterile, e.g. surgical instruments. Sterile single-use disposable, e.g. needles
Medium-risk	Items that have contact with mucous membranes or are contaminated by microbes which are easily transmitted	Disinfect or sterilize	Autoclave (not in packs) e.g. vaginal speculum Chemically disinfect e.g. endoscopes Pasteurize e.g. bedpans, crockery
Low risk	Items used on intact skin	Clean	Wash with detergent and hot water and dry, e.g. washbowls, mattresses

chemicals and should be used wherever feasible. Quality control is more easily achieved in a Central Sterile Supply Department (CSSD) and if possible, equipment should be decontaminated there.

The risk of transmitting infection on equipment depends on how the item is used. If the skin is penetrated, normally sterile body areas are entered or there is contact with broken mucous membranes, then the risk of introducing infection is high and the items used must be sterile. Medium risk items are those that come into contact with mucous membranes or that may be contaminated by micro-organisms which are easily transmitted to others. Disinfection is usually adequate for these items, although sterilization is preferable as it reliably removes contamination. Equipment used on intact skin presents a low risk and is unlikely to transmit infection and can be decontaminated by cleaning.

Special decontamination procedures for instruments used on patients known to be infected with **pathogens**, for example blood-borne viruses, are not usually necessary. Many patients may not be identified as infected and the method used for routine decontamination must destroy pathogens if cross-infection is to be avoided.

Inactivation of *Mycobacterium*

Mycobacteria are inactivated by sterilization but can also be destroyed by heating in water to a temperature of around 80°C; the time taken will vary according to the temperature. Contaminated equipment or linen can be safely decontaminated in a washer–disinfector or washing machine, respectively. Glutaraldehyde (2%) can be used to destroy most mycobacteria in approximately 20 min. An immersion time of 2 h is recommended for *M. avium-intracellulare*, which is more resistant to glutaradehyde (Collins, 1986).

Inactivation of Human Immunodeficiency Virus (HIV) and Hepatitis B Virus

These viruses are destroyed by sterilization in an autoclave or by boiling for 5 min (Ayliffe, 1986). Glutaraldehyde (2%) and hypochlorite disinfectants (10 000 ppm available chlorine) will also destroy the virus rapidly, although the time taken will depend on the amount of blood or body fluid present (Bloomfield *et al.*, 1990). HIV is an enveloped virus and although susceptible to 70% alcohol, this is not a reliable method of decontamination unless equipment has been thoroughly cleaned beforehand (Hanson *et al.*, 1989).

Inactivation of the Creutzfeld–Jakob Disease Virus-like Agent

Transmission of this disease has been associated with neurosurgical electrodes (Benoulli *et al.*, 1977). The virus-like agent is thought to be particularly resistant to sterilization and special measures must be taken to decontaminate surgical instruments used on patients with this disease (DHSS, 1984; DOH, 1992).

Methods of Decontamination
Cleaning

Cleaning is important for two reasons, firstly in its own right as a method of decontaminating low-risk items and secondly prior to disinfection or sterilization processes. Many pieces of equipment classed as low risk can be safely decontaminated between patients by this method, for example washing bowls, cots, beds and commodes.

Detergent is essential for effective cleaning. It breaks up grease and dirt and improves the ability of water to remove soil. Approximately 80% of micro-organisms will be removed during the cleaning procedure (Ayliffe *et al.*, 1967). However, drying the equipment after it has been cleaned is also extremely important to prevent any bacteria that remain from multiplying. The importance of thoroughly drying equipment before storage was demonstrated by Greaves (1985). Thiry-four per cent of washing bowls were not dried completely before storage and over 50% of these damp bowls were found to be contaminated with large numbers of **Gram-negative bacilli**. These bacteria could be transmitted readily to another patient when the bowl was next used.

Cloths used for cleaning also become heavily contaminated with bacteria, which are readily transferred to hands and equipment (Scott and Bloomfield, 1990) and they should be discarded after each use.

Gram-negative bacilli can survive in solutions of detergent and, where possible, items should not be left to soak in bowls of detergent (Werry *et al.*, 1988).

Blood and body fluids must be completely removed from instruments before they are subjected to a disinfection or sterilization process. Thorough cleaning with detergent and water removes a significant proportion of the micro-organisms and increases the efficiency of disinfection. Organic material such as blood is coagulated by heat or chemicals and consequently difficult to remove after sterilization. Hollow tubing is particularly difficult to clean effectively and requires the use of special brushes or high-powered water jets. Most tubing is single-use and disinfection of this type of item should not be attempted because of the difficulty of ensuring complete decontamination and the risk of subsequent cross-infection (Anderton and Nwoguh, 1991).

Decontamination by Heat

Heat is the best method of decontamination for medical equipment. Its effects are predictable and it is easily controlled. The process is most efficient in the presence of water because the heat will be conducted evenly to all parts of an object.

The number of micro-organisms destroyed depends on the temperature and the period of exposure; the higher the temperature the shorter the period of exposure. Additional time should be allowed for all parts of the item to reach the selected temperature.

There are a number of decontamination methods based on the use of heat, the most commonly used are described below.

Pasteurization

In this process items are heated to temperatures between 65 and 80°C at which many micro-organisms are destroyed provided that they are exposed for a sufficient length of time. The higher the temperature the shorter the exposure period required. Pasteurization is used to disinfect a variety of medium-risk equipment, but cannot be used to sterilize.

Examples of pasteurization used in a clinical setting are: bedpan washers at 80°C for at least 1 min; the disinfection of linen at 71°C for not less than 3 min during the wash cycle (DHSS, 1987); and dishwashers.

Boiling

Although not commonly used in hospitals, boiling can be used to disinfect medium-risk equipment. Most bacteria and viruses are destroyed by boiling for a few minutes; however, sterilization by this method is not possible as some bacterial spores will not be destroyed.

Boiling is relatively easily controlled visually. Instruments are added to the boiling water, the 5-min immersion period should be timed from when the water returns to boiling point.

Water boilers are still used in some general practice surgeries for the decontamination of vaginal specula, ear syringes, etc. They must not be used to decontaminate surgical instruments or other equipment used for high-risk procedures.

Steam Under Pressure (Autoclave)

The use of steam under pressure is the most reliable method of sterilizing equipment. At atmospheric pressure water boils at 100°C, which is not sufficient to destroy bacterial spores. Water boils at a higher temperature if the atmospheric pressure is increased, for example at 1.03 bar (15 lb/inch^2) it boils at 121°C and at 2.2 bar (32 lb/inch^2) at 134°C. Steam at these higher temperatures destroys **spores** in 15 and 3 min respectively, and these times and pressures are most commonly used in **autoclaves**.

The steam must come into contact with all surfaces of the item requiring sterilization. Sterilization occurs when steam condenses on to the surface of the instrument, releasing its latent heat. Instruments placed inside an autoclave (except porous-load autoclaves) should therefore not be piled up but separated out so that steam can reach all surfaces.

Autoclaves are the most common method of sterilization for high- and medium-risk equipment. Instruments used for medium-risk procedures require pathogens from one patient to be removed before use on another and can be used again in a clean, but not necessarily sterile, condition. They should be stored in a clean, covered container after autoclaving (e.g. vaginal speculae). Instruments used in high risk procedures *must* be sterile at the point of use. To prevent contamination of these instruments on removal from the autoclave, they must either be autoclaved inside a sealed packet or autoclaved immediately prior to use. Paper or linen wrapping will protect instruments from contamination indefinitely, provided that they remain intact and do not become wet.

Steam is unable to reach the surface of instruments if they are placed inside packs in a simple autoclave. Autoclaves used in CSSD have an extra stage in the sterilization cycle. A vacuum is created in the chamber prior to the injection of steam, to ensure that steam penetrates porous materials such as paper or linen rather than condensing on the surface of the pack before sterilization takes place. The packs must be dry before removal from the autoclave, as wet wrappings would allow micro-organisms to pass through. Autoclaves with these facilities are called *porous-load* autoclaves.

Fig. 13.1
A small autoclave.

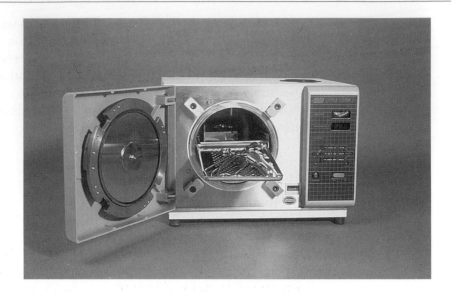

Small, simple autoclaves, such as the one illustrated in Fig. 13.1, do not include a pre-vacuum stage in the sterilization cycle. They are therefore not suitable for the sterilization of packed or wrapped instruments. If this type of autoclave is used to process high-risk instruments, these should be used immediately, placed in a sterile container or covered with sterile paper and used within 3 h.

Staff responsible for processing instruments in autoclaves must be properly trained in their use and in the preparation and loading of instruments (see Guidelines for Practice).

There are a number of small, relatively inexpensive autoclaves which are suitable for processing unwrapped instruments for use in clinics or general practitioners surgeries (NHS Procurement Directorate, 1990).

Hot Air Ovens

Hot air can also be used to sterilize, but higher temperatures and longer exposure times are necessary because air does not conduct heat as efficiently as steam. Sterilization can be achieved by holding at a temperature of 170°C for 1 h; however, instruments must reach the required

Guidelines for Practice

Using Small Autoclaves

- Use an autoclave with an automatic cycle and temperature and pressure indicators
- Clean instruments/equipment thoroughly with detergent and water prior to sterilization
- Separate instruments in the chamber so that all surfaces are exposed to steam
- Wash cleaning brushes after use and store dry
- Ensure the autoclave is serviced regularly

temperature before commencing timing and must be allowed to cool before removal. This limits their use to those instruments that can withstand high temperatures and to situations where a rapid turnround of equipment is not essential (UK Health Departments, 1994).

Instruments must be thoroughly cleaned before sterilization as organic matter will be baked on to the surface and become very difficult to remove.

Ethylene Oxide

Equipment easily damaged by heat cannot be sterilized in an autoclave or hot air oven and for these items, a lower temperature can be used with ethylene oxide gas.

Ethylene oxide is not corrosive, but it is irritant and toxic. It is absorbed into many materials and will then gradually leach out, causing harm to patient and staff in contact with the equipment. After exposure, therefore, items must be completely aired to remove all traces of the chemical. This can take up to 7 days. Items must be thoroughly cleaned before sterilization.

Ethylene oxide is flammable and can be explosive when mixed with air in certain concentrations. It is harmful at far lower concentrations than can be detected by smell and the gas must be safely vented from the area. Ethylene oxide sterilization requires the use of specialist facilities and the process must be closely controlled by trained operators. There are few items that require sterilization by this method and ethylene oxide facilities are not available in most hospitals.

Ionizing Radiation

This method is not used in hospitals but is widely employed commercially for the sterilization of plastic, disposable items such as syringes, cannulae, etc. The process may alter plastic materials and resterilization of disposable equipment should not be attempted.

Tests for the Effectiveness of Sterilization

An autoclave which is not functioning correctly may not sterilize instruments. The internal controls should indicate when the process has failed. They must be properly maintained and should be checked by a sterilizer engineer every 6–12 months, or as recommended by the manufacturer.

Autoclave tape should be used to indicate that an item has been through an autoclave rather than as a guarantee of sterility. The quality assurance of sterilization should be through monitoring the process not the product. For porous-load autoclaves, a record of the temperatures and pressures achieved in the chamber must be recorded for each cycle and these closely monitored. The machines must be regularly maintained and checked by a sterilizer engineer weekly.

Decontamination by Chemicals

A variety of chemicals are used for the decontamination of skin, equipment and the environment. Most are not active against bacterial spores and have limited activity against mycobacteria. Most can only be used to disinfect, not sterilize, equipment. Some viruses with lipid membranes are easily destroyed whilst those without are more resistant.

Always check the hospital disinfection policy or with the infection control nurse, that the method of disinfection that you have selected is appropriate, will reliably kill micro-organisms, and will not corrode the equipment.

Chemical disinfection has considerable disadvantages (see Table 13.3). Many disinfectants are corrosive and highly irritant, and disposable gloves and aprons should be worn to handle them. After disinfection, equipment usually needs to be rinsed in water to remove traces of the irritant chemical. Disinfectants must be used at the correct dilution; too high a concentration may be corrosive, toxic and irritant, too low a concentration may be ineffective. Diluted disinfectants are often unstable and lose activity enabling some bacteria, particularly *Pseudomonas*, to grow in the solution.

Effective disinfection cannot be achieved unless the solution is in contact with a surface for a reasonable period of time. Some solutions have a very rapid antimicrobial action, for example alcohols and hypochlorite disinfectants, and on clean surfaces kill microbes within a few minutes. Other disinfectants may take longer, for example immersion in glutaraldehyde for several hours is required to destroy bacterial spores. The important principles for using chemical disinfectants are summarized in the Guidelines for Practice.

Table 13.3
Disadvantages of chemical disinfectants

- Most are not active against all micro-organisms
- Tubercle bacilli and spores not easily destroyed
- Variable ability to destroy viruses
- Poor penetration of blood, pus and other organic material
- May be inactivated by organic material, detergent, rubber or plastics
- May be unstable, particularly if diluted, and may support the growth of some micro-organisms
- Often corrosive, toxic or irritant
- Variable exposure time required to achieve disinfection

Using Chemical Disinfectants for Decontamination of Equipment

- **Don't** use a chemical disinfectant unless you have to
- **Do** completely remove blood and body fluid with detergent and water before disinfection
- **Do** ensure that disinfection is necessary and that you are using the correct disinfectant
- **Do** check the COSHH assessment before using a disinfectant
- **Do** wear disposable gloves, apron and eye protection if indicated
- **Do** immerse for the correct time - use a timer
- **Do** rinse equipment with water after disinfection
- **Do** discard disinfectant solution after use, clean container and store dry
- **Don't** dilute a disinfectant by guesswork

Decontamination by heat is a considerably more reliable process and should be used in preference to chemicals wherever possible. This may mean the purchase of additional instruments to enable processing by CSSD or using single-use equipment.

COSHH Regulations and the Use of Chemical Disinfectants

The Control of Substances Hazardous to Health (COSHH) Regulations require employers to assess the risks presented by the use of hazardous substances. Chemical disinfectants may be inflammable, toxic if inhaled or ingested, and irritant to eyes or skin. Even detergent can damage the skin but can be used quite safely if the proper precautions are followed. Table 13.4 lists the factors which should be considered when assessing the risk of a chemical disinfectant.

This information should be provided in the form of a **risk assessment** and a copy kept in each area where the chemical is used. A risk assessment must be made for each chemical used in the department. The pharmacy or supplies department can often help to draw up risk assessments. The risk of injury from disinfectants is minimized provided the staff who use the chemicals are properly trained and follow the guidelines for use of the chemical described in the assessment.

Table 13.4
Control of substances hazardous to health – factors to be considered for risk assessment

- Establish how the chemical is used
  e.g. how often, what for, in what amounts, is it necessary?
- Potential harmful effects of the chemical
- How to prevent and control exposure
  e.g.   use of protective clothing
         covered containers
         ventilation
         restricted use
- Inform and train users
- Health surveillance (if appropriate)
  e.g. glutaraldehyde

Occupational Exposure Standards (OES)

These are the maximum concentrations of a substance in air to which people may be exposed without suffering harmful effects. The Health and Safety Executive recommends an OES for a number of disinfectants, including glutaraldehyde, chlorine gas, phenol, iodine and alcohol (EH 40/92), as these chemicals may irritate the eyes, skin or mucous membranes and should not be used in large quantities in poorly ventilated areas.

Properties of Common Chemical Disinfectants

Alcohol

Examples: 70% industrial methylated spirit (IMS), 70% isopropyl alcohol solution, alcohol handrub, alcohol impregnated wipes.

Alcohol rapidly destroys both bacteria and **fungi**, although it has no effect on bacterial spores. Isopropyl alcohol has poor activity against some **viruses**, IMS at a concentration of 90% is effective against most viruses. Alcohol does not penetrate protein-based organic matter and should only be used on clean surfaces. It damages some materials (e.g. lens cement) and is inflammable. It is not a suitable disinfectant for most equipment but its rapid action and volatility make it useful for skin disinfection and it is often used for this in combination with other chemicals such as chlorhexidine.

Alcohol-impregnated wipes are widely used to disinfect surfaces but because of the short contact time are unlikely to have much effect and their use is probably unnecessary (Thompson and Bullock, 1992).

Chlorhexidine

Examples: handwash solution (Hibiscrub, Hibisol), chlorhexidine in 70% alcohol, aqueous chlorhexidine (Savlon, Savlodil, Hibidil).

Gram-positive bacteria are more susceptible to chlorhexidine than **Gram-negative** organisms, but it has no effect on tubercle bacilli or spores and little effect on viruses. Chlorhexidine is mainly recommended as a skin disinfectant, either combined with a detergent in a handwash solution or with alcohol as a preoperative skin disinfectant or handrub. It has the advantage of being highly effective against the resident microbial flora of the skin, with an action persisting for several hours after the initial application. Although not an irritant to intact skin some studies have suggested that chlorhexidine is toxic to fibroblasts and may interfere with the healing of wounds (Neidner and Schöpf, 1986).

Its limited spectrum of activity, inactivation by organic matter and expense make chlorhexidine an unsuitable disinfectant for most equipment. It is sometimes used for the disinfection of low-risk equipment (e.g thermometer, aural speculum) in combination with alcohol, although the alcohol is the primary disinfectant. Solutions used to immerse equipment may become contaminated by bacteria after time and should be discarded immediately after use. Savlon, an aqueous chlorhexidine preparation, is often used for cleaning equipment prior to decontamination. However, general purpose detergent is just as effective and considerably cheaper. The main use of chlorhexidine is in surgical scrubs, but these are not recommended for routine handwashing in most ward areas, where soap is a cheaper and more suitable solution (see Chapter 6).

Glutaraldehyde

Examples: Cidex, Asep, Totocide.

Glutaraldehyde has a wide range of antimicrobial activity. It kills bacteria, fungi and viruses rapidly, tubercle bacilli within 60 min and bacterial spores in 3–10 h. Glutaraldehyde does not corrode metal and is not seriously inactivated by organic material although it only penetrates it slowly. Protein material will be coagulated on to the surface therefore blood or other organic material must be completely removed before immersion.

Once activated, alkaline solutions of glutaraldehyde remain active for 14–28 days (depending on brand) although they should be replaced if organic matter builds up and if the solution becomes cloudy.

Unfortunately, glutaraldehyde is highly irritant to skin and mucosa and extensive exposure has been associated with sensitization reactions, including dermatitis, running nose and eyes and asthma. As a result, most hospitals restrict the use of glutaraldehyde to equipment that cannot be decontaminated by heat or other chemicals and where destruction of a broad spectrum of micro organisms is essential. The best example of such equipment is fibre-optic endoscopes which, because they are used on mucous membranes, may result in cross-infection if not decontaminated after each use.

Where there is no alternative disinfection method to glutaraldehyde, precautions must be used to ensure minimal exposure to the user. Nitrile gloves (e.g. household gloves) and eye protection must always be worn to handle the solution. It must be kept in a container with a fitted lid and good ventilation provided to remove glutaraldehyde vapour from the atmosphere. After immersion, the equipment must be thoroughly rinsed with water.

Hydrogen Peroxide

Examples: hydrogen peroxide, Virkon, peracetic acid.

These solutions have a wide range of activity against bacteria, viruses and fungi. Some destroy spores (e.g. peracetic acid) and mycobacteria. Hydrogen peroxide has a low toxicity and irritancy but may be corrosive to some metals.

Hypochlorites (and other Chlorine-based Disinfectants)

Examples: Milton, Chloros, Domestos, sodium dichloroisocyanurate (NaDCC) – Presept, Haz–Tabs.

Hypochlorites are inexpensive and effective disinfectants. They are active against most micro-organisms, including HIV and hepatitis B, and may also destroy bacterial spores and mycobacteria. Although probably the best general purpose disinfectant, hypochlorites have a number of disadvantages which make them unsuitable for the decontamination of instruments. Particular problems are the corrosive effect on some metals and ready inactivation by organic material.

To prevent corrosion of surfaces, hypochlorite should be washed off with detergent and water and should not be used on fabric or carpets since it will bleach out the colour. Hypochlorites should not be mixed with large volumes of acidic substances (e.g. urine) in confined spaces because of the release of harmful chlorine gas (DOH, 1990).

Dilute solutions of hypochlorite lose their activity quite rapidly and fresh solution should be made up daily. The concentration of hypochlorite solutions is often expressed as parts per million of available chlorine (ppm av. Cl). A 1% hypochlorite solution, which contains 10 000 ppm av. Cl, is recommended for the treatment of blood and body fluid spills. At this concentration the available chlorine is less likely to be inactivated by the organic matter. A granular form of NaDCC is useful for decontamination of body fluid spills as the spill is absorbed and can be removed more easily (Coates and Wilson, 1989). A 0.1% solution of hypochlorite contains 1000 ppm av. Cl. and is recommended for the disinfection of surfaces (e.g. laboratories) and a 125 ppm av. Cl. solution can be used for the disinfection of infant feeding bottles. Domestos and most other thick bleaches contain 100 000 ppm av. Cl. and should be diluted before use.

Making the correct dilution of hypochlorite solutions can be difficult but the addition of NaDCC tablets (e.g. Presept, Haz–Tabs) to water, provides the easiest method of making up solutions of the required strength.

Non-abrasive powders which contain hypochlorite are sometimes used to clean baths although whether these powders have any advantage over detergent is debatable.

Phenolics

Examples: Hycolin, Clearsol, Stericol.

The phenolics are active against most bacteria, including mycobacteria but have little effect on bacterial spores and a variable activity against viruses, particularly those without lipid membranes. Although inexpensive, stable and not readily inactivated by organic material, phenolic disinfectants are no longer widely used for environmental disinfection. Their spectrum of activity is not wide enough to enable them to be used to disinfect equipment. In addition, phenolics are absorbed by rubber and plastics and are irritants. They should therefore not be used to disinfect equipment that is used on skin or mucous membranes.

Re-use of Single-use Equipment

The re-use of equipment intended for use by one patient only is sometimes practised within hospitals often in the name of economy. Although it may seem wasteful to discard these often expensive items, their decontamination and re-use raises a number of issues.

Firstly, the decontamination process may cost more in staff time and materials than the item itself. Secondly, the decontamination procedure may damage the item and cause it to malfunction on subsequent use. Thirdly, if a user reprocesses items intended for single-use then the user takes on the liabilities of the manufacturer.

In general, re-use of single-use items is not economical and if re-use is considered feasible then these factors should be carefully considered (Pickersgill, 1988).

Decontamination of Equipment Prior to Service or Repair

Equipment that has been in contact with patients or their blood or body fluids may transmit infection to staff involved in servicing and repair. To avoid placing them at risk and to comply with the Health and Safety at Work Act (1974), such equipment must be thoroughly decontaminated before it is inspected or repaired. Guidance issued by the NHS Management Executive in 1993, states that a certificate demonstrating the method of decontamination should accompany any item requiring servicing or repair. This includes equipment that is returned to the manufacturer. An example of a decontamination certificate is shown in Fig. 13.2.

Decontamination of the Environment

Furniture, Floors and Walls

The purpose of cleaning is to remove dust which may contain bacteria resistant to desiccation (e.g. *Clostridium difficile*, *Staphylococcus aureus*) and to keep equipment and surfaces dry. A surface that is clean and dry will not support the growth of most bacteria, and hospital infections are rarely

Fig. 13.2
*A decontamination
certificate.*

DECONTAMINATION CERTIFICATE

For issue prior to inspection, service or repair of any medical or laboratory equipment.

TO (Works dept/Manufacturer): ....

Description of equipment ....

Serial No .... Unit .... Date ....

Tick box A if applicable, otherwise complete sections B and C.

A.   ☐   **This equipment has not been in contact with blood, body fluid, respired gases or pathological specimens.**

B.   **Has this equipment been exposed to hazardous material?**

Blood, body fluids, respired gases
pathological specimens   Yes/No

Chemicals or substances hazardous
to health   Yes/No

Other hazards   Yes/No

Provide details of contamination: ....

C.   **Has this equipment been cleaned and decontaminated?**

Yes/No   Method..

If No, state why ....

*Note: equipment which has not been decontaminated must not be returned/presented
without prior agreement of recipient.*

I declare that I have taken all reasonable steps to ensure the accuracy of the above
information.

Signature .... Name .... Position ....

acquired from furniture, walls or floors (Maki *et al.*, 1982). Most of the micro-organisms found on floors and other horizontal surfaces are from dust particles that have settled and the majority are **coagulase**-negative staphylococci (Collins, 1988). Those present on floors are not easily dispersed into the air and are unlikely to be a significant source of infection. Bacteria are rarely found on vertical surfaces such as walls and these only require spot cleaning to remove splashes or stains (Ayliffe *et al.*, 1967). Dust particles are largely composed of skin scales, respired droplets and fibres from clothing or linen of which a small proportion carry micro-organisms. The most important component of an effective cleaning programme is the regular removal of dust from horizontal surfaces either by a vacuum cleaner or a dust control mop. Removal of dust is more sensible than wiping floors with a damp mop which redistributes bacteria in dust rather than removing them.

Mopping with detergent and water removes most micro-organisms and is of value when surfaces are soiled or exposed to spillages. Ayliffe *et al.* (1967) demonstrated that although disinfectants removed more bacteria from floors than detergent, recontamination of the floor occurred within an hour of treatment (Fig 13.3). Mopping of the floors several times a day will have a minimal impact on the number of bacteria present. Disinfectants are used for spills of body fluid which may contain micro-organisms. Chlorine-based granules can be used to soak up the

Fig. 13.3
Disinfectants are not deodorants.

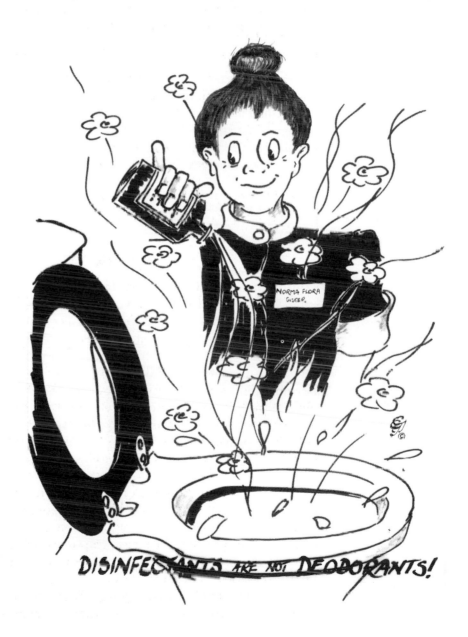

DISINFECTANTS ARE NOT DEODORANTS!

fluid and destroy micro-organisms present, reducing the risk of infection to the person clearing it up (Coates and Wilson, 1989).

There is no evidence that carpets present a greater risk of infection than hard floors. They should be vacuum cleaned daily to remove bacteria in dust and spillage of body fluid should be removed with detergent and water, preferably by a cleaning machine. For practical reasons, it is probably not advisable to fit carpets to areas where frequent spillage is anticipated. Carpets fitted in clinical areas must be washable and the fibres short and water-repellant to enable spills to be dealt with more easily.

Mops

Some bacteria multiply on a wet, dirty mop, stored in a bucket of dirty water for long periods. Such mops are more likely to deposit bacteria on floors than to remove them. The water used for mopping should be changed regularly during cleaning and discarded after use. Mop heads should be laundered and dried daily and not disinfected with chemicals which are unlikely to be effective.

Baths, Washbasins and Toilets

Bacteria are able to survive more easily in these moist environments; however, the routine use of disinfectants is not justified since they do not present a major source of micro-organisms (Levin et al., 1984). Bacteria **colonizing** washbasins and taps are usually environmental organisms and unlikely to cause disease in humans even if transferred to vulnerable sites on the patients (Ayliffe et al., 1974). Toilet seats do not become heavily contaminated by faecal bacteria and are an unlikely route of cross-infection (Newsom, 1972). Regular cleaning with detergent will remove pathogens and reduce the risk of cross-infection. Baths may become contaminated with pathogenic bacteria after use by a patient with a large, open wound. They should be thoroughly cleaned with detergent between patients. Non-abrasive powders containing a disin-fectant can be used but may damage the surface and increase the ability of bacteria to adhere. Bath hoists may become easily contaminated with bacteria and should be thoroughly cleaned with detergent after each use (Murdoch, 1990). Washbowls have been associated with outbreaks of infection by Gram-negative bacilli when not washed and dried properly after use (Joynson, 1978).

Beds and Mattresses

Bedframes accumulate dust and should be cleaned regularly. Babies' incubators should be cleaned routinely with detergent and water. If disinfection is required a dilute solution of hypochlorite (125 ppm av. Cl.) is suitable but should be rinsed off. Some incubators have an integral humidifier. These should be disinfected by raising the temperature of the water to at least 70°C for 10 min or removed and autoclaved (Ayliffe *et al.*, 1993).

Mattresses with an intact, impermeable cover do not support the growth of bacteria if clean and dry. If contaminated with body fluid, they should be cleaned with detergent and water and the surface thoroughly dried. Some chemical disinfectants (e.g. phenol) can damage mattress covers and their use should be avoided. The mattress cover should be carefully inspected for signs of wear or loss of impermeability. Outbreaks of infection caused by *Pseudomonas aeruginosa* and *Acinetobacter* have been associated with damaged mattresses (Fujita *et al.*, 1981; Sherertz and Sullivan, 1985).

Decontamination of Flexible Endoscopes

Flexible, fibre-optic endoscopes are difficult to clean as they contain narrow channels and valves and are usually damaged by high temperatures. Inadequate cleaning and disinfection of endoscopes has resulted in outbreaks of infection (Earnshaw *et al.*, 1985). The most common method of decontamination is immersion in glutaraldehyde, for a period depending on the type of endoscope (Table 13.5). Thorough cleaning of the external and internal surfaces of the scope with detergent and water is essential to maximize the efficacy of disinfection. All channels should be brushed and flushed with detergent and water. Biopsy forceps and other accessories should be ultrasonic cleaned to ensure that all debris is removed. Automatic washer–disinfectors do not eliminate the need for

Table 13.5
Immersion times for flexible endoscopes

Type of scope	Immersion time (between patients) (min)
Operative endoscopes	
Arthroscope	10[a]
Laparoscope	10[a]
Cystoscope	10[a]
Choledochoscope	10[a]
Colonoscope	4
Sigmoidoscope	4
Gastroscope	4
Bronchoscope	20[b]

[a] 3 h of immersion required to achieve sterility.
[b] 90–120 min if atypical mycobacteria suspected.

an initial cleaning process but improve the quality of disinfection and reduce exposure of staff to glutaraldehyde. These machines must be cleaned and maintained regularly to prevent contamination by micro-organisms.

Endoscopes that are used in the gastrointestinal tract may transfer enteric pathogens or blood-borne viruses from patient to patient. Decontamination should remove these micro-organisms and an immersion in glutaraldehyde for 4 min between each patient is considered sufficient (British Society of Gastroenterology, 1988). Longer immersion times of 20 min are recommended at the beginning and end of each list as bacteria multiply in the damp channels whilst the endoscope is stored.

The main infection risk associated with bronchoscopes is the transmission of respiratory pathogens, particularly mycobacteria and blood-borne viruses. Decontamination between patients is by immersion in glutaraldehyde for 20 min after each patient (British Thoracic Society, 1989). Provided the bronchoscope has first been thoroughly cleaned, this immersion time should be adequate to destroy mycobacteria if the scope is used on patients suspected of having tuberculosis (Ayliffe *et al.*, 1993). *Mycobacterium avium-intracellulare* is more resistant to chemical disinfectants and an immersion of 90–120 min is recommended after use on a patient with known or suspected infection (Collins, 1986).

Operative flexible endoscopes (e.g. laparoscopes, arthroscopes, cystoscopes) enter a sterile body area and should be sterilized between each patient. In practice, it is usually impractical to immerse them for 3 h after each use and high level disinfection by immersion for 10 min is considered acceptable (Ayliffe *et al.*, 1992).

After immersion, endoscopes must be rinsed with water to remove glutaraldehyde which could irritate mucous membranes, tissues or the operator. Sterile or filtered water should be used to rinse the channels as tap water may contain mycobacteria which can contaminate the scope and cause misleading laboratory results from specimens.

The extensive use of glutaraldehyde in endoscopy units can expose staff to serious health risks and adequate facilities must therefore be available. The health of the staff should be monitored by the occupational health department.

Decontamination of Respiratory Therapy Equipment

The main risk of infection associated with this type of equipment is from the use of humidifiers or nebulizers which create a moist environment in which bacteria can multiply. Glutaraldehyde is not recommended for use on respiratory equipment as it may be absorbed by the equipment and cause irritation to the respiratory mucosa.

Ventilators and Anaesthetic Machines

Contamination should be prevented by a filter on the expiratory circuit.

Tubing

Use disposable tubing and discard every 48 h or protect with a heat–moisture exchange filter at the patient end of the circuit. If non-disposable tubing is not protected by a filter it should be decontaminated in an automatic washer, preferably with a tube drying facility. Face masks should be cleaned with detergent and water

Humidifiers

These should be cleaned, dried and re-filled with sterile water every 48 h. Cascade humidifiers can be heat disinfected by increasing the water temperature to 70°C.

References

Anderton A, Nwoguh CE (1991) Re-use of enteral feeding tubes – a potential hazard to the patient? A study of the efficacy of a representative range of cleaning and disinfection procedures. *J. Hosp. Inf.* **18**: 131–8.

Ayliffe GAJ (1986) Viruses, specula and vaginal cancer. *Lancet* **1**: 158.

Ayliffe GAJ, Collins BJ, and Lowbury EJl. (1967). Ward floors and other surfaces as reservoirs of hospital infection. *J. Hyg.(London)* **2**: 181.

Ayliffe GAJ, Babb JR, Collins BJ *et al.* (1974) *Pseudomonas aeruginosa* in hospital sinks. *Lancet* **ii**: 578–81.

Ayliffe GAJ, Babb JR, Bradley CR (1992a) Sterilisation of arthroscopes and laparoscopes *J. Hosp. Inf.* **22**: 265–70.

Ayliffe GAJ, Coates D, Hoffman PN (1993) *Chemical Disinfection in Hospital.* PHLS, London.

Benoulli C, Siegfried J, Baumgartner G *et al.* (1977) Danger of accidental patient-to-patient transmission of Creutzfeldt–Jakob disease by surgery. *Lancet* **i**: 478–9.

Bloomfield SF, Smith-Burchnell CA, Dalgleish AG (1990) Evaluation of hypo-chlorite-releasing disinfectants against the human immunodeficiency virus (HIV). *J. Hosp. Inf.* **15**: 273–8.

British Society of Gastroenterology (1988). Cleaning and disinfection of equipment for gastrointestinal flexible endoscopy: interim recommendations of a working party. *Gut* **29**: 1134–51.

British Thoracic Society Research Committee (1989) Bronchoscope and infection control. *Lancet* **ii**: 270–1.

Cefai C, Richards J, Gould FK *et al.* (1990) An outbreak of *Acinetobacter* respiratory tract infection resulting from incomplete disinfection of ventilatory equipment. *J. Hosp. Inf.* **15**: 177–82.

Coates D, Wilson M (1989) Use of dichloroisocyanurate granules for spills of body fluids. *J. Hosp. Inf.* **13**: 241–52.

Collins BJ (1988) The hospital environment: how clean should a hospital be? *J. Hosp. Inf.* **11(Suppl. A)**: 53–6.

Collins FM (1986) Bactericidal activity of alkaline glutaraldehyde solution against a number of atypical mycobacterial species. *J. Appl. Bact.* **61**: 247–51.

Department of Health (1990) Spills of urine: potential misuse of chlorine-releasing disinfecting agents. *SAB* **59** (90): 41.

Department of Health (1992) *Neuro and Ophthalmic Procedures on Patients With or Suspected to Have, or at Risk of Developing, Creuzfeldt–Jakob Disease (CJD), or Gerstmann–Straussler-Scheinker Syndrome (GSS)*. PL(92)CO/4. HMSO, London.

Department of Health and Social Security (1984) *Management of Patients with Spongiform Encephalopathy (Creutzfeld–Jakob Disease (CJD)*. Circular DA(84)16. HMSO, London.

Department of Health and Social Security (1987) *Hospital Laundry Arrangements for Used and Infected Linen*. HC(87)30. HMSO, London

Earnshaw JJ, Clark AW, Thom BT (1985) Outbreak of *Pseudomonas aeruginosa* following endoscopic retrograde cholangiopancreatography. *J. Hosp. Inf.* **6**: 95–7.

Fujita K, Lilly HA, Kidson A et al. (1981) Gentamicin-resistant *Pseudomonas aeruginosa* infection from mattresses in a burns unit. *Brit. Med. J.* **283**: 219–20.

Greaves A (1985) We'll just freshen you up, dear. *Nursing Times* **March** 6 (Suppl.): 3–8.

Hanson PJV, Gor D, Jeffries DJ et al. (1989) Chemical inactivation of HIV on surfaces. *Brit. Med. J.* **298**: 862–4.

Health and Safety Executive (1988) *Control of Substances Hazardous to Health Regulations*. HMSO, London.

Health and Safety Executive. *Occupational Exposure Standards*. Guidance note EH40/92. HMSO, London.

Joynson DHM (1978) Bowls and bacteria. *J. Hyg.* **80**: 423–4.

Kolmos HJ, Thuesen B, Nielsen SV et al. (1993) Outbreak of infection in a burns unit due to *Pseudomonas aeruginosa* originating from contaminated tubing used for irrigation of patients. *J. Hosp. Inf.* **24**: 11–22.

Levin MH, Olsen B, Nathan C et al. (1984) Pseudomonas in the sinks of an intensive care unit: relation to patients. *J. Clin. Path.* **37**: 424–7.

Maki DG, Alvarado CJ, Hassemer CA et al. (1982) Relation of the inanimate environment to endemic nosocomial infection. *New. Engl. J. Med.* **307**: 1562–6.

Murdoch S (1990) Hazards in hoists. *Nursing Times* **86**(49): 68–70.

Neidner R, Schöpf R (1986) Inhibition of wound healing by antiseptics. *Br. J. Derm.* **115**(S31): 41–4.

Newsom SWB (1972) Microbiology of hospital toilets. *Lancet* **ii**: 700–3.

NHS Management Executive (1993) *Decontamination of Equipment Prior to Inspection, Service or Repair*. HSG(93)26. HMSO, London.

NHS Procurement Directorate (1990) *A Further Evaluation of Transportable Steam Sterilizers for Unwrapped Instruments and Utensils*. Health Equipment Information 196. HMSO, London.

Pickersgill F (1988) The case against re-use. *Nursing Times* **84**(44): 45–8.

Scott E, Bloomfield SF (1990) The survival and transfer of microbial contamination via cloths, hands and utensils. *J. Appl. Bact.* **68**: 271–8.

Sherertz R, Sullivan M. (1985) An outbreak of infections with *Acinetobacter calcoaceticus* in burn patients: contamination of patients' mattresses. *J. Inf. Dis.* **151**: 252–8.

Skaliv P, Sciple GV, Savannah GA (1964) Survival of staphylococci on hospital surfaces. *Arch. Envr. Health* **8**: 636–41.

Thompson G, Bullock D (1992) To clean or not to clean? *Nursing Times* **88**(34): 66–8.

UK Health Departments (1994) Dry heat sterilisers: purchase, maintenance and use. *SAB* (94) 23, HMSO, London.

Werry C, Lawrence JM, Sanderson PJ (1988) Contamination of detergent cleaning solutions during hospital cleaning. *J. Hosp. Inf.* **11**: 44–9.

Further Reading   Atwell C (1990) Control of substances hazardous to health. *Surg. Nurse* **3**(6): 10–13.

Ayliffe GAJ, Lowbury EJL, Geddes AM, Williams JD. (1992b) *Control of Hospital Infection – a Practical Handbook*, 3rd edn. Chapman & Hall Medical, London.

British Medical Association (1984) *A Code of Practice for the Sterilisation of Instruments and Control of Cross Infection.* BMA, London.

Coates D (1988) Household bleaches and HIV. *J. Hosp. Inf.* **11**: 95–6.

Department of Health (1987). *Decontamination of Equipment, Linen or Other Surfaces Contaminated With Hepatitis B or Human Immunodeficiency Virus.* Health Notice HN(87)1. HMSO, London.

East J (1992) Implementing the COSHH regulations. *Nursing Stand.* **6**(26): 33–5.

Gibbs J (1990) Glutaraldehyde: handle with care. *Nursing Times* **86**(21): 52–3.

Medical Devices Directorate (1993) *Sterilisation, Disinfection and Cleaning of Medical Equipment.* Guidance from the Microbiology Advisory Committee to the Department of Health Medical Devices Directorate. HMSO, London.

Hoffman PN (1987) Decontamination of equipment in general practice. *The Practitioner* **231**: 1411–15.

Morgan DR, Lamont TJ, Dawson JD *et al.* (1990) Decontamination of instruments and control of cross-infection in general practice. *Brit. Med. J.* **300**: 1379–80

Nystrom B. (1981) The disinfection of baths and showers trolleys in hospitals. *J.Hosp.Inf.* **2**: 93–5.

Russell AD, Hugo WB, Ayliffe GAJ (Eds) 1992. *Principles and Practice of Disinfection, Preservation and Sterilisation*, 2nd edn. Blackwell Scientific, Oxford.

Ward K (1990) All that glisters . . . *Nursing Times* **86**(24): 32–4.

Wicks J (1994) Handle with care. *Nursing Times* **90**(13)(Suppl.): 67–70.

Appendix A Policy for the Decontamination of Equipment.

Adapted from Sterilization and Disinfection Policy, Riverside Health Authority and reprinted with permission

Item	Method	Frequency
Ambu-bags	Protect with filter	Change filter after each patient
	Autoclave	After each patient
Auriscopes	Clean	After each use
Baby bottles	Use presterilized feeds if possible	
	Clean, immerse in 125 ppm av. Cl. hypochlorite for 1 h or boil for 5 min	After each use
Baby scales	Clean	After each use
Baths	Clean	After each use
	If patient has large open wounds or bathwater contaminated by body fluid, wipe with hypochlorite (1000 ppm av. Cl) after cleaning	
Bath hoists	Clean	After each use
Bedpans	Washer–disinfector	After each use
	Disposables – macerate, clean carriers	
Bowls (washing)	Clean, dry and store inverted	After each use
Commodes	Clean	When visibly soiled
Duvets		
PVC covered	Clean	After each patient
Fabric	Launder	Every 3 months
Duvet cover	Launder	After each patient and when soiled
Incubators	Clean	After each patient
Instruments	Autoclave or hot air oven	After each use
Jugs	Washer–disinfector or clean and dry or CSSD	After each use
Laryngoscopes		
Blades	Clean and autoclave or washer–disinfector	After each use
Handles	Clean	After each use
Mattresses	Clean, allow to dry before turning	After each patient and when visibly soiled
	Ensure cover intact	
Mops	Launder	Daily
Nail-brushes	Use sterile, send to CSSD or discard	After each use
Nebulizers (medicine)	Clean and dry	After each use
	Discard	After each patient
Ophthalmic prisms	Clean, immerse in hydrogen peroxide for 10 min	After each use

Item	Method	Frequency
Pillows	Clean	After each patient and when visibly contaminated
	Ensure cover intact	
Razors		
Electric	Brush out hairs, Immerse head in alcohol for 10 mins	After each use
Specula		
Vaginal	Autoclave or boil	After each use
	Use sterile speculum for IUD insertion	
Spirometer	Change mouthpiece	After each patient
Suction		
Bottles	Clean or autoclave if possible	After each use
Tubing	Single-use	Change between patients
Filter		Change when discoloured and every 3 months
Temperature probes	Use a plastic sleeve,	For each use
	Clean, wipe with alcohol, store dry	After each patient
Thermometers	Wipe with alcohol or use a plastic sleeve	After each use For each use
	Clean, immerse in alcohol for 10 min and store dry	After each patient
Thermometer holders	Clean	After each patient
Toys		
Hard	Clean	When soiled
Soft	Launder	
Tracheostomy tubes (silver)	Autoclave	After each patient
Trollies		
Dressing	Clean	Daily
Urinals	Washer–disinfector	After each use
	Macerate disposables	

Clean = wash with detergent and water, then dry.

The Management of the Infectious Patient

- Introduction
- Historical Perspective
- The Principles of Isolation Precautions
- References and Further Reading
- Appendix: Routes of Transmission for Common Infections

Introduction

Micro-organisms cause a wide variety of **infections**, some of which are described in Chapter 3. Many take advantage of a host who is susceptible to invasion but do not spread from that person to another person. A few micro-organisms cause infections which can spread easily from person to person and are called **contagious** or **infectious** diseases.

The traditional approach to an infectious disease is to exclude the individual from contact with others. In the community this usually means exclusion of the individual from school or work and sometimes if the infection is very serious and the patient very ill, admission to hospital. In hospital, patients with infectious diseases present additional problems because the frequency of contact with staff, and other patients made vulnerable by illness, can enable the infection to spread easily. Special procedures called **isolation precautions** or **barrier nursing** are used to prevent the transmission of these micro-organisms from an infected patient to other patients or to staff. Isolation precautions are sometimes referred to as 'source isolation' to indicate that the patient is the **source of infection**.

Whilst the need for some precautions in the care of infectious patients is usually recognized they have never been thoroughly evaluated and there is considerable controversy about their value. Many isolation procedures in use today are based on tradition not scientific evidence and few studies have tested their efficacy or cost-effectiveness (Jackson and Lynch, 1985). These procedures are usually diagnosis-driven, that is they are only implemented when a particular infection or disease is diagnosed. Frequently, the patient will be infectious for several days before the clinical illness becomes apparent or the micro-organism is detected. For example, a patient may carry a **methicillin-resistant S.**

aureus for many days before a swab result indicates its presence. Although all health care workers with direct patient contact could transmit infectious diseases, isolation procedures are generally regarded as the sole responsibility of nurses and are often not addressed in medical textbooks.

Historical Perspective

The fear of infectious disease was recorded long before microbes were discovered in the late nineteenth century. Isolation was an early remedy for infection and segregation of infected individuals has been practised for at least 4000 years. The oldest comprehensive isolation system is set out in the bible, in the book of Leviticus and the principles applied throughout the Middle Ages, particularly for leprosy and plague (Selwyn, 1991).

Isolation procedures were first introduced in hospitals in the early twentieth century. To cope with the lack of single rooms or cubicles two approaches were employed: barrier nursing and 'bed isolation'. Barrier nursing involved the use of special procedures to prevent the spread of micro-organisms, for example gloves and gowns as a barrier for patient contact. Bed isolation involved the segregation of the infected patient to one part of the ward. Frequently the bed was surrounded by a partition, wire screen or a curtain soaked in disinfectant (Glenister, 1991). The purpose of the screen was to keep the patient away from other patients and to remind the staff to take barrier precautions. Many workers, including Florence Nightingale in her concept of 'fever nursing' for the care of patients with infection, realized that infection was rarely transmitted by the air or from the environment but that contact with body fluids was usually responsible and transmission could be prevented by the use of barrier precautions. This was an early recognition of the importance of basing isolation precautions on the **epidemiology** of the infecting micro-organism; that is, how it spreads from person to person.

More recently, two different isolation systems that take account of how different micro-organisms spread have been described: disease-specific isolation precautions and categories of isolation precautions (Garner and Simmons, 1983).

Disease-Specific Isolation Precautions

In this system only the precautions needed to prevent transmission of a particular infection are used. For example, Hepatitis A is a gastrointestinal infection that spreads by contact with faeces. The precautions necessary to prevent the spread of infection are the use of protective clothing for direct contact with faeces and handwashing after contact with the patient.

The advantage of this system is that it eliminates unnecessary practices and can be incorporated into the plan of care for the individual patient. The disadvantage is that staff have to identify the relevant precautions and make more decisions, so mistakes are more likely to occur.

Categories of Isolation Precautions

This system groups diseases that require similar isolation precautions into separate categories. Commonly used categories are *Strict* isolation for highly infectious disease such as Lassa fever; *Respiratory* for tuberculosis, viral respiratory infections; *Wound and Skin* for infected or **colonized** wounds; and *Enteric* for gastrointestinal **pathogens** such as *Salmonella* (Control of Infection Group, 1974).

The disadvantage of this type of system is that some precautions may be used unnecessarily and because not all infections in the category may spread in exactly the same way, patients will not receive individualized care. In addition, the spread of some **antibiotic**-resistant bacteria may not be controlled by a single category of isolation as they may colonize many parts of the body. The advantage is that staff need to learn a few isolation procedures and are less likely to make mistakes.

Universal Blood and Body Fluid Precautions

These precautions were originally recommended because of concerns about the risks of transmission of blood-borne viruses to health care workers (CDC, 1987, 1988). However, many infection control specialists have recognized that the adoption of these precautions into routine care has an impact on the requirements of isolation precautions (Lynch *et al.*, 1987; Wilson and Breedon, 1990). For example, if gloves are routinely worn for contact with excreta then this advice need not be specifically included in the isolation precautions for patients with a gastrointestinal infection.

When universal blood and body fluid precautions form part of routine infection control practice (see Chapter 7) simplified disease-specific isolation precautions can be used for patients with infectious disease (Fig. 14.1). This approach has been referred to as 'Body Substance Isolation' (Lynch *et al.*, 1987). The advantage of this system is that it enables individualized patient care, but because precautions are taken with all body fluids additional precautions are not required for those patients identified as infectious. It also helps to prevent the transmission of infection even before infection has been diagnosed. The disadvantage is that the greater use of gloves and aprons increases costs and some workers have suggested that it is difficult to maintain the routine use of precautions with all patients. A lapse in use of precautions (e.g. not changing gloves between patients) could increase the risk of cross infection. (Garner and Hierholzer, 1993).

The Principles of Isolation Precautions

Despite the controversy surrounding the use of isolation precautions the underlying aim of preventing an infectious agent spreading from one person to another should be remembered. Whenever possible nursing care should be planned for individual patients, using precautions necessary to prevent the spread of the particular infection, eliminating unnecessary precautions and taking into account of the needs of the patient and of other patients. The Infection Control Nurse should always be involved when considering isolation of a patient. He or she will be able to advise on appropriate precautions and identify unnecessary practices. Figure 14.1 illustrates a simple isolation procedure which should be used in conjunction with the Routes of Transmission of Common Infections described in the Appendix to this chapter.

Single Room Accommodation

Patients with infections that are transmitted in the air by respiratory droplets or skin scales require physical separation from others to prevent the spread of infection. Infections spread by this route are relatively uncommon in hospital but include respiratory viruses, tuberculosis, and methicillin-resistant *Staphylococcus aureus* (MRSA) if the patient is shedding excessive amount of skin scales or has infection of the respiratory tract (see Chapter 5). Special ventilation of isolation rooms has been recommended (Fig. 14.2). The ventilation should ensure that air flows into the room from the corridor and out of the room directly to the outside (Garner and Simmons, 1983). However, there is little evidence to support the efficacy of ventilation in isolation precautions and many consider natural ventilation to be adequate (George, 1984).

Patients suspected to be suffering from one of the viral haemorrhagic fevers (e.g. Lassa fever, Marburg or Ebola viruses) are considered to be highly infectious and must be transferred to one of the special isolation units in London, Glasgow or Liverpool where they will be cared for in a plastic isolator (Bowell, 1986).

Single rooms are not essential to prevent the transmission of infections spread by direct contact, but if the patient is in a private room isolation procedures are probably more likely to be observed. Sometimes a single room is advisable because the patient is particularly likely to contaminate the environment (e.g. faecal incontinence, severe vomiting, profuse

Fig. 14.1
An isolation policy.

Indication

Isolation is necessary when a patient has or is suspected to have a communicable infection

Check the list of communicable infections to find out if isolation is necessary and what material from the patient is infectious

Remember: Universal precautions must be used with all patients including those in isolation

Aims

- To prevent the transmission of micro-organisms from an infected patient to others
- To provide psychological support and reassurance to the patient whilst he/she is in isolation
- To ensure that all staff are aware of the correct precautions to take and that unnecessary precautions are avoided

Equipment

- Single room with a washbasin
- Remove excess equipment from the room before patient is isolated

  Hand soap
  Disposable gloves
  Paper towels
  Yellow waste bag
  Plastic aprons
  Alcohol handrub

Practice	Rationale
Patient: explain reason for isolation and provide reassurance	To reduce anxiety and gain patient's co-operation
Aprons: wear plastic apron for contact with body fluid and infectious material, discard before leaving the room	To protect clothing from contamination
Gloves: wear for contact with body fluids and infectious material. Discard before leaving the room and between procedures	To prevent contamination of hands To prevent cross-infection
Masks: not usually necessary	There is no evidence that they protect from respiratory infections
Hands: always wash hands and forearms before leaving the room.	To prevent transfer of micro-organisms to other patients
Faeces/urine/vomit: discard directly into bedpan washer/macerator or toilet	Prompt disposal essential to prevent transmission
Linen: place in an alginate bag, then into a red nylon outer bag	To prevent dissemination of micro-organisms and protect laundry staff
Disposable items: discard used or soiled items into a yellow plastic bag	To ensure waste is incinerated
Equipment: clean/disinfect before removing from the room (see disinfection policy/ contact ICN)	To prevent the spread of micro-organisms

Fig. 4.1
Continued

Practice	Rationale
Crockery: use normal utensils and return to main kitchens in usual way	Risk of cross-infection from crockery is minimal. Washing in hot water and detergent is sufficient
Visitors: must be instructed to wash their hands before leaving the room. Children and susceptible visitors should be discouraged from visiting	For most infections the risk to visitors is minimal as they do not have contact with body fluids
Other departments: avoid visits to other departments. If necessary, the department should be notified in advance and the patient seen at the end of the list. Porters need not wear protective clothing but should be instructed to wash their hands on completion of the journey	To keep contact with other patients to a minimum and enable the department to take appropriate precautions
Cleaning: inform domestic supervisor that the patient is being isolated. A mop, bucket and cleaning cloths will be provided for the room. Ask the domestic to wear gloves and apron to clean and discard on leaving the room	To maintain a clean environment and minimize risk of spread
In case of death: follow the usual last offices procedure. Body bags are usually required for patients known to be infected with blood-borne viruses	Body fluids leaking after death may present a risk to mortuary staff. The use of body bags for infected patients is indicated in DOH guidance (1991)
Duration of isolation: refer to list of communicable infections or contact ICN	Isolation can be distressing for the patient and should not be continued for longer than necessary

Termination of isolation

See above for treatment of bed linen, disposable items and equipment. It is not necessary to discard unused packets of disposable equipment

Cleaning – all furniture and surfaces, including the mattress and bed frame should be cleaned with detergent and water. Once cleaned the room may be re-used immediately

Special points

Chickenpox, shingles (Herpes zoster), measles

Patients with these infections must not be looked after by staff unable to give a definite history of the infection or appropriate vaccination

Pulmonary tuberculosis (smear positive)

Visitors, apart from immediate family should be discouraged from visiting for the first week of antituberculosis treatment

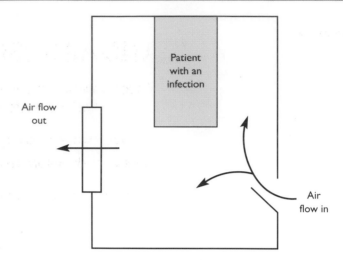

Fig. 14.2
Ventilation for source isolation.

bleeding or, in the case of children or the mentally confused, poor hygiene).

There is no reason why patients with an infection that is spread by direct contact should not be allowed to leave their room periodically, for example as part of their rehabilitation programme.

In outbreaks, patients infected with the same organism can be nursed together in one ward or ward bay rather than in individual rooms. This approach, called **cohorting,** helps the nursing management of infected patients.

Notices at the entrance of the room or displayed by the patient's bed can indicate to visitors and staff, particularly those who may not work regularly on the ward, that special precautions are being observed (Fig. 14.3).

Handwashing

Hands are a very effective method of transmitting infection from patient to patient (see Chapter 7). Handwashing is the single most important means of preventing the spread of infection (Garner and Hierholzer 1993).

Micro-organisms can be acquired on the hands by contact with infectious material from the patient, from contaminated equipment or from the patient's environment. Careful handwashing after any contact with infectious patients or their environment is essential. To ensure that no organisms remain on the hands before contact with another patient, hands should be washed after protective clothing is removed and before leaving the patient's room or bed area.

As the organisms are acquired transiently on the skin, they can be removed easily by thorough washing with soap and water. However,

STANDARD ISOLATION

Visitors please check with nurse
before entering

- Remove white coats before entering
- **Wash hands before leaving**

For further information refer to Isolation Policy

some antibiotic resistant **Gram-negative bacilli** appear to be particularly resistant to removal by soap and water and antiseptic soap solutions may be recommended to prevent their spread (Wade *et al.*, 1991).

Alcohol handrub provides a quicker alternative to soap and water for hands that are physically clean, for example where a patient history has been taken but there has been no direct contact with the patient (Makintosh and Hoffman, 1984).

Protective Clothing

It is illogical to wear a whole range of protective clothing each time the room is entered regardless of the purpose of the visit. The choice of protective clothing should be dictated by the anticipated contact with the infectious material which varies according to the type of infection. The Appendix illustrates the source of infectious material for a number of infections commonly encountered in hospital.

If protective clothing is worn routinely for contact with blood and body fluid, then in many instances additional protective clothing will not be required for infectious patients, since body fluids are the main source of infectious material.

Protective clothing should be readily available both outside and inside the isolation room (Fig. 14.4).

Gloves

Disposable gloves are worn to reduce the contamination of hands with micro-organisms. They should be worn for direct contact with infectious material and changed between procedures to ensure that bacteria from a infected or colonized site on the patient are not transferred to a susceptible site such as a wound or urine catheter. Gloves should be discarded

Fig. 14.4
An isolation room.

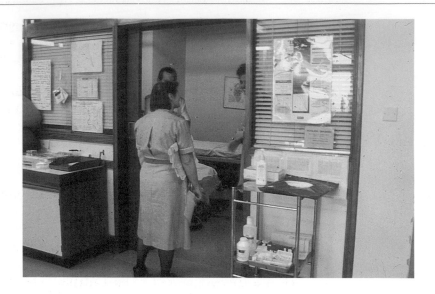

before leaving the room or before initiating care on another patient. Hands are easily contaminated during the removal of gloves and should therefore be washed after gloves have been discarded (Olsen *et al.*, 1993).

Gowns and Aprons

Contamination of clothing during patient care has been reported, particularly after procedures involving heavily contaminated sites such as infected wounds and burns (Speers *et al.*, 1969; Hambraeus, 1973). The number of organisms actually transferred to the clothing is quite small and most will not survive there for very long periods. The front, the part that has most direct contact with patients and their immediate environment, becomes most contaminated (Babb *et al.*, 1983).

Example in Practice	*Mrs Jones has been admitted with gastroenteritis caused by* Salmonella. *She has frequent diarrhoea and is receiving intravenous fluids, but is mostly able to care for herself.*
	To prevent the transmission of *Salmonella* to other patients on the ward, gloves and a plastic apron should be worn by anyone who has direct contact with faeces, commodes or bedpans. For any other care, such as adjusting Mrs Jones' intravenous therapy or assisting her with daily hygiene, gloves and apron are not necessary. Staff should always wash their hands before leaving the room, although an alcohol handrub can be used if the hands are not soiled.

Micro-organisms can pass through fabric gowns, particularly when they are wet (Hoborn, 1990). Plastic aprons are less likely to become contaminated with bacteria and because they are impermeable provide the most practical form of protection for the parts of the clothing most likely to become contaminated (Babb *et al.*, 1983). They should be worn when contact with infectious material is anticipated. The re-use or **disinfection** of aprons is impractical and not cost-effective.

Masks

Although masks are often recommended to protect staff from infections spread by an airborne route, there is little evidence to support their efficacy (Taylor, 1980). Many respiratory infections are more likely to be transmitted on hands than in airborne droplets (Ansari *et al.*, 1991).

To protect the wearer from respiratory tract infection the mask must act as a barrier to very small particles able to reach the lungs. These microscopic droplets may pass through the fabric of the mask, whilst other particles may be inhaled in around the sides (Masden and Masden 1967; Rogers, 1980). To compound the problem, masks worn for prolonged periods become damp, reducing the ability of the material to filter out particles.

An effective means of preventing transmission of certain airborne infections to health care workers is to ensure that they are protected by **immunization**. For example, masks are unlikely to confer additional protection if the staff caring for a patient with tuberculosis have evidence of adequate immunity to tuberculosis (British Thoracic Society, 1990).

Naturally acquired **immunity** through previous exposure to an infection can also provide protection for staff. For example, approximately 90% of adults in the UK have acquired immunity to chickenpox following infection in childhood. Staff with a history of previous infection can therefore safely have contact with a patient with chickenpox or shingles and the use of a mask is unnecessary. Since chickenpox is highly transmissible, staff who are not immune are very likely to acquire the infection through contact with an infectious patient whether they wear a mask or not and should therefore not care for the patient.

Masks may help reduce the risk of transmission during some procedures when there is close contact with respiratory secretions (e.g. bronchial suction, intubation) and they should be worn to protect staff when there is risk of blood or body fluid splashing into the mouth.

Excreta

Safe disposal of excreta from patients with infections transmitted by the faecal–oral route is particularly important but excreta from all patients should be treated as potentially infectious and disposed of in the same way. Excreta may be discarded into a toilet, into a bedpan washer or macerator. Bedpans can be taken out of an isolation room wearing gloves and plastic apron and emptied directly into the bedpan washer. Protective clothing can then be discarded into a yellow waste bag and hands washed. There is no risk of cross-infection if the nurse has no direct contact with other patients until gloves and aprons have been removed and hands washed. The practice of attempting to remove intestinal **pathogens** from excreta with **disinfectants** is illogical since more pathogens enter the sewage system in domestic waste than from hospitals.

Pathogens on re-usable bedpans are destroyed provided the bedpan washer achieves a temperature of 80°C for at least 1 min during the wash cycle. Most modern bedpan washers have a temperature display to enable the temperature to be checked.

Spillage of excreta should be cleaned up promptly, preferably with disposable wipes and using gloves and a plastic apron. Toilets splashed with excreta from patients with intestinal infections may in theory present a risk to others. This risk can be eliminated by regular cleaning of the toilet with detergent.

Waste Material and Linen

Waste generated by caring for the infected patient may be contaminated with infectious material and care must therefore be taken to ensure that it is disposed of safely. In the UK all waste contaminated with blood or body fluid should be destroyed by incineration (Health and Safety Executive, 1992). Waste from an infectious patient does not require any special labelling, but should be discarded into yellow waste bags. A national colour coding system dictates that yellow bags are incinerated. The outer surfaces of waste bags do not become significantly contaminated and there is no reason to enclose them inside a second bag before disposal (Maki et al., 1986).

Linen may transmit infection to laundry workers who sort it prior to washing. To minimize this risk, it has been recommended that linen used by patients with infectious diseases should not be sorted until it has been disinfected by washing. Infected linen should be sent to the laundry in water-soluble or water soluble stitched bags which can be placed directly into a washing machine and split open in the water. Micro-organisms on linen are removed by detergent and the dilution of the water and destroyed by the water temperature of at least 71°C during the wash cycle (DHSS, 1987).

Equipment

Micro-organisms potentially transmitted between patients on equipment can be removed by careful decontamination. In most cases, normal decontamination procedures are sufficient and are discussed in Chapter 13.

Items that are likely to become contaminated by infectious material, such as a commode used by a patient with enteric infection, should be cleaned with detergent after each use. It may, however, be more practical to allocate such equipment for sole use by the patient and clean thoroughly when no longer required.

Items that do not become contaminated with infectious material do not require special cleaning and it is not usually necessary to discard unused disposable items in the room after the patient has been discharged or taken out of isolation.

Disposable crockery and cutlery for infectious patients is not necessary. Crockery and cutlery are unlikely to become contaminated with significant numbers of pathogens and bacteria will not be able to survive and multiply on the surface of clean, dry plates or cutlery. After use they should be washed in hot water and detergent, preferably in a dishwasher which has a rinse temperature of approximately 80°C, and allowed to dry before storage or re-use.

Cleaning

The environment is not a significant factor in the transmission of most infections because most micro-organisms cannot survive for long on clean, dry surfaces. Some bacteria are able to survive for prolonged periods in dust as they form spores or are extremely resistant to desiccation (e.g. *Clostridium difficile, Mycobacterium tuberculosis*). The spores of *Cl. difficile* have been found to persist in the environment for 5 months and large numbers are dispersed from patients with diarrhoea (Hoffman, 1993). The contamination of the environment has been associated with outbreaks of *Cl. difficile* (Cartmill *et al.*, 1994). Although the **spores** are difficult to remove, disinfectants do not appear to be more effective than detergents for cleaning. (Hoffman 1993). Contamination of the environment is not implicated in the spread of mycobacteria. Very few organisms are released into the environment from an infected patient. Transmission occurs only after direct, and usually prolonged, contact with an infectious person (British Thoracic Society, 1990).

Equipment and surfaces should be kept clean and dry to prevent micro-organisms accumulating. The room or bed area of the infected patient should be cleaned in the same way as other areas. Disinfectants for cleaning are unnecessary. Disposable cleaning cloths should be used and discarded. Some hospitals designate a separate mop and bucket to clean the room.

Domestic staff do not have direct contact with the patient and the risk of their acquiring infection from a patient is even less than nursing or medical staff. To reduce the risk to a minimum they should be instructed to wear protective clothing to clean the room and to remove it and wash their hands before leaving. Careful reassurance is essential as they may be extremely concerned about acquiring infection from the isolated patient and as a result the standard of cleaning may suffer.

After an isolated patient has been discharged the room should be cleaned before the next patient is admitted. A thorough clean to remove all dirt and dust is sufficient using normal detergent-based cleaning agents. Afterwards the next patient can be admitted. Leaving isolation rooms for a period of time to air is unnecessary, since most infections are not spread by an airborne route and bacteria do not survive in significant numbers on surfaces that have been cleaned.

Visitors

Visitors are unlikely to have contact with infectious material, such as faeces or respiratory secretions and unlike staff they will not usually be able to transmit infection through contact with other patients on the ward. Visitors should be advised to wash their hands before leaving the patient's room but there is usually no reason for them to wear protective clothing. Where appropriate children and elderly visitors, who may be more susceptible to the infection, should be advised of the risks of visiting whilst the patient remains infectious (e.g. if the patient has chickenpox, RSV, etc.).

For patients with tuberculosis, where possible visiting should be restricted to close relatives for the first few days of treatment. They have already been exposed to the infection prior to the patient's admission but will be followed up by the Public Health Department to establish if they have acquired the infection.

Psychological Effects of Isolation

Isolation affects individual patients in different ways and as social beings, humans generally do not like being isolated from others (Fig. 14.5). The combination of isolation and fear of being infectious can be particularly stressful for some patients. Carers must be sensitive to actions that increase anxiety, such as the use of excessive protective clothing or an inconsistency in the use of protective clothing which can be confusing. A nurse who understands how the infection is transmitted can reassure and explain things to the patient.

Psychological disorders have been reported in patients who have been isolated (e.g. anxiety, time-disturbance, hallucinations) (Denton, 1986). Some become extremely demanding, fussy or irritable and the nurse

Fig. 14.5
The isolated patient.

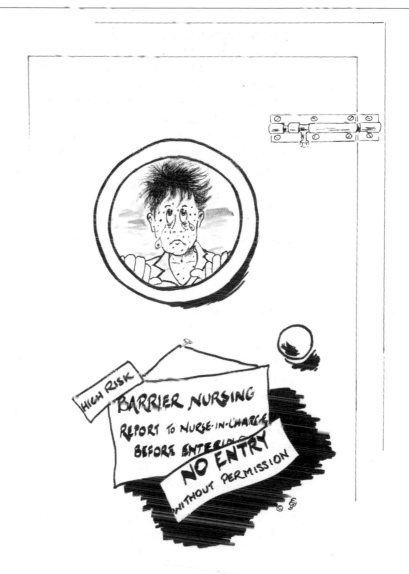

should recognize this behaviour as a response to isolation rather than that of a 'difficult' patient. Knowles (1993) studied eight patients in isolation. Many expressed feelings of loneliness, abandonment, inferiority and boredom (Table 14.1). Although the nurses often understood the patient's response to isolation, they did not take account of these problems and change the nursing care that they gave.

Patients with an infectious disease are often isolated for far longer than necessary. The recommended period of isolation varies for each infection but usually precautions can be stopped once the symptoms have resolved, for example when diarrhoea has stopped, or for some infections after a short course of appropriate antimicrobial therapy (see Appendix).

For many infections, where transmission only occurs through direct

Table 14.1
Patients' response to isolation and nurses' perception of their situation. From Knowles (1993)

Patient	Patients' response to isolation	Nurses' perception of patients' response
A	Feels 'browned off' and isolated Feels confined and frustrated by lack of progress Feels lonely, misses company of others No meaningful activities when alone	Is depressed, feels isolated Is neglected and stigmatized Dislikes being alone
B	Feels neglected and imprisoned Feels inferior, stigmatized	Gets forgotten by staff Feels cut off
C	Feels isolated and abandoned Feels physically separate from the ward Makes sleeping and pastimes easier	Feels isolated Appreciates quiet
D	Feels enclosed Makes pastimes more pleasurable Values own company, not lonely	Gets forgotten by staff Values quiet, facilitates pastimes
E	Feels neglected, shunned, inferior Feels shut in Lack of meaningful activity when alone Misses company of others	Feels neglected, isolated, lonely Feels shut in Easier access to television
F	Is bored Values privacy Feels isolated, enclosed, imprisoned, stigmatized, punished Lacks information and control, feels anxious as a result	Is bored Values privacy

contact with the infectious material, the stress of isolation can be relieved by allowing the patient out of the room. Isolation procedures should not interfere with rehabilitation, for example physiotherapy or occupational therapy.

Patient Education

The role of the nurse as a health educator can be of particular importance when the patient has an infectious disease.

For example, a patient with *Salmonella typhi* may continue to excrete the organisms in his or her stool for several weeks after the symptoms have resolved. To ensure that the infection is not transmitted to other members of the patient's family the nurse should discuss the importance of handwashing after using the toilet and before preparing any food (see Chapter 12).

References

Ansari SA, Springthorpe S, Sattar SA *et al.* (1991) Potential role of hands in the spread of respiratory infections: studies with human parainfluenza virus 3 and rhinovirus 14. *J. Clin. Micro.* **29**: 2115–19.

Ayliffe GAJ, Collins BJ, Lowbury EJL *et al.* (1967) Ward floors and other surfaces as reservoirs of hospital infection. *J. Hyg* **65**: 515–36.

Babb JR, Davies JG, Ayliffe GAJ (1983) Contamination of protective clothing and nurses uniforms in an isolation ward. *J. Hosp. Inf.* **4**: 49–57.

Bowell E (1986) Nursing the isolated patient: lassa fever. *Nursing Times* **33**(17 Sept): 72–81.

British Thoracic Society, Joint Tuberculosis Committee (1990) An updated code of practice. *Brit. Med. J.* **30**: 995–1000.

Cartmill TDI, Panigrahi H, Worsley MA *et al.* (1994) Management and control of a large outbreak of diarrhoea due to *Clostridium difficile. J. Hosp. Inf.* **27**: 1–16.

Centers for Disease Control (1987) Recommendations for the prevention of HIV transmission in health care settings. *MMWR* (Aug 21) **36**: (2S).

Centers for Disease Control (1988) Update: universal precautions for the prevention of human immunodeficiency virus, hepatitis virus and other blood-borne pathogens in health care settings. *MMWR* (June 24) **37**: 24.

Control of Infection Group, Northwick Park Hospital and Clinical Research centre (1974) Isolation system for general hospitals. *Brit. Med. J.* **2**: 41–6.

Denton P (1986) Psychological and physiological affects of isolation. *Nursing* **3**(3): 88–91.

Department of Health (1991) *Safe Working and Prevention of Infection in Clinical Laboratories.* HMSO, London.

Department of Health And Social Security (1987) *Hospital Laundry Arrangements for Used and Infected Linen.* HC(87)30. HMSO, London.

Garner JS, Hierholzer WJ (1993) Controversies in isolation policies and practice. In *Prevention and Control of Nosocomial Infections*, 2nd edn (RP Wenzel, Ed.), pp. 70–81. Williams and Wilkins, Baltimore MD.

Garner JS, Simmons BP (1983) Guideline for isolation precautions in hospitals. *Inf. Contr.* **4**: 245–325.

George RH (1984) Tuberculosis in hospital. *J. Hosp. Inf.* **5**: 109–17.

Glenister H (1991) Surveillance methods for hospital infection. PhD Thesis, Surrey University.

Hambraeus A (1973) Transfer of *Staphylococcus aureus* via nurses' uniforms. *J. Hyg. (Camb).* **71**: 799–814.

Health and Safety Executive (1992) *Safe Disposal of Clinical Waste.* HMSO, London.

Hoborn J (1990) Wet strike through and transfer of bacteria through operating barrier fabrics. *Hyg. Med.* **15**: 15–20.

Hoffman PN (1993) *Clostridium difficile* and the hospital environment. *PHLS Micro. Digest* **10**(2): 91–2.

Jackson MM, Lynch P (1985) Isolation practices: a historical perspective. *Am. J. Inf. Contr.* **13**(1): 21–31.

Knowles HE (1993) The experience of infectious patients in isolation. *Nursing Times* **89**(30): 53–6.

Lynch P, Jackson MM, Cummings MJ *et al.* (1987) Re-thinking the role of isolation practices in the prevention of nosocomial infections. *Ann. Intern. Med.* **107**: 243–6.

Mackintosh CA, Hoffman PN (1984) An extended model for transfer of micro-organisms via the hands: differences between organisms and the effect of alcohol disinfection. *J. Hyg.* **92**: 345–55.

Maki DG, Alvarado C, Hassemer C (1986) Double bagging of items from isolation rooms is unnecessary as an infection control measure: a comparative study of surface contamination with single and double bagging. *Inf. Contr.* **7**: 535–7.

Masden PO, Masden PE (1967) A study of disposable surgical masks. *Am. J. Surg.* **114**: 432–5.

Olsen RJ, Lynch P, Coyle MB *et al.* (1993) Examination gloves as barriers to hand contamination in clinical practice. *J. Am. Med. Ass.* **270**(3): 350–3.

Rogers KB (1980) An investigation into the efficiency of disposable face masks. *J. Clin. Path.* **33**: 1086–91.

Selwyn S (1991) Hospital infection – the first 2500 years. *J. Hosp. Inf.* **18** (Suppl. A): 5–65.

Speers R, Shooter RA, Gaya H *et al.* (1969) Contamination of nurses' uniforms with *Staphylococcus aureus*. *Lancet* **ii**: 233–5.

Taylor L (1980) Are face masks necessary in operating theatres and wards? *J. Hosp. Inf.* **1**: 173–4.

Wade JJ, Desai N, Casewell MW (1991) Hygienic hand disinfection for the removal of epidemic vancomycin-resistant *Enterococcus faecium* and gentamicin-resistant *Enterobacter cloacae*. *J. Hosp. Inf.* **18**: 211–18.

Wilson J, Breedon P. (1990) Universal precautions. *Nursing Times* **86**(37): 67–70.

Further Reading

Bowell B (1992) A risk to others. *Nursing Times* **88**(4): 38–40.

Curran ET (1993) Taking down the barriers; a new approach to barrier nursing. *Prof. Nurse* **9**(7): 472–8.

Grazier S (1988) The loneliness barrier. *Nursing Times* **84**(41): 44–5.

Webster O, Bowell E (1986) Thinking prevention. *Nursing Times* **82**(23): 68–74.

Appendix. Routes of transmission for common infections

Infection	Infective material	Isolation	Duration of infectivity (isolation)
AIDS	Blood, body fluids	None	Indefinitely
Campylobacter	Faeces	Yes	Whilst symptomatic
Chickenpox	Oral/lesion, secretions	Yes	Until lesions are crusted
Cholera	Faeces	Yes	Whilst symptomatic

Clostridium
    difficile
	Faeces	Yes	Isolate for duration of
			    diarrhoea

perfringens	Faeces and lesion secretions	None	
Creutzfeldt–Jakob disease	Blood, brain tissue	None	Indefinitely
Croup (usually viral)	Respiratory secretions	Yes	Duration of symptoms
Cryptosporidium	Faeces	Yes	Duration of diarrhoea
Cytomegalovirus	Urine, respiratory secretions	None	

Diarrhoea,
    unknown origin
	Faeces	Yes	Isolate for duration of
			    diarrhoea

Diphtheria
    pharyngeal
	Oral/nasal secretions	Yes	Until two nose/throat
			    cultures negative

cutaneous	Lesion secretions	Yes	Duration of lesions
Enteropathic *E. coli* (infants)	Faeces	Yes	Duration of symptoms
Gas gangrene	(see *Clostridium perfringens*)		
Gastroenteritis			Isolate for duration of
viral e.g. SRSV	Faeces, vomit	Yes	symptoms
unknown		Yes	Isolate for duration of symptoms
Gonorrhoea	Discharge	None	Until 24 h antibiotic treatment
Hepatitis A	Faeces	Yes	Until onset of jaundice
Hepatitis B	Blood and body fluids	None (unless uncontrolled bleeding)	Until HbsAg negative
Herpes simplex (severe)	Lesion secretions	Yes	Duration of lesions
Herpes zoster	Lesion secretions	Yes	Until lesions have crusted
Human immunodeficiency virus	Blood and body fluids	None	Indefinitely
Impetigo	Skin lesions	Yes	Duration of lesions
Influenza	Nasal/oral secretions	Yes	Duration of illness

Lassa fever	Blood and body fluids,
	    oral secretions
		Seek advice immediately from infection
		    control nurse/doctor	

Legionnaires' disease		None	
Lice			
head	Hair	None	Until treated
body	Clothing	None	Until clothing washed
crab	Coarse body hair	None	Until treated
Listeria			
neonate		Yes	Duration of illness
adult		None	

Appendix
Continued

Infection	Infective material	Isolation	Duration of infectivity (isolation)
Malaria		None	
Measles	Nasal/oral secretions	Yes	7 days after onset of rash
Meningitis			
meningococcal	Respiratory secretions	Yes	Until 24–48 h of antibiotic treatment
haemophilus	Respiratory secretions	Yes	Until 48 h of antibiotic therapy
pneumococcal		None	
viral		None	
unknown cause		Yes	
Methicillin-resistant *Staphylococcus aureus*	See multi-resistant bacteria		
Multiresistant bacteria	Body fluids, lesions, sometimes skin	Yes	Seek advice from infection control nurse/doctor
Mumps	Oral secretions	Yes	Until 9 days after onset of symptoms
Paratyphoid	Faeces/urine	Yes	Isolate for duration of illness (may excrete organism for several more weeks)
Pertussis	Oral secretions	Yes	Until 7 days after start of treatment
Pneumonia	Respiratory secretions	None (usually)	
Poliomyelytis	Faeces	Yes	Until 7 days after onset of symptoms
Rabies	Saliva	Seek advice immediately from infection control nurse/doctor	
Respiratory syncitial virus	Oral/respiratory secretions	Yes	Isolate for duration of illness
Rotavirus	Faeces	Yes	Isolate for duration of symptoms
Rubella			
congenital	Urine and oral	Yes	Duration of hospitalization and for any admission until 1 year
acquired	Oral secretions	Yes	Until 5 days after onset of rash
Salmonella	Faeces	Yes	Isolate for duration of symptoms (may excrete organism for several more weeks)
Scabies	Skin	None (usually)	Until treated
Shigella	Faeces	Yes	Isolate for duration of diarrhoea

Appendix
Continued

Infection	Infective material	Isolation	Duration of infectivity (isolation)
Staphylococcus aureus			
extensive lesions	Pus	Yes	Until culture negative
MRSA	Lesions and skin	Yes	Seek advice from Infection Control Nurse/Doctor
Streptococcus			
(Groups A, C, G)	Lesions	Yes	Until 48 h of antibiotic treatment or culture negative
erysipelas	Skin	Yes	
cellulitis	Skin	Yes	
puerperal fever	Vaginal secretions	Yes	
pharyngitis	Oral secretions	Yes	
scarlet fever	Oral secretions	Yes	
Tetanus		None	
Toxoplasmosis		None	
Tuberculosis			
pulmonary (open) (smear positive)	Oral/respiratory secretions	Yes	Until clinical improvement (1–2 weeks after antibiotic therapy)
other site/organ		None	
Typhoid	Faeces/urine	Yes	Isolate for duration of symptoms (may excrete organism for several more weeks)
Typhus		None	
Viral haemorrhagic fevers	Blood and body fluids, oral secretions	Seek advice immediately from Infection Control Nurse/Doctor	
Whooping cough	See pertussis		

Ectoparasitic Infections and Environmental Infestations

Introduction

This chapter examines the problem of infections and infestations by arthropods and other animals, firstly by discussing a number of **parasites** which can infect the human skin and secondly by looking at infestation of the health care environment by a variety of pests.

Ectoparasitic Infections

The prospect of a close encounter with lice or scabies usually induces a sense of panic in even the most composed nurse. In reality, most of these infections can be eradicated easily and the risk of staff or other patients acquiring the offending parasite is slight. An understanding of how the parasite is transmitted is essential if the treatment is to carried out with the minimum of precautions and the maximum sensitivity to the patient's feelings. In addition to topical treatment of the parasite, education of the patient and treatment of other members of the family should also be considered. The health visitor, school nurse and medical social worker may be able to assist in this process.

Lice (Pediculosis)

Lice can be caught only by close contact, they cannot jump or fly but need to be close enough to walk on to another host. They feed from the host, usually taking blood about five times a day. An allergic reaction develops to the bites causing them to itch. This allergic reaction can take up to 3 months to develop and carriers easily become desensitized and therefore no longer notice the bites. Lice found off the body on bedding, chairs, floors, etc. are either dead, dying or injured and would not be able to crawl on to another host.

There are about 500 different species of lice but only three of these use humans as their host and each lives on a specific part of the body.

The Head Louse (*Pediculus humanus capitis*)

This species lives on head and eyebrow hair and is between 1 and 4 mm long (Plate 15.1). The female louse lays about eight eggs in a night and sticks them on to the base of hairs where it is warmest. The eggs hatch after 7–10 days leaving the egg-cases or nits so firmly stuck to the hair that they can remain attached until the hair falls out (Plate 15.2). Once hatched the louse moults three times before reaching adulthood and lives for about 3 weeks. Transmission to another host occurs when two heads are in direct contact and the louse crawls on to a new head. Lice are sensitive to temperature, preferring temperatures of at least 31°C. This keeps them close to the scalp and their source of food. Consequently lice are not easily passed to others unless heads are in contact for a minute or more allowing time for the hair to warm up and the lice to pass across (Maunder, 1993). Lice prefer a clean head of hair where they can move around easily. They are able to cling on tightly to hairs and are not removed by washing. Frequent combing is a useful method of control as injured lice cannot regenerate damaged parts and die.

Head lice are invariably acquired from family members or close friends. A third of louse infections occur on adults and remain undetected for long periods (Maunder, 1993). The infection is difficult to detect in its early stages. Lice use a local anaesthetic to make the feeding process painless. The eggs are not visible until they have hatched because they are only the size of a grain of sugar and the louse disguises them by matching the colour to that of the skin. The empty eggshell is white and this, rather than incubating eggs, is usually removed during fruitless nit-combing activity. The most obvious evidence of head lice is the appearance of skin casts or small black flecks of faeces on bedding.

Treatment

There are many products available for the treatment of lice which can be obtained from the pharmacist with or without a prescription. The conventional treatments are based on the insecticides malathion, an organophosphate (e.g. Prioderm, Suleo-M and Derbac-M) or carbaryl (e.g. Carylderm, Derbac and Suleo-C). A single application of lotion to dry hair and left on the scalp for 12 h is usually sufficient to eradicate the lice. As some of the products are alcohol-based a hairdryer should not be used. After 12 h the hair should be washed, fine-tooth combing is not necessary. Shampoos are also available but although they contain a higher concentration of insecticide they are not as effective as they are diluted during washing. Three separate treatments with shampoo are therefore necessary to eradicate the lice.

Two new products have become available recently: a pyrethroid, phenothrin (Full Marks), lotion which should be applied to dry hair and left in contact for 2 h before washing. Permethrin (Lyclear) is a lotion applied after the hair has been washed.

Prolonged exposure to insecticides may cause resistant lice to emerge and to prevent this, health authorities recommend only one type (an organophosphate, carbonate or pyrethroid) at a time, alternating every 3 years.

Close family or friends who have had sufficient contact to enable transmission of lice should also be checked for infection. Head lice cannot be transmitted to others on clothing or linen and therefore no special precautions are necessary. Patients with head lice need not be **isolated**, except on paediatric wards where close contact between children may transmit the lice.

Crab (Pubic) Lice (*Pthirus pubis*)

Crab lice are far more common than head lice. They live on coarse body hair, particularly pubic and axillary hair, but also on chest and facial hair and eyelashes. They are much broader and flatter than head or body lice and have large claws on the second and third legs (see Fig. 15.1). The female louse if under clothing lays her eggs on the shaft of the hair rather than at the base and after hatching the lice take 17 days to mature. It can

Fig. 15.1
Adult crab (pubic) louse.

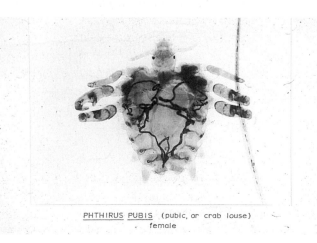

PHTHIRUS PUBIS   (pubic, or crab louse)
female

take a minimum of 4–6 weeks for the host to react to the bite of the lice during which time they usually remain undetected but once sensitized the itching around the anus and vagina is severe. Crab lice are transmitted by close physical contact frequently, but not always, by sexual contact. Children may acquire crab lice through close contact with their mother (e.g. axillary hair). They may be passed easily where people are living in crowded conditions but can not be transmitted on inanimate objects (**fomites**), except perhaps on shared towels.

Treatment

The treatments for crab lice are aqueous-based to enable them to be applied to delicate parts of the body. Lindane (quellada) is very effective but may be absorbed through the skin and is toxic. It should not be given to pregnant women, breast feeding mothers, epileptics or people with a very low body weight. Malathion (Derbac M) and carbaryl (Derbac C) are also effective. As with head lice, the recommended treatment is changed regularly to discourage resistance. The treatment should be applied to all hair on the body except for the head.

Crab lice on clothing or bedding are not transmitted to other people and can be removed by washing. **Isolation precautions** are not necessary.

Body Louse (*Pediculus humanus humanus*)

The body louse is very similar to, but slightly larger than the head louse. It lives in clothing, not hair and goes on to the body only to feed. It usually lays its eggs in the seams of clothing and produces up to 300 during its 3-week lifespan. Bite marks usually occur opposite seams such as under the collar or waistband, are extremely itchy and usually result in characteristic long, linear scratch marks on the torso. If the host is sensitized to louse faeces, this may cause a generalized rash and sneezing may sometimes result. Transmission occurs in overcrowded conditions by contact with infested clothing.

To survive, body lice depend on the same clothes being worn for prolonged periods, washed in cool water and then re-worn immediately. Body lice are therefore nowadays associated with low temperature washing powders, although traditionally they were associated with poverty, war or other disasters and were frequently found on vagrants.

Body lice are easy to eradicate as they will die if the clothing is not worn for 3 days and provided the clothes are changed once a week the young lice will not be able to feed when they hatch out of the eggs. Lice are also destroyed by washing clothes in hot water and hot tumble-drying destroys both lice and eggs.

The human body louse is responsible for the transmission of a number of serious **infectious** diseases. *Borrelia recurrentis* causes European relapsing fever which is characterized by bouts of fever lasting several weeks. It is a spirochaete which multiplies in the body of the louse and is transmitted to human hosts when the lice feeds. Typhus, caused by *Rickettsia prowazeki* is a severe fever associated with a death rate of 10–20% and is transmitted by louse faeces entering a cut on the skin. Epidemics of typhus and relapsing fever are associated with cold, lack of fuel, overcrowding, famine and war; conditions that are conducive to louse infestation.

Treatment

Clothing should be washed in hot water (60°C or more) and be changed at least once a week. Fifteen minutes in a hot tumble-dryer is sufficient to destroy both lice and eggs. No treatment of the skin or isolation precautions are necessary.

Scabies

Scabies is caused by a small mite, *Sarcoptes scabiei* (Fig. 15.2). The mites live in the deeper layers of the epidermis, moving up to 5 mm a day by burrowing horizontally through the skin. The burrows which can only be seen on a minority of patients, appear as tiny, white lines, 15–30 cm long, with the female mite appearing as a small brown spot of less than 0.5 mm at one end. To an experienced eye these are diagnostic of scabies, but the absence of visible burrows does not exclude the disease.

The female mite lives for about 6 weeks and lays two or three eggs a day in the burrow. The eggs hatch after 3 days, and the larvae construct new burrows off the maternal burrow. After 10 days and three moults females become adults, mate and establish new burrows. The male mite is much smaller, moults only twice and does not make burrows once an adult.

Fig. 15.2
The scabies mite Sarcoptes scabiei *(dorsal view of female).*

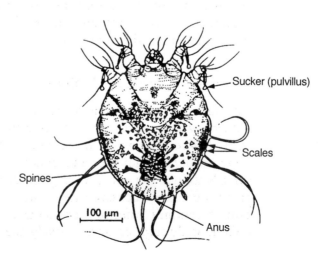

Sucker (pulvillus)

Scales

Spines

100 μm

Anus

The mites are usually found on the inner surface of the wrist and between the fingers, although they may also occur on the feet, groins, buttocks, elbows and axillae, and around the nipples in women and penis in men. They do not commonly spread to the head and neck except in the elderly or immune-deficient patients and are unusual on the soles of the feet and palms of the hands, except in children (Taplin, 1986).

Despite the conventional view of scabies as a highly infectious disease, it is not easily transmitted from person to person and is not easily spread by social contact. The mite moves extremely slowly and therefore prolonged contact is required for it to move on to another host. It can be transmitted between family members and sexual partners and in hospital is often seen in care of the elderly and psychiatric settings where holding hands may be more common. The incidence of scabies fluctuates, with **epidemics** occurring every 30 years. In the UK a major increase in scabies appears to have begun in 1991 (Barrett and Morse, 1993).

The severe itching and rash associated with scabies is not caused directly by the mite, but is the result of the host's allergic response to it. Consequently, the reaction does not appear immediately, but develops between 4 and 6 weeks after infection. The itch and rash do not necessarily coincide with the site of the mites. The rash tends to appear on the hands, arms, legs, sides of the trunk and around the waist (Maunder, 1983) and the itching becomes more severe at night. If the person has been infected with the scabies mite previously then the body responds rapidly, and itching develops within hours as a response to an immune counter-attack on the mite, which may then be killed before it can re-establish an infection.

The appearance of a generalized rash or itch may be diagnosed as scabies, but because of the implications of contact tracing and treatment of contacts it is important to make a definite diagnosis. A dermatologist can usually confirm a diagnosis of scabies and skin scrapings can be examined in the laboratory for evidence of mites and their eggs, or more likely their faecal pellets.

Norwegian (Crusted) Scabies

This form of scabies occurs when the scabies mite infects a person with a deficiency of their immune system, either caused by disease or **immunosuppressive** therapy. In the absence of a normal immune system the body cannot control the mite infection, the mite multiplies rapidly and spreads all over the body, causing the skin to appear dry and crusted. The crusts are heavily contaminated with dead and dying mites. Individuals cannot transmit infection on their clothes or bedding but are very infectious through contact. Usually the infection will not be associated with itching. Outbreaks of scabies, spread from an unrecognized index case of Norwegian scabies, commonly spread through nursing homes or elderly care units. Particular problems are associated with wards caring for a high proportion of patients with acquired immune deficiency syndrome (AIDS), where rapid spread may occur and several cases of Norwegian scabies may develop as a result (Sirera *et al.*, 1990). Contacts with a normal immune system may develop conventional scabies.

Treatment

There are three main forms of treatment for scabies: gamma benzene hexachloride (lindane), malathion and permethrin. All are applied to the whole body except the scalp and left on for up to 24 h. The lotion should be reapplied to the hands when they are washed. Lindane is not recommended for babies, very young children or nursing mothers as it is absorbed through the skin and can harm the nervous system. Permethrin is a reletively new treatment which has a low toxicity and high cure rate.

Patients should be a warned that itching persists for some time after treatment because it takes a few days for the allergic response to subside even though the mites have been killed. Re-treatment is not indicated unless itching persists for longer than a week.

All close contacts of the person should be treated, even if they are asymptomatic because of the long delay between infection and development of symptoms.

Extensive experimentation has demonstrated that scabies is not transmitted by clothes or bedlinen and these items do not require not special treatment (Robinson, 1986; Maunder, 1992).

Patients with scabies do not require isolation as actual skin-to-skin contact is required to transmit infection. However patients with Norwegian scabies are highly **contagious** and isolation precautions are recommended until treatment has been completed. No special treatment of clothing, bedding or the environment is required (Maunder, 1992).

Infestation of the Environment

Health care premises provide an ideal environment in which pests can flourish. They are warm and full of people whose habits inevitably provide a constant source of food. Pests can be described as animals or insects that cause damage, annoyance or in some cases present a risk of infection.

Pests that most commonly infest hospitals are cockroaches, Pharaoh's ants, fleas, birds, rodents and cats. Although It is unlikely that all pests could be totally eradicated from hospitals or other centres of health care, an effective and continuous strategy to control their numbers is essential.

Nurses have a crucial role to play in the reporting of pests or signs of infestation and should be aware of the system of reporting and treating infestations that occur in their place of work. Pests frequently only appear at night and are not easily observed. Even small signs should be reported. The sighting of a single cockroach, egg-case or mouse dropping is probably indicative of an infestation problem.

The Department of Health recommends that each hospital or unit of management should nominate a pest control officer (PCO) with responsibility for all aspects of pest control (NHS Management Executive, 1992). These individuals should be trained in the recognition of pests and methods of controlling them, keep a record of pest sightings, investigate reports and ensure that appropriate action is taken. Most hospitals have a contract with a pest control servicing company that will treat infestations and inspect the site regularly for pests. The pest control officer is responsible for liaison with the contractor and monitoring the contract. This may involve periodic inspections of the site at night when the activity of many pests is at its greatest. In large complex buildings, information on pest sightings from staff is particularly valuable.

Cockroaches

Cockroaches have existed for millions of years and there are over 3000 different species. The two most common species in the UK are the German (*Blattella germanica*) and oriental (*Blatta orientalis*) cockroach, American (*Periplaneta americana*) and brown banded cockroaches are only rarely seen. Any large building that is warm is prone to infestation.

Cockroaches feed on an enormous variety of meat and vegetable matter including sewage and organic waste. They also need a supply of water and cavities in which to hide. They can live in tiny cracks and crevices and behind wall and floor tiles and, because they are strongly nocturnal, infestation often goes unnoticed until the population is very large. The life cycle of the cockroach includes three stages: the eggs are enclosed within a capsule; they hatch out as nymphs – smaller, wingless versions of the adult insect which after several moults mature into adults. Some species hide their eggs in cracks; German cockroaches carry them until nearly ready to hatch; while Oriental cockroaches abandon them. Both German and oriental adult cockroaches have wings but do not fly.

The German cockroach is the smallest, about 12 mm long and accounts for about 10% of cockroach infestations. Its common name is the 'steamfly' as it prefers warm and humid conditions and is therefore most commonly found in kitchens. It is good at climbing and can be found in heated trollies, vending machines, refrigerator motors and behind false ceilings. The oriental cockroach is larger, about 25 mm long and accounts for about 90% of all cockroach infestations in heated

Fig. 15.3
(a) Adults and nymphs of the oriental cockroach feeding on a courgette discarded in a kitchen yard. (b) Mixture of oriental and German cockroaches on a kitchen wall. Notice also the slugs!

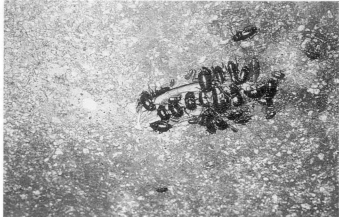

(a)

(b)

buildings (Fig. 15.3a). However, it can tolerate cooler conditions and so may be found outside, around the perimeter of buildings and in drains and underground ducting. The American cockroach is the largest species found in the UK, about 35 mm long. It needs access to water and warm conditions of between 24 and 33°C and is usually found in large heated greenhouses and in ports and airports where it is introduced from abroad on ships or aeroplanes.

Many hundreds of cockroaches can live in gaps behind tiles gaining access through breaks or cracks (Fig. 15.3b). Nursing staff can help to discourage infestation in ward areas by employing simple preventative measures: storing food in tight-fitting containers and secure cupboards, not leaving out prepared food, discarding waste food and refuse promptly and ensuring that leaking pipes and damaged surfaces are repaired (DHSS, 1984; Smith, 1988).

Millions of bacteria have been isolated from the bodies and faecal droppings of cockroaches which they probably acquire through feeding on food, decaying matter and faeces. The microbes they carry reflect the microbial flora of the environment in which they live (Fotedar *et al.*, 1991; Bennett, 1993). Although it is difficult to prove that cockroaches are responsible for particular cases of infection, they could in theory transmit infection if allowed to crawl over working surfaces or prepared food. Circumstantial evidence for transmission of infection by cockroaches was provided by Graffar and Mertens (1950) who reported an outbreak of *Salmonella typhimurium* in a Brussels children's ward. Cockroaches were observed running over the children and their bedclothing by a night nurse. *Salmonella typhimurium* was isolated from one of the captured insects and the outbreak came to an end once the infestation had been eradicated.

Ants

Garden ants, attracted by food debris, may occasionally cause a minor problem in buildings but are easily controlled by treatment with insecticide. Far more serious problems can be caused by Pharaoh's ants, tiny insects 1–2 mm long which can invade equipment and contaminate food (Fig. 15.4). Originally introduced from tropical countries, they can survive easily in centrally heated buildings in temperate climates. Nest colonies each containing several thousand worker ants are sited in almost any concealed area, for example behind tiles, light fittings and in brickwork. Nests have been found in heated food trollies, drink-vending machines and **autoclave** units. They eat both meat and vegetable matter but prefer meat and sweet substances. They can chew through plastic and have been found in intravenous fluid administration sets and sterile packs. (Beatson, 1973). They will also search out suppurative lesions and feed on the discharge from the wound.

Infestation in operating theatres or central sterile supply departments enables ants to invade sterile packs. In intensive care units worker ants

Fig. 15.4
Pharoah's ants trapped in the filter of an administration set

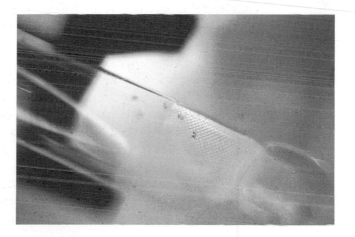

have been found in intravenous tubing and resuscitation equipment (Beatson, 1972). Infestation in the laundry or other service departments results in ants being transferred throughout the hospital. They can also spread through ducting.

There is some evidence that these ants can transmit infection and indeed they are more likely to be found in contact with patients and their equipment than more shy insects, such as cockroaches. A large range of bacteria, including *Pseudomonas* spp., staphyloccoci and *Enterobacter*, have been isolated from the surface of their bodies (Beatson, 1972). Their affinity for moist areas such as sinks, toilets and sluices means they could acquire **pathogenic** bacteria on their bodies and transfer them onto food, into sterile packs or on to patients' wounds.

Suspected infestation with Pharaoh's ants should be reported promptly to the PCO so that extensive treatment by a professional pest control company can be carried out without delay.

Fleas

There are over 1000 species of flea and although they feed on any warm-blooded animal, they require a specific host on which to breed. Human fleas are now rarely encountered. They dislike the warm, dry environment of modern homes and are usually only found in association with vagrants or homeless people. They live in the environment, feeding infrequently from their hosts and should be treated by washing infested clothing and applying insecticide to the environment.

The cat and dog flea (Fig. 15.5) are responsible for most flea bites on humans (Watkins and Wyatt, 1989). They thrive in the warm, dry environment of the domestic home and live in furniture and carpets, jumping on to passing animals and humans for food. The bites are

Fig. 15.5
Mixture of cat and dog fleas caught in 1 h on selotape in a radiography department

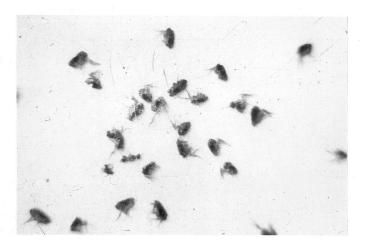

commonly seen on the ankles and lower legs, although many people become desensitized to them and will not develop an immune response to the bite. Infestations in hospitals may originate from colonies of feral cats or animals kept as pets and can be very troublesome. Feral cats living in ducting or basements can support a large population of fleas which may then gain access to the building. Cat flea infestations have even been responsible for the closure of an operating department and a laundry (Baker, 1981). If infestation with fleas is suspected in a hospital department the pest control officer should be contacted who will arrange for the source of the infestation to be identified and treated with insecticides.

Preventing flea infestations depends on control of feral cat populations by neutering. Pet animals should be sprayed regularly with insecticide and bedding should also be treated. The Environmental Health Department of the local authority or a company specializing in pest control can be called in to treat severe infestation with fleas in the home.

Birds

Birds, particularly pigeons and house sparrows, become pests when their population is large enough to cause a nuisance, either by fouling, noise or secondary pests such as mites and fleas. Roosting can be deterred by nets, wires, spikes, etc. and they should be prevented from gaining access to buildings. To avoid attracting birds refuse must be carefully sited, spillages cleared up promptly and deliberate feeding discouraged.

Rodents

The main rodent pests are rats and mice. They can cause damage to furnishings, spoil food and may also carry pathogenic bacteria. They are often detected by evidence of damage or droppings. Rodents can be discouraged by storing food in tightly closing containers or secure cupboards and discarding waste promptly. Waste for disposal should not be stored for prolonged periods and the storage area should be kept clean and tidy.

References

Baker LF (1981) Pests in hospital. *J. Hosp. Inf* **2**: 5–9.
Barrett NJ, Morse DL (1993) The resurgence of scabies. *CDR* **3**(2): R32–3.
Beatson SH (1972) Pharaohs ants as pathogen vectors in hospitals. *Lancet* **i**: 425–7.
Beatson SH (1973) Pharoah's ants enter giving sets. *Lancet* **i**: 606.
Bennett G. (1993) Cockroaches as carriers of bacteria. *Lancet* **i**: 732

Department of Health and Social Security (1984) *An Introduction to Pest Control in Hospitals*. Domestic Services Management Advice Notes. HMSO, London.

Fotedar R, Shrinivas U, Banerjee U *et al.* (1991) Nosocomial infections: cockroaches as possible vectors of drug-resistant klebsiella. *J. Hosp. Inf.* **18**: 155–9.

Graffar M, Mertens S (1950) Le role des blattes dans la transmission des salmonelloses. *Ann. Inst. Pasteur* **79**: 654–60.

Maunder J. (1983) The increase in scabies. *Postgrad. Doctor* **6**: 198–202.

Maunder J. (1987) Lousy news for lice. *Community Outlook* **August**: 20.

Maunder J (1992) The scourge of scabies. *Chemist and Druggist* **Jan 11**: 54–5.

Maunder J (1993) An update on headlice. *Health Visitor* **66**(9): 317–18.

NHS Management Executive (1992) Pest Control Management for the Health Service. HSG (92)35.

Roberts C. (1987) A lousy life. *Community Outlook* **August** 16–19.

Robinson R (1986) Scratching the surface. *Nursing Times* **34** (Dec 3): 71–2.

Sirera G, Ruis F, Romeu J *et al.* (1990) Hospital outbreak of scabies stemming from two AIDS patients with Norweigan scabies. *Lancet* **335**: 1227.

Smith P (1988) An unpleasant case of cracked tiles. *Health Services Journal* **26 May** (S): 6.

Taplin D (1986) Cutaneous infestations. In *Modern Management of Skin Diseases* pp. 18–25. (CFH Vickers, Ed.) Churchill Livingstone, Edinburgh.

Watkins M, Wyatt T (1989) A ticklish problem; pest infestation in hospitals. *Prof. Nurse* **May**: 369–92.

Willis J (1990) Common pests. *Community Outlook* **Sept**. 24–9.

Further Reading

Health Service Pest Control (1988) *Health Services Journal* (Suppl.) **26th May**.

Henderson C (1991) Community control of scabies. *Lancet* **337**: 1548.

Lane RP, Crossley RW (1993) *Medical Insects and Arachnids*, pp. 517–28, Chapman and Hall, London.

Lice and scabies – diagnosis and treatment. Produced by Derbec product licence holder. Bengue and Co., Maidenhead.

Glossary

Abscess	a localized collection of pus.
Acid	a substance that when dissolved in water dissociates into hydrogen ions H^+ and negative ions.
Acquired immunity	immunity which develops in response to a stimulus, e.g. an infection.
Adenine	an organic base found in DNA, RNA and elsewhere.
Adenosine triphosphate (ATP)	a chemical compound which contains energy-rich bonds and serves as the main 'energy currency' of the cell. It breaks down into adenosine diphosphate and phosphate ion, releasing energy.
Aerobe	a microbe that grows in the presence of oxygen. A strict aerobe requires oxygen. *See* anaerobe.
Agar	a polysaccharide made from seaweed and used in solidifying bacteriological media.
Agglutinate	to stick to one another, clump (of particles, red cells, etc); the result is agglutination.

$$\text{= ethanol, } H-\overset{\displaystyle H}{\underset{\displaystyle H}{C}}-\overset{\displaystyle H}{\underset{\displaystyle H}{C}}\ \ O-H$$

Alcohol	(the reason for the intoxicating effect of beer, wine etc).
Algae	photosynthetic microbes; the blue-green algae are procaryotes and the others eucaryotes.
Alkali	a substance that, when dissolved in water, dissociates into OH^- ions and positive ions.
Allergic response	an exaggerated immune response to an antigen resulting in histamine release, inflammation and tissue damage anaphylaxis. The effects may be localized (e.g. asthma, hay fever) or systemic (e.g. anaphylactic shock).
Amino acid	an organic acid occurring in proteins and elsewhere. It has the structure

$$R-\overset{\displaystyle }{\underset{\displaystyle NH_2}{C}}-COOH$$

	where R may be any one of various chemical groups.
Amoeba	a eucaryotic organism that lacks a rigid cell wall and moves by pseudopods.
Anabolism	the formation of new compounds from simple molecules.
Anaerobe	a microbe that grows in the absence of oxygen. A strict anaerobe will not grow in the presence of oxygen, a facultative anaerobe grows in the presence or absence of oxygen.
Anaphylaxis	*See* allergic response
Antibiotic	a substance which is toxic for certain microbes; the first antibiotics to be

used were produced by microbes, but many are now partly or wholly synthesized by pharmaceutical chemists (= antimicrobial agent).

Antibody   a protein which appears in the body fluids of an animal after contact with a foreign molecule, 'antigen', and which combines specifically with that antigen.

Antigen   any substance, usually proteins, which the body regards as foreign and produces antibodies against.

Antimicrobial agent   *See* antibiotic.

ATP   *See* adenosine triphosphate.

Attenuated   a microbe that is *attenuated* has lost its virulence and may be suitable for use as a vaccine.

Autoclave   a machine in which materials can be exposed to steam under pressure and therefore at a temperature higher than that of boiling water.

Bacillus   any rod-shaped bacterium; also the name of a genus of bacteria, Gram-positive rods which are often found in soil and dust.

Bacteraemia   presence of bacteria in the blood.

Bacteria   *see* bacterium

Bactericidal   capable of killing bacteria.

Bacteriophage   an 'eater of bacteria', a bacterial virus which enters a bacterial cell and multiplies within it by directing the bacterial metabolic machinery to manufacture bacteriophage components.

Bacteriostatic   ability to inhibit or slow down the growth of bacteria.

Bacterium   a procaryotic microbe.

Bacteriuria   the presence of bacteria in the urine without symptoms of infection.

Barrier nursing   *see* isolation precautions.

Base   an ion or molecule capable of accepting a hydrogen ion. Bases normally produce OH^- ions when dissolved in water.

Base pair   two nitrogenous bases linked by hydrogen bonds in the double-stranded DNA molecule. Adenine–thymine and guanine–cytosine are the only two possible pairings.

Basophil   a white cell of the blood, so called because it takes up basic dyes; in the usual stains for blood films, basophils have large black granules.

B cell (lymphocyte)   one of the two main cell types of the immune system, chiefly involved in the production of antibodies.

Binary fission   division of one cell into two daughter cells, the usual method of reproduction in bacteria.

Biochemistry   the science dealing with chemical processes in living organisms.

Biofilm   a film of proteins and micro-organisms which frequently covers the surface of foreign material when it is in contact with tissue.

Biosynthesis   the synthetic processes carried out by living cells.

Bronchitis (acute)   inflammation of the bronchi caused by bacteria or viruses. In chronic bronchitis excessive mucus is secreted by bronchial glands and the condition is frequently exacerbated by acute infection.

Capsid	the protein layer enclosing the nucleic acid of a virus.
Capsule	a slimy substance, usually polysaccharides, which forms a protective layer around some bacterial cells.
Carbohydrate	a compound of carbon, hydrogen and oxygen, the hydrogen and oxygen being present in a ratio of 2 : 1; e.g. glucose $C_6H_{12}O_6$ is a carbohydrate.
Carriage	*See* carrier.
Carrier	an individual who persistently excretes a microbe or who has a body surface colonized by a microbe, but who is not obviously ill with this infection.
Catabolism	the breakdown of large and complicated compounds into their constituent molecules, releasing energy.
Catalyst	a substance that increases the rate of a chemical reaction, but is itself unaltered when the reaction is complete.
Cell-mediated immunity	a form of immune response carried out by T-lymphocytes.
Cellular immune system	the part of the immune system controlled by the T-lymphocytes (= cell-mediated immune system).
Cellulose	a carbohydrate composed of glucose molecules. An important constituent of plant cell walls.
Cell wall	the rigid outer layer of most procaryotic cells and of some eucaryotic ones.
Centriole	a small particle found near the nucleus of cells and involved in the separation of chromosomes during cell division.
Chemotaxis	movement of a cell in response to the presence of a chemical.
Chemotherapy	treatment of disease with chemicals; in practice, this means antibiotics.
Chlorophyll	a green pigment found in plants and some bacteria which absorbs light to provide energy for the synthesis of carbohydrates from water and carbon dioxide (photosynthesis).
Chromosome	this contains the genetic information of the cell. It is composed of a long thread of DNA and associated proteins.
Cilia	hair-like structures which beat rhythmically in a co-ordinated fashion.
Clinical waste	waste material from health care premises or veterinary practices which may be infectious, toxic or hazardous. This waste must usually be destroyed by incineration.
Clone	a group of organisms descended from a single parent by asexual reproduction and therefore exact copies of it. The term is now extended to the production of copies of DNA molecules.
Coagulase	an enzyme which clots plasma.
Coccus	a bacterium that is spherical in shape
Cohort	a group of people. *Cohorting* is a term used to describe a method of controlling outbreaks of infection in hospital by grouping affected patients together.
Colonization	a microbe that establishes itself in a particular environment such as a body surface without producing disease or symptoms is said to 'colonize' the site.

Colony	when a bacterial cell (or a few cells) multiplies on a solid medium until the group is visible to the naked eye, the group is called a *colony*. A typical colony contains 10–100 million cells.
Commensal	a commensal organism lives in association with another, without benefiting or harming it. Many members of the gut flora appear to be commensals.
Communicable	a disease that can be transmitted from one person to another is communicable (= contagious, = infectious).
Community-acquired infection	an infection acquired in the general community, not as a result of treatment in hospital.
Complement	a complex of proteins in the blood; reactions between the component proteins promote the movement of phagocytes and the phagocytosis and killing of bacteria.
Conjugation	the transfer of genetic material from one bacterial cell to another by cell-to-cell contact.
Contagious	*see* communicable.
Counterstain	a stain used to enhance contrast in a differential stain.
Cross-infection	*see* exogenous.
Culture	a culture of microbes is the result of inoculating a medium with them and incubating it until large numbers are present.
Cutaneous	relating to the skin.
Cyst	a stage in the lifecycle of some protozoan parasites, in which the organism is encased in a tough outer wall.
Cytoplasm	in a procaryote, everything inside the cytoplasmic membrane; in a eucaryote, everything inside the cytoplasmic membrane, except the nucleus.
Cytoplasmic membrane	the membrane which constitutes the outer boundary of the cell except for the cell wall (when one is present) and which prevents the escape of the large and small molecules making up the cytoplasm of the cell.
Cytosine	an organic base found in DNA, RNA and elsewhere.
Deoxyribonucleic acid (DNA)	the large molecule in which genetic information is encoded, the genetic material. The component nucleotides contain the sugar deoxyribose.
Diploid	a diploid cell contains two copies of each chromosome. The body cells of most eucaryotic organisms are diploid.
Disinfectant	chemicals which can be used to achieve disinfection.
Disinfection	a process which reduces the number of micro-organisms to a level at which they are not harmful but which does not usually destroy spores.
DNA	*see* deoxyribonucleic acid.
Ectoparasite	a parasite that lives on the outer surface of its host e.g. lice.
Electron	a negatively-charged particle in orbit round the nucleus of an atom.
Electron microscope	a microscope in which a beam of electrons is used instead of light rays to produce an image.

ELISA (*enzyme-linked immunosorbent assay*)	a technique for detecting and estimating antigens and antibodies, in which a coloured compound is formed by the enzyme linked to the detector antibody.
Encephalitis	inflammation of the brain.
Endemic	if a disease is endemic, cases regularly appear in the population. *See* epidemic.
Endocarditis	an inflammation, especially one due to infection, of the lining of the heart, including its valves.
Endogenous	arising within the body (= self-infection); an *endogenous* infection is caused by the normal flora.
Endoplasmic reticulum	a complicated membrane system extending throughout the cytoplasm of the eucaryotic cell. During protein synthesis, ribosomes are often attached to it.
Endotoxin	part of the outer membrane of Gram-negative cells: it consists of various sugars and a lipid (lipopolysaccharide) and possesses toxic properties, causing activation of complement, inflammation, blood clotting and fever.
Envelope	in some viruses, an outer coat that surrounds the capsid and may be derived partly or wholly from the host cell.
Enzyme	a protein which catalyses a biochemical reaction.
Eosinophil	a white blood cell, so called because it takes up the dye eosin; in the usual stains for blood films, eosinophils have large orange-red granules.
Epidemic	in an epidemic of a disease, many cases appear in a short time and then the number decreases for months or years.
Epidemiology	the study of the occurrence of diseases, how and when they occur, how they are transmitted, etc.
Epiglottitis	inflammation of the tissue at the entrance to the larynx (the epiglottis). Swelling can cause obstruction of the air flow into the lungs.
Epithelization	the healing of a wound by the formation of new granulation tissue and micro-circulation.
Erythema	a flushing of the skin caused by dilation of capillary blood vessels, often a sign of inflammation or infection.
Eucaryotic cell	one of two chief types of living cells, in which the nucleus is delimited from the cytoplasm by a membrane.
Exogenous	derived from outside the body (= cross-infection); compare '*endogenous*'.
Exotoxin	Substances produced by bacteria which diffuse out of the cell. They can be highly toxic and have a specific effect on the host eg. muscle spasm or paralysis.
Extracellular	outside the cell.
Facultative	an organism which is not restricted to a particular way of life; thus a facultative anaerobe can live in the absence or presence of oxygen.
Facultative anaerobe	*see* anaerobe.
Fat	a substance containing fatty acids (triglycerides) and used to store energy in the body.

Fermentation	production of energy from carbohydrates in the absence of oxygen. The electrons generated are passed to organic molecules.
Fertilization	fusion of a male (spermatozoon) and female (ovum) cell to form a zygote.
Fibrin	an insoluble protein which links together to form a mesh and seal damaged blood vessels. It is the final product of blood coagulation and is made by the action of the enzyme thrombin on the precursor, fibrinogen.
Flagellum	an organ attached to the surface of the cell and used for locomotion.
Fluorescent antibody technique	a technique for detecting microbes in which the antibody is tagged with fluorescent dyes and thus rendered visible when viewed with a special microscope (fluorescence microscope) in which ultraviolet light is used.
Fomites	Inanimate objects which may have been contaminated with microbes, and could transfer infection to others. Common fomites are towels, bedclothes, furniture and crockery.
Fungus	a simple plant which lacks chlorophyll.
Gangrene	Death of body tissue such as a limb, because of interference with the blood supply.
Gene	a 'unit of heredity', a segment of DNA that encodes the structure of a protein.
Genetics	the science of heredity.
Genetic code	the information carried by DNA. It determines the sequence of amino acids in proteins and therefore governs the nature of all proteins in the cell.
Genome	the genetic information of an organism.
Genus	in biological nomenclature the *genus* is the larger grouping and is written with a capital; the *species* is the smaller grouping. Both words are modern Latin and are printed in italics.
Glycocalyx	a more or less diffuse layer outside the cell wall of procaryotes; it consists of polysaccharide, polypeptide or both.
Glycogen	a polysaccharide stored by animals and some bacteria.
Golgi body	an organelle present in the cytoplasm of eucaryotic cells; it is involved in the secretion of proteins from the cell.
Gram-negative	*see* Gram stain.
Gram-positive	*see* Gram stain.
Gram stain	a staining procedure that distinguishes two types of procaryotes, Gram-positive and Gram-negative.
Granulocytes	phagocytic cells of the immune system which circulate in the blood. There are three types: neutrophils (the largest proportion); basophils and eosinophils.
Guanine	an organic base found in DNA, RNA and elsewhere.
Haemolysin	a molecule that lyses red cells. Many bacteria produce haemolysins.
Helix, helical	spiral.
Histamine	a molecule released by mast cells; it causes inflammation, increased permeability of blood vessels, asthma.
HLA antigens	*see* human leucocyte antigen system.

Hospital-acquired infection	an infection acquired as a result of treatment in hospital or during a period of hospitalization.
Human leucocyte antigen system	the main group of histocompatibility antigens, cell-surface antigens involved in many aspects of immunological recognition of "self". They are the main antigens recognized in the rejection of grafts.
Humoral immune system	the production of antibody by B-lymphocytes.
Hydrogen bond	a type of chemical bond, relatively weak in nature.
Hypersensitivity	an exaggerated or inappropriate immune response, leading to inflammation or tissue damage (= allergic response).
Icosahedron	a solid figure with 12 (vertices) corners and 20 triangular faces.
Immunity	the result of infection by a particular microbe or of immunization against that microbe.
Immunization	the process of artificially inducing immunity to infection by a particular microbe.
Immunocompromised	*see* immunodeficiency.
Immunodeficiency	impairment of the immune response rendering the host particularly susceptible to infection. May be caused by genetic disorder, underlying illness, chemotherapy or certain viral infections (= immunocompromised).
Immunoglobulin	an antibody.
Incidence	the number of new cases occurring in a particular population over time.
Incubation period	the interval between contact with the microbe and the development of the symptoms and signs of infection.
Infection	entry of a harmful microbe into the body and its multiplication in the tissues.
Infectious	*see* communicable.
Inflammation	a response to infection or other injury characterized by swelling, heat, redness and pain (= inflammatory response).
Inoculum	material (containing bacteria) added to a growth medium to initiate a culture; hence *inoculate*.
Inorganic ions	small molecules present in living creatures and also in non-living materials; they do not usually contain carbon.
Interferon	a lymphokine produced by T-lymphocytes which promotes the activity of natural killer cells.
Intracellular	inside cells.
Intravascular (IV) device	cannula or catheter inserted into a vein or artery.
Isolation precautions	special procedures used to prevent the transmission of micro-organisms from an infectious patient to other patients or staff (= barrier nursing). *See* protective isolation.
Latent infection	a condition in which the clinical signs of infection are absent and the causative organism may be temporarily undetectable; under certain conditions the infection may again become obvious.

Leucocyte white blood cell.

Lipid a fat, a molecule made up of glycerol and fatty acids.

Lipopolysaccharide a constituent of the Gram-negative bacterial cell-wall, in which chains of various sugars are linked to lipid A. They can act as endotoxin.

Live-attenuated vaccine vaccines made of live micro-organisms which have been altered to prevent them causing infection.

Lymph fluid derived from blood, similar composition to plasma but contains lymphocytes. Lymph is carried in the vessels of the lymphatic system and passes through a series of lymph nodes before returning to the bloodstream via the thoracic duct.

Lymph nodes composed of lymphoid tissue, they produce lymphocytes and filter foreign particles from lymph preventing them entering the blood stream.

Lymphatic system network of vessels which carry electrolytes, water and proteins (lymph) between the tissues and blood.

Lymphocyte a type of white blood cell present in the blood, lymph system, gut wall and bone marrow. They are involved in the immune response and can be divided into B lymphocytes which produce antibodies and T lymphocytes which are responsible for cell-mediated immunity.

Lymphokines polypeptides released chiefly by T cells and activating macrophages.

Lysosome an intracellular organelle, a bag of enzymes.

Lysozyme an enzyme that can dissolve the cell walls of certain bacteria.

Malaise a general feeling of being unwell.

Macrophage a type of phagocyte.

Mast cell a cell involved in the hypersensitivity response. In appearance it closely resembles the basophil. It contains histamine and other substances the release of which causes inflammation.

Meiosis a form of cell division, characteristic of eucaryotic cells which results in male and female gametes.

Memory cell cells of the immune system which produce specific antibodies able to persist in the blood for many years. When an antigen enters the blood it is recognized by the memory cell which begins immediate production of antibody against it.

Meningitis inflammation of the meninges (membranes which enclose the brain and spinal cord) caused by infection.

Mesosome an infolding of the cell membrane in bacterial cells associated with the DNA and involved in cell division.

Messenger RNA the transcript of the DNA from which a polypeptide is synthesized by the ribosome.

Metabolism a general term for all the biochemical processes that occur in a living cell.

Methicillin-resistant *Staphylococcus aureus* a strain of *S. aureus* that is resistant to many antibiotics, including flucloxacillin which is usually used to treat infection caused by *S. aureus*.

Microbe a creature too small to be seen with the naked eye (or only just visible);

the term includes bacteria, fungi, protozoa, some of the algae and the viruses (= micro-organism).

Microbicide an agent which destroys micro-organisms

Micrometre (μm) a unit of length, 10^{-6} metres.

Micro-organism *see* microbe.

Microscope an instrument used to provide a greatly enlarged image of an object.

Mitochondrion an intracellular organelle that contains the energy-generating systems of eucaryotic cells.

Mitosis division of a eucaryotic cell into two daughter cells.

Monocytes phagocytic white blood cells which are found in tissues.

Mononuclear macrophages phagocytic cells of the immune system found in the tissues.

Mould a fungus that forms a mycelium which may be seen as a 'furry' growth on the surface of e.g. bread or fruit.

MRSA *see* methicillin-resistant *Staphylococcus aureus*

Mycelium an intertwined mass of filaments (hyphae), typical of the growth of moulds.

Myocarditis inflammation of the heart muscle.

Natural killer cells large lymphoid cells capable of killing cells with the appropriate receptors on the surface.

Necrotic tissue tissue which has died through injury, disease or impaired blood supply.

Neutrophil a white blood cell, actively phagocytic.

Normal flora the community of microbes that colonizes a body surface.

Nosocomial *see* hospital-acquired infection.

Nuclease an enzyme which catalyses the breakdown of nucleic acids.

Nucleic acid the organic acids DNA and RNA present in all living cells as genetic information.

Nucleolus an area in the nucleus of a eucaryotic cell where RNA is synthesized.

Nucleotide a constituent of DNA or RNA, made up of a sugar, an organic base and a phosphate group.

Nucleus the part of the cell that contains the genetic material.

Obligate an obligate organism is restricted to a particular way of life; e.g. an obligate parasite cannot live free without a host.

Obligate aerobe/ anaerobe *see* aerobe, anaerobe.

Opportunistic pathogen a micro-organism which only causes infection in a host with an impaired immune system.

Opsonize a process by which foreign cells are marked by proteins to distinguish them from host cells enabling them to be removed by phagocytosis.

Organelle a distinct structure within the cytoplasm of a eucaryotic cell that possesses a separate function; e.g. the mitochondria, Golgi body.

Organic an organic compound is one that contains carbon.

Osmosis the movement of a solvent (e.g. water) from a less concentrated to a more concentrated solution through a semi-permeable membrane (allows passage of some molecules but not others).

Otitis media   inflammation, usually caused by infection, of the middle ear (the chamber behind the eardrum).

Outbreak of infection   the occurrence of two or more related cases of the same infection or where the number of infections is more than would normally be expected.

Oxidation   the addition of oxygen to, or the removal of electrons from, a substance.

Pairs of bases   *see* base pair.

Pandemic   a worldwide outbreak of an infectious disease.

Parasite   an organism that lives in or on another creature and obtains food and shelter without benefiting the host. Hence *parasitism*. *See* commensal *and* symbiosis.

Parenteral   administered by injection directly into the tissues.

Passive immunity   immunity conferred on the host animal by antibodies made in another host.

Pathogen   a microbe capable of causing disease.

Pathogenicity   the ability of a microbe to invade and cause disease.

Peptide   a chain of amino acids.

Peptidoglycan   a major structural component of bacterial cell walls, consisting of chains of sugars cross-linked by peptides.

Pericarditis   inflammation of the membranous sac (pericardium) surrounding the heart.

Peritonitis   inflammation of the peritoneum – the membrane lining the walls of the abdomen and covering the abdominal organs.

pH   the symbol denoting hydrogen ion concentration; the pH ranges between 0 and 14 and its value indicates the relative acidity or alkalinity of a solution.

Phage   *see* bacteriophage.

Phagocyte   a cell capable of phagocytosis.

Phagocytosis   the ingestion of material by a cell either in order to destroy foreign matter or for its own nutrition.

Phospholipid   a lipid made up of glycerol, two fatty acids and a phosphate group.

Photosynthesis   the use of solar energy by green plants and some bacteria to synthesize carbon compounds from CO_2 and water.

Plasma   the liquid portion of blood.

Plasma cell   a cell that develops from a B-cell and that manufactures a specific antibody.

Plasmid   a double-stranded circle of DNA which may be present in the cytoplasm of a microbial cell; it may be able to bring about conjugation between bacterial cells and it may carry genes for antibiotic resistance, for virulence and for various biochemical pathways.

Pneumonia   inflammation of the lung caused by bacteria in which the alveoli fill up with pus, excluding the air and causing the lung to become solid (consolidation).

Polymorphonuclear leucocyte   blood contains three polymorphonuclear leucocytes, neutrophils, eosinophils and basophils.

Polypeptide a chain of at least four, and usually more amino acids.

Polysaccharide a carbohydrate formed from many sugars joined into long chains. Used as structural elements of the cell and for the storage of energy (e.g. starch and glycogen).

Precipitate the result of a reaction between two soluble substances to form an insoluble material that 'falls' out of solution.

Prevalence the number of cases occurring within a particular population at any one time.

Primary intention healing this occurs in wounds where there is no loss of tissue and the two surfaces are sutured together e.g. surgical wounds.

Primary response the production of antibody in response to the first contact with the antigen.

Procaryotic cell one of two chief types of living cells, in which the nucleus is not delimited from the cytoplasm by a membrane. In general procaryotic cells are smaller and of less complex structure than eucaryotic cells.

Prophylaxis treatment which is intended to prevent disease rather than cure it after it has developed; e.g. prophylactic antibiotic therapy.

Prostaglandin a group of hormones present in a wide variety of tissues and body fluids.

Protective isolation special precautions used to protect immune-deficient patients from infection (= reverse barrier nursing).

Protein a large molecule, one of the main constituents of living matter; it consists of one or more polypeptide chains.

Protozoa microscopic single-celled eucaryotic microbes; some are free-living, others are important parasites.

Pseudo-membranous colitis a severe infection of the bowel caused by the bacterium *Clostridium difficile*.

Puerperal sepsis a septicaemia originating from streptococcal infection of the uterus during childbirth.

Pus an accumulation of fluid due to infection; it consists of living and dead microbes, phagocytes and tissue cells, together with the fluid that has accumulated in the tissue because of inflammation.

Reservoir of micro-organisms the place where they live and multiply; e.g. the reservoir of *Salmonella* is the intestine of chickens where they are carried asymptomatically.

Respiration the generation of energy by the conversion of organic compounds to carbon dioxide and water. The energy generated is stored as ATP.

Restriction endonucleases enzymes that cut DNA strands at points determined by bases and which therefore always yield the same fragments from a given DNA.

Reverse transcriptase an enzyme that works 'in reverse', synthesizing DNA from an RNA template. The human immunodeficiency virus contains a reverse transcriptase.

Ribonucleic acid (RNA) a nucleic acid in which the component nucleotides contain the sugar ribose. The ribonucleic acids of cells are messenger RNA, transfer RNA and ribosomal RNA; in addition the genome of some viruses consists of RNA.

Ribose   a five-carbon sugar present in the nucleotides of RNA.

Ribosomal RNA   RNA which forms part of the ribosome.

Ribosome   the protein-synthesizing 'factory' of the cytoplasm.

Risk assessment   systematic identification of hazards or risks to health; e.g. assessing the requirement for protective clothing according to the anticipated risk of exposure to body fluid. Risk assessment can also be used to identify patients who are particularly likely to develop infection and target preventive measures accordingly.

RNA   *see* ribonucleic acid.

Secondary intention healing   this occurs in wounds where there has been loss of tissue and involves the gradual closing of the gap by the formation of new tissue at the base of the wound.

Self-infection   *see* endogenous

Sense strand   the strand of DNA that carries the genetic message.

Septicaemia   bacteria in the bloodstream accompanied by symptoms and signs of infection and illness.

Seroconversion   the production of specific antibodies in response to an antigen.

Serology   the study of blood serum and particularly the constituents which protect the body against disease.

Serotype   a strain of a bacterial species which can be differentiated by the antigens present on its surface; these are detected by antibodies (*serological* methods).

Serum   the liquid which remains when plasma clots.

Sex pilus   small tubes used by bacteria to transfer DNA between cells.

Skin commensal   *see* commensal.

Slough   dead tissue which separates from healthy tissue after inflammation or infection.

Solute   molecules in a solution.

Source of infection   the place from which a micro-organism causing a particular infection originates. Not all reservoirs of micro-organisms are sources of infection e.g. sinks are a reservoir for many bacteria but are unusual sources of infection.

Species   *see* genus

Spore   a resistant casing which some bacteria use to enclose their cells in adverse environmental conditions. When conditions improve the spores germinate and the cell begins to multiply.

Sterilization   a process which removes or destroys all micro-organisms including spores.

Strain (of a bacterium)   a group of bacteria of the same species but which have distinguishing properties. Some strains can be detected by special laboratory techniques called 'typing'.

Subclinical infection   an infection which produces no symptoms or signs of disease; most infections are subclinical.

Subcutaneous	beneath the skin.
Surveillance	the systematic observation of the occurrence of disease in a population, with analysis and dissemination of results.
Symbiosis	an obligate association between two species in which there is mutual benefit.
Systemic	involving the whole body.
T cell	*see* lymphocyte.
T lymphocyte	one of the two main cell types of the immune system, responsible for cell-mediated immunity.
Teichoic acid	a polymer of an alcohol, phosphate and other molecules found in Gram-positive cell walls.
Template strand	the strand of DNA complementary to the sense strand; both the sense strand and the messenger RNA are synthesized on the template strand.
Thymine	an organic base found in DNA.
Titre	a means of expressing the concentration of an antibody.
Topical	a drug that is applied directly to the affected part (e.g. skin or eye) is applied *topically*.
Toxin	any poisonous substance produced by a living organism, especially a microbe.
Toxoid	a microbial toxin treated (usually with dilute formaldehyde) so that its toxic activity is destroyed, but it is still capable of stimulating the production of antibodies which react with and inactivate the parent toxin.
Trace element	a chemical element required for growth, but only needed in very small amounts.
Transcription	copying the sense strand of the DNA into messenger RNA.
Transduction	the introduction into a bacterial cell, by a bacteriophage, of new genes which are not bacteriophage genes and which are derived from the bacterium in which the phage previously replicated.
Transfer RNA	RNA molecules which carry individual amino acids to the ribosome.
Transformation	the introduction of new genes into a cell by the uptake of DNA from solution.
Translation	synthesizing a polypeptide chain from the messenger RNA template.
Transposon	a 'jumping gene', a segment of DNA which can move from one DNA molecule to another, or from one site to another in the same DNA molecule.
Tuberculin test	a skin test used to detect infection by mycobacteria.
Uracil	an organic base found in RNA.
Vaccination	the process of inducing immunity by administering a vaccine.
Vaccine	a preparation of killed microbes, inactivated microbial toxins or microbial antigens used to induce immunity.
Virulence	the ability to cause disease.
Virus	a micro-organism only capable of reproduction within living cells.
White blood cell (leucocyte)	any blood cell that contains a nucleus. They are divided into granulocytes, monocytes and lymphocytes.
Yeast	a unicellular fungus.

Index